Digital Design and Manufacturing of Medical Devices and Systems

Rajkumar Velu • Karupppasamy Subburaj •
Anand Kumar Subramaniyan
Editors

Digital Design and Manufacturing of Medical Devices and Systems

Springer

Editors
Rajkumar Velu
Additive Manufacturing Research Laboratory, Mechanical Engineering
Indian Institute of Technology Jammu
Jammu, Jammu and Kashmir, India

Karupppasamy Subburaj
Mechanical and Production Engineering
Aarhus University
Aarhus, Denmark

Anand Kumar Subramaniyan
Additive Manufacturing Research Laboratory, Mechanical Engineering
Indian Institute of Technology Jammu
Jammu, Jammu and Kashmir, India

ISBN 978-981-99-7099-5 ISBN 978-981-99-7100-8 (eBook)
https://doi.org/10.1007/978-981-99-7100-8

This Springer imprint is published by the registered company Springer Nature Singapore Pte Ltd.
The registered company address is: 152 Beach Road, #21-01/04 Gateway East, Singapore 189721, Singapore

Preface

A transformation is underway in the rapidly evolving landscape of biomedical engineering, where technology and healthcare converge. Over the past 50 years, the intersection of technology and healthcare has given rise to innovative design solutions that had and have the potential to reshape patient care, accessibility, and affordability. Various disruptive technologies have driven this transformation, promising to enhance the design, development, and manufacturing of medical devices and systems. As engineers, scientists, and healthcare professionals, we find ourselves at the cusp of a new era where the boundaries between innovation and application are blurring, and the promises of cutting-edge technology translate into reality.

The motivation behind this book, *Digital Design and Manufacturing of Medical Devices and Systems*, lies in recognizing the urgent need for a comprehensive resource that delves into the world of disruptive technologies shaping the biomedical landscape. As technology continues to redefine healthcare, it becomes increasingly essential for professionals across various domains to grasp the potential of these technologies and harness their power for designing advanced biomedical devices. This book aims to bridge the gap between the intricate intricacies of these technologies and their practical applications, empowering researchers, engineers, clinicians, and students to explore, innovate, and collaborate in digital health.

We have organized the contents of this book to offer a structured exploration of the myriad disruptive technologies underpinning the design and manufacturing of medical devices and systems. Beginning with a comprehensive overview of the current state-of-the-art and market trends in the field, the book sets the stage for an in-depth journey through the world of advanced technologies. Chapters are devoted to futuristic biomaterials tailored for 3D-printed healthcare devices, integrating sensors in prosthetic sockets, the synergies between augmented reality and additive manufacturing, design methodologies, and 3D printing applications in tissue engineering. Cutting-edge topics such as 3D-printed smart implants, embedded electronic subsystems, and AI-powered pharmaceutical product development reflect the diverse spectrum of technologies at the forefront of biomedical innovation.

The sequence of chapters mirrors the chronological journey from fundamental concepts to advanced applications, guiding readers through a seamless learning progression. Each chapter is designed to offer insights into the latest advancements, techniques, and methodologies, providing readers with both the theoretical foundation and practical insights necessary to navigate the complexities of digital design and manufacturing in the medical domain.

The development of this book was a collaborative effort that brought together the expertise of numerous individuals from biomedical engineering, materials science, manufacturing, and clinical practice. We thank the scholars, researchers, and professionals who have contributed their time, knowledge, and insights to make this endeavor possible. We are indebted to our colleagues and mentors who have guided and supported us throughout the process of curating this comprehensive resource. We express our sincere appreciation to Mr. Mohit Teacher, who handled the administration of the project, including working with the contributors and reviewers to ensure the chapters and reviews were carried out on time.

As you embark on this journey through the pages of *Digital Design and Manufacturing of Medical Devices and Systems*, we invite you to explore the boundless possibilities that emerge at the intersection of technology and healthcare. May this book serve as a beacon of knowledge, inspiration, and collaboration, guiding you toward unlocking the full potential of disruptive technologies in the service of humanity's well-being.

Jammu, Jammu and Kashmir, India — Rajkumar Velu
Aarhus, Denmark — Karupppasamy Subburaj
Jammu, Jammu and Kashmir, India — Anand Kumar Subramaniyan

Contents

Editors and Contributors

About the Editors

Rajkumar Velu, PhD is an Assistant Professor at the Indian Institute of Technology, Jammu and 2023 visiting research associate at the University of Michigan (UoM), USA. Priorly worked as a Research Fellow at the Center for Laser Aided Intelligent Manufacturing (CLAIM), UoM, USA, and as a Postdoctoral Research Fellow at the Digital Manufacturing and Design Centre (DManD), Singapore University of Technology and Design, Singapore. He completed his PhD thesis in selective laser sintering of specific biopolymer composites for biomedical application at the Auckland University of Technology, New Zealand. Dr. Velu also receives academic awards for his academic performances at the university level. Consequently, he has considerable insights and knowledge of different polymer, polymer composites, metal alloys, and advanced materials used explicitly for additive manufacturing. More than 40 publications were generated from his research activities, and he received a scientific research award at an international conference conducted by Philadelphia University, Amman, Jordan, in 2010. Also, he was a recipient of the "Young Scientist Award" 2018 at the Annual Conference on 3D Printing and Bioprinting in Health Care, Singapore. Dr. Velu's research interests encompass engineering design, optimization, and developing advanced manufacturing processes (Additive Manufacturing) and materials for designing and fabricating fuel cell, biomedical and aerospace applications. Moreover, based on his current research practice, he is involved in developing Artificial Intelligence into an additive manufacturing process to fabricate end-use products and eliminate post-mortem analysis.

Karupppasamy Subburaj, PhD is an Associate Professor of Biomechanical Engineering in the Department of Mechanical and Production Engineering at Aarhus University in Denmark. He leads an interdisciplinary research group, Medical Engineering and Design (MED), focusing on developing data-driven engineering solutions for healthcare, including medical devices, methodologies, and analysis tools for diagnosing, predicting, monitoring, and treating musculoskeletal disorders and disabilities. He tackles critical challenges from the complexity of realizing them in biological and clinical settings to bringing them to the bedside through collaborations with healthcare institutions and industry. Before moving to Aarhus University, he was a founding design faculty in the Engineering Product Development Pillar at the Singapore University of Technology and Design (SUTD) and led Healthcare Engineering and Design Track. In parallel, he served as an adjunct faculty at the Changi General Hospital, where he implemented a pathway for clinicians to work with students to develop engineering product design solutions for their clinical needs. He received his postdoctoral research training in Musculoskeletal Biomechanics from the University of California San Francisco (UCSF). His publication portfolio includes 4 international patents, 5 books, and over 150 articles and presentations in international journals and conferences. In 2020, he received the Outstanding Education Award—Excellence in Teaching from SUTD for his pedagogical contribution to design-based healthcare engineering education.

Anand Kumar Subramaniyan, PhD is an Assistant Professor in the Department of Mechanical Engineering at the Indian Institute of Technology Jammu. He has over 10 years of product development targeting biomedical, aerospace, and automobile applications. Further, his research interests include additive manufacturing, digital twin of systems, surface engineering, materials characterization, tribology, fatigue, and fracture. He has published over 100 original research papers in peer-reviewed international journals and conferences. He obtained his PhD from the Indian Institute of Technology-Madras. Further, he has postdoctoral work experience of a couple of years at Tamkang University, Taiwan. He worked as a Principal Engineer at TSMC, Taiwan.

Contributors

S. Mohammed Adhil Amrita Hospital, Faridabad, Haryana, India

K. A. Arirajan Department of Mechanical Engineering, Thiagarajar College of Engineering, Madurai, India

G. Sahaya Dennish Babu Department of Physics, Chettinad College of Engineering and Technology, Karur, Tamil Nadu, India

T. Berman Department of Electrical and Electronic Engineering Science, University of Johannesburg, Johannesburg, South Africa

Sridhar Chandrasekaran School of Electronics Engineering, Vellore Institute of Technology, Chennai, Tamil Nadu, India

K. Chockalingam Department of Mechanical Engineering, Thiagarajar College of Engineering, Madurai, India

C. Dhavamani Department of Aeronautical Engineering, Mahendra Engineering College (Autonomous), Namakkal, Tamil Nadu, India

Koyeli Girigoswami Faculty of Allied Health Sciences, Chettinad Academy of Research and Education, Chettinad Hospital and Research Institute, Kelambakkam, Chennai, Tamil Nadu, India

M. Gololo Department of Electrical and Electronic Engineering Science, University of Johannesburg, Johannesburg, South Africa

Rahul Gorka All India Institute of Medical Sciences Vijaypur, Jammu, Jammu and Kashmir, India

Arunkumar Jayakumar Department of Electrical and Electronics Engineering, St. Peter's Institute of Higher Education and Research, Chennai, Tamil Nadu, India

Pauline John Division of Engineering, New York University Abu Dhabi, Abu Dhabi, UAE

Manigandan Kannan Department of Mechanical Engineering, University of Akron, Akron, OH, USA

Brahmansh Kaushik Department of Mechanical Engineering, Northwestern University, Evanston, IL, USA

Anand Kumar Subramaniyan Additive Manufacturing Research Laboratory, Mechanical Engineering, Indian Institute of Technology Jammu, Jammu, Jammu and Kashmir, India

Surinder Kumar Acharya Shri Chander College of Medical Sciences (ASCOMS) and Hospital, Jammu, Jammu and Kashmir, India

L. Lebea Department of Mechanical and Mechatronic Engineering, Central University of Technology, Free State, Bloemfontein, South Africa

S. Stella Mary Department of Physics, St. Peter's Institute of Higher Education and Research, Chennai, Tamil Nadu, India

Ahmed O. Mosleh Faculty of Engineering, Benha University, Cairo, Egypt

Saraswathi Nagaraj Faculty of Allied Health Sciences, Chettinad Academy of Research and Education, Chettinad Hospital and Research Institute, Kelambakkam, Chennai, Tamil Nadu, India

F. J. Nemavhola Faculty of Engineering and the Built Environment, Durban University of Technology, Durban, South Africa

H. M. Ngwangwa Department of Mechanical Engineering, University of South Africa, Johannesburg, South Africa

K. Ouahada Department of Electrical and Electronic Engineering Science, University of Johannesburg, Johannesburg, South Africa

T. Pandelani Department of Electrical and Electronic Engineering Science, University of Johannesburg, Johannesburg, South Africa
Unisa Biomechanics Research Lab, Department of Mechanical Engineering, School of Engineering, College of Science Engineering and Technology, University of South Africa, Pretoria, South Africa
Faculty of Engineering and the Built Environment, Durban University of Technology, Durban, South Africa

Mohit Pant Department of Mechanical Engineering, National Institute of Technology Hamirpur, Hamirpur, Himachal Pradesh, India

Mitali Pareek Mahatma Gandhi Dental College and Hospital, Jaipur, Rajasthan, India

Jairam Raigar Department of Mechanical Engineering, Indian Institute of Technology Jammu, Jammu, Jammu and Kashmir, India

Murali Krishnan Ramachandran Department of Mechanical Engineering, University of Akron, Akron, OH, USA

S. Rimer Department of Electrical and Electronic Engineering Science, University of Johannesburg, Johannesburg, South Africa

Arun Karthick Selvam Department of Biomedical Engineering, Sri Sivasubramaniya Nadar College of Engineering, Kalavakkam, Tamil Nadu, India

Paramasamy Shanmugam Department of Mechanical Engineering, Sethu Institute of Technology, Pulloor, Kariapatti, Tamil Nadu, India

Sneha Sharma The University of Texas at Dallas, Richardson, TX, USA

Yojana Sharma Department of Mechanical Engineering, National Institute of Technology Hamirpur, Hamirpur, Himachal Pradesh, India

Parnika Shrivastava Department of Mechanical Engineering, Dr. B.R. Ambedkar National Institute of Technology, Jalandhar, Punjab, India

M. Shunmathi Department of Mechanical Engineering, Thiagarajar College of Engineering, Madurai, India

Mohit Teacher Additive Manufacturing Research Laboratory (AMRL), Indian Institute of Technology Jammu, Jammu, Jammu and Kashmir, India

Mannat Uppal HealthCubed India Private Limited, Bengaluru, Karnataka, India

Rajkumar Velu Additive Manufacturing Research Laboratory, Mechanical Engineering, Indian Institute of Technology Jammu, Jammu, Jammu and Kashmir, India

State-of-the-Art Overview and Recent Trends in Biomedical Devices Using Digital Manufacturing: Opportunities, Limitations, and Current Market

1

Murali Krishnan Ramachandran, Jairam Raigar, Manigandan Kannan, and Rajkumar Velu

Contents

Abstract

Digital manufacturing involves creating, modifying, and optimizing manufacturing processes using computer-aided design (CAD) software and

M. K. Ramachandran (✉) · M. Kannan
Department of Mechanical Engineering, The University of Akron, Akron, OH, USA

J. Raigar
Department of Mechanical Engineering, Indian Institute of Technology Jammu (IIT - Jammu), Jammu, Jammu and Kashmir, India

R. Velu
Additive Manufacturing Research Laboratory, Mechanical Engineering, Indian Institute of Technology Jammu, Jammu, Jammu and Kashmir, India

R. Velu et al. (eds.), *Digital Design and Manufacturing of Medical Devices and Systems*, https://doi.org/10.1007/978-981-99-7100-8_1

other additive manufacturing technologies. Additive manufacturing, specifically 3D printing, has transformed the biomedical device industry by enabling the development of patient-specific implants, prosthetic limbs, and surgical instruments. This chapter examines how recent digital manufacturing technologies such as Artificial Intelligence (AI) & Machine Learning (ML), Augmented Reality (AR), Virtual Reality (VR), and Internet of Medical Things (IoMT) have altered biomedical devices to produce extremely accurate and individualized devices for patients. Ultimately, the legislative and ethical concerns, cost-effectiveness, and scaling challenges have been addressed for future research and developments. Overall, the outcome of this study allows the researchers to build a more sustainable healthcare system, additionally directing them to focus on developing materials by integrating various digital manufacturing technologies, thereby improving the customization and personalization of biomedical equipment.

Keywords

Digital manufacturing · Healthcare · IoT/IoMT · AI and ML

1.1 Introduction

The development of digital manufacturing technology has had a considerable impact on the field of biomedical devices recently. Digital manufacturing is the creation, modification, and optimization of manufacturing processes using computer-aided design (CAD) software and other digital technologies (Velu et al. 2023a). It is possible to create digital representations of products that can subsequently be utilized as guidance for automated manufacturing procedures like 3D printing, CNC machining, and laser cutting. Using this technology in the context of biomedical equipment permits the construction of intricate and unique devices that may be catered to the requirements of a specific patient. Additionally, it enables quicker and more effective production procedures, which can lower expenditures and increase access to medical devices. The significance of digital manufacturing in biomedical devices is shown in Table 1.1.

Digital manufacturing techniques enable the development of sophisticated tissue-like structures, which are useful in biodevice fabrication, disease modeling, and drug testing. Processability, cell compatibility, and structural integrity of biomaterials employed in biomedical device fabrications are all affected by their qualities (Zaeri et al. 2022). To overcome this, research has been progressing to associate digital manufacturing with intelligence technologies, such as Machine learning (ML) and Internet of Medical Things (IoMT). ML, a subfield of Artificial Intelligence (AI), enables computers to learn from data, make predictions, and improve performance. In terms of flexibility, adaptability, and prediction accuracy, ML models outperform classical physics-based models. The decision between physics-based and ML models is determined by the task at hand, with ML excelling in cases where direct

Table 1.1 Significance of digital manufacturing in biomedical devices

Significance	Definition	Pros	Cons	Application	Ref.
Design and customization	Allows for precise design and customization biomedical devices to fit the specific needs of individual patients	• Customization of medical devices to fit an individual's unique anatomy	• Expensive to produce than standard devices, leading to higher costs for patients	• Customized prosthetics, dental implants	Velu et al. (2019)
Precision	Using technologies such as 3D printing and CNC machining offers higher precision and accuracy compared to traditional methods	• Reduced material waste • Faster production times • More consistent production quality • Ability to create devices with tight tolerances	• Higher initial investment costs • Limited materials and production sizes	• 3D-printed surgical tools • CNC-machined orthopedic implants	Velu et al. (2019)
Design flexibility	Enables complex and intricate designs, as well as the ability to make changes to designs quickly and easily	• Creation of custom-fit devices • Reduced need for secondary surgeries • Ability to optimize design for functionality and aesthetics	• Higher production costs • Longer production times	• 3D printed implants, customized surgical tools	Velu et al. (2023a)
Advanced materials	Utilize advanced materials such as biodegradable polymers and shape-memory alloys for better performance and biocompatibility	• Improved device biocompatibility • Enhanced device functionality	• Higher material costs • *Limited material availability*	• Biodegradable implants • Shape-memory alloy stents	Velu et al. (2023b)
Integration with technologies	Integrated with other technologies such as AI, IoMT, and AR/VR to create smarter and more innovative devices	• Improved functionality and efficiency • Reduced risk of errors	• Increased need for skilled personnel • Higher development costs	• Smart prosthetics with IoMT sensors • AR-assisted surgery planning	Velu et al. (2023a)

(continued)

Table 1.1 (continued)

Significance	Definition	Pros	Cons	Application	Ref.
Quality control	Allows for greater control over the production process, resulting in higher quality devices that meet rigorous regulatory requirements	• Improve device safety • Consistent and accurate production of medical devices	• Proper validation and testing of processes required to ensure product safety and efficacy	• 3D printed medical models and implants	Velu et al. (2023a)
Cost reduction	Reduce the need for expensive tooling and molds and can produce devices in small quantities	• Eliminate the need for expensive tooling and molds • Increased affordability • Improved access to care	• High initial costs of equipment and technology can offset the cost savings	• 3D printed prosthetics • Customized dental devices	Velu et al. (2023a, b)

information is restricted but there are plenty of training examples available. While machine learning has been successfully used to optimize 3D printing processes, its applicability in 3D bioprinting is currently limited. In the future, ML-driven bioprinting holds promise for safer drug testing, less reliance on animal testing, and potential organ repair or replacement. Increased research emphasis on ML-based bioprinting has the potential to expedite progress in regenerative medicine. On the other hand, the IoMT, a subclass of Internet of Things (IoT) technology, focuses on interconnected medical devices for healthcare monitoring. IoMT devices allow for remote monitoring of patients' health parameters and make medical data gathering, processing, and transmission easier. This wireless monitoring aids in the prevention of needless hospital visits and the reduction of associated expenditures (Bandyopadhyay et al. 2021). This chapter provided an overview of the fact that digital manufacturing technologies such as AI and Machine Learning (ML), Augmented Reality (AR), Virtual Reality (VR), and the Internet of Medical Things (IoMT) have altered biomedical devices to produce extremely accurate and personalized devices for patients. Finally, the legislative and ethical problems, cost-effectiveness, and scaling issues for future research and development have been addressed. Overall, the findings of this study enable researchers to create a more sustainable healthcare system and to direct their efforts toward generating materials through the integration of multiple digital manufacturing technologies, thereby boosting the customization and personalization of biomedical equipment.

1.2 Digital Manufacturing Technologies for Biomedical Devices

1.2.1 3D Printing

Additive manufacturing, denoted as 3D printing, is the development of three-dimensional objects from digital models. This technology has transformed the biomedical device industry by enabling the development of patient-specific implants, prosthetic limbs, and surgical instruments with complex geometries and structures that would be difficult to produce using traditional manufacturing methods (Velu et al. 2023b).

Customization aside, 3D printing is a very adaptable and flexible manufacturing process that can work with a variety of materials, notably biocompatible and biodegradable materials. As a result, it can be used to create a variety of biomedical devices, from surgical tools to tissue engineering scaffolds to drug delivery systems (Velu et al. 2019; Rajkumar et al. 2020).

1.2.1.1 Stereolithography

A technique of 3D printing called stereolithography (SLA) selectively cures liquid photopolymer resins layer-by-layer using a UV laser to produce three-dimensional objects, as schematically represented in Fig. 1.1. Given that it enables the manufacture of highly accurate and precise parts with a resolution of up to nanometers—

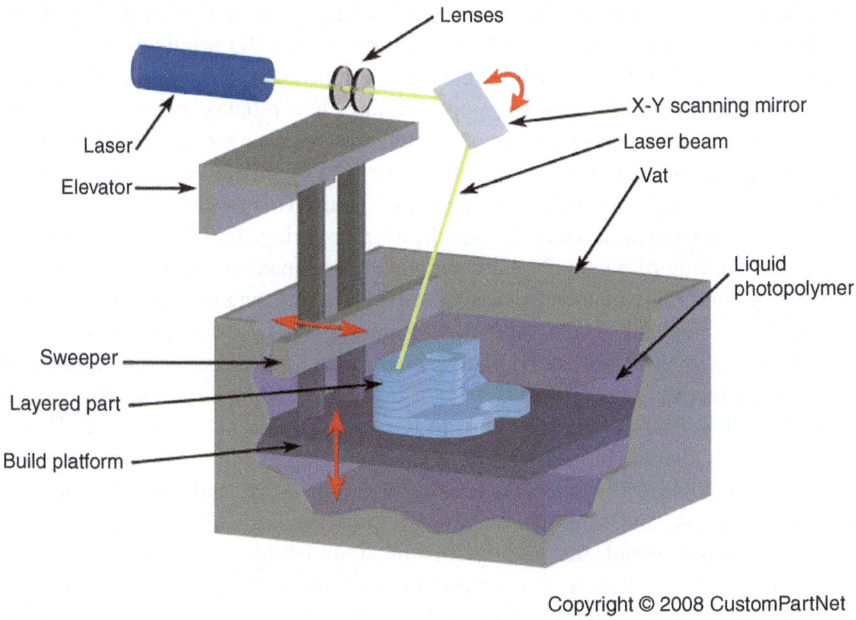

Fig. 1.1 Schematic diagram for stereolithography (CustomPartNet 2023a)

significantly higher than other 3D printing technologies like FDM or SLS. Venkata Siva Gummaluri et al. demonstrated the use of SLA to create structures that are suitable for random lasing. On a photo resin chip, the researchers create vertical cylindrical microchannels that are randomly dispersed. They then inject liquid optical gain medium into the channels to adjust the peak lasing wavelength, threshold, and lowest feasible line width. With slight adjustments to the microchannels' diameter, a wavelength tunability of about 22 nm is possible (Gummaluri and Vadakke Matham 2023). Qingchuan Song et al. discussed the use of multi-material stereolithography to fabricate customized pneumatic actuators for microactuators, soft robots, and biomedical engineering applications. Vat-based stereolithography is utilized to combine materials with different Young's moduli, resulting in multimaterial actuators having a resolution up to 200 μm. In terms of deformation controllability and ease of construction, multi-material actuators outperform single-material actuators (Song et al. 2023).

Ishak Ertugrul et al. described the design and testing of a 3D-printed strain sensor made from photopolymer-based conductive and flexible UV resin components. The sensor was created using a stereolithography-based printer and was composed of two parts: conductive channels and a flexible bottom base comprised of different materials. Experiments revealed a linear relationship between the strain sensor and the measured resistance value, and the sensor's flexible nature makes it suited for use in soft applications. Tensile test specimens were also created to study behavior and offer data on sensor placement. It is constructive when making tiny, complex components for biological equipment such as dental implants, hearing aids, and microfluidic gadgets. A smooth surface finish fabrication procedure is perfect for biomedical equipment that need biocompatibility and cleaning simplicity. The smooth texture is also less likely to encourage bacterial adherence, making it perfect for uses like implants or surgical equipment (Ertugrul et al. 2023).

1.2.1.2 Fused Deposition Modeling

Figure 1.2 shows the schematics of Fused Deposition Modeling (FDM). FDM is a sort of 3D printing technology that builds three-dimensional objects by melting a material via a nozzle and depositing it one layer at a time. It is especially helpful for developing prototypes and small-batch production runs from surgical tools to prosthetic limbs, using a variety of materials with various mechanical properties that satisfy unique medical needs. The mechanical characteristics of the finished product can also be adjusted by changing printing settings including layer height, infill density, and print orientation. It is essential for biomedical equipment, such as prosthetic limbs, to be able to create objects with varied degrees of stiffness, flexibility, and durability.

Izabella Rajzer et al. developed a composite filament modified with bioglass and zinc-doped bioglass, which was used to create 3D-printed scaffolds for osteochondral implants. The bioglass-modified filaments were strong and flexible, and the scaffolds showed good biological properties, including cell attachment and

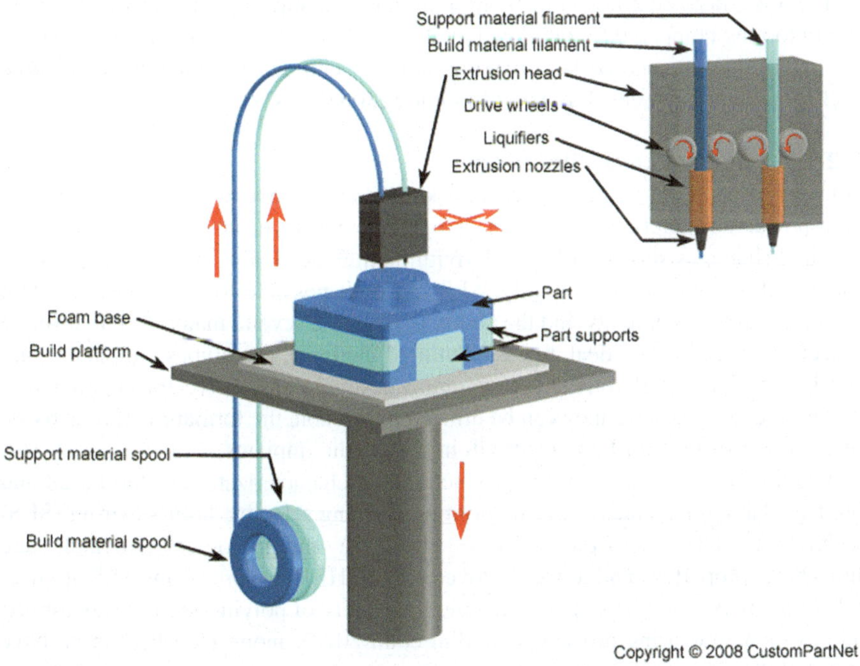

Fig. 1.2 Schematic of fused deposition modeling (CustomPartNet 2023b)

proliferation. Due to the existence of a spatial microstructure, the scaffolds also exhibited lower mechanical characteristics. In vitro mineralization investigations revealed that apatite formed on bioglass-modified scaffolds after 7 days of immersion in simulated bodily fluid, whereas zinc slowed apatite production. Overall, the innovative composite filaments have potential for use in creating bioactive scaffolds for tissue engineering applications (Rajzer et al. 2023). Raffaele Pertusio et al. aimed at creating a 3D-printed housing for thin-film sensors such as FlexiForce® used for measuring forces in biomedical studies and clinical trials. The housing is designed to protect the sensor, enhance accuracy, and increase repeatability of measurements by shielding it, thereby encountering the effects of the surface material. Using existing medical-grade printing materials and 3D printers, the 3D-printed housing may be adapted to demands and manufactured fast and affordably (Pertusio and Roatta 2023). Stanislav Y. Shilov et al. employed fused deposition modeling (FDM/FFF) to create cylindrical plates of polylactide (PLA), polyethylene terephthalate glycol (PETG), and polyetheretherketone (PEEK) to evaluate the adherence of rat bone marrow and peritoneal cells. The number of attached cells and polymer sample weight varied substantially (44–119% and 0.61–2.18%, respectively) based on surface roughness adjusted by nozzle diameter and printing layer height. The results showed that more cells attached to PLA materials with a higher nozzle diameter and layer height, but adherence was greater with a smaller nozzle diameter for PEEK samples. The variation in outcomes between polymers is due to their chemical structure (Shilov et al. 2022).

FDM is a fast and efficient method of producing complex geometries without the use of tooling compared to traditional method such as CNC machining, as a result it eliminates the time and costs of making molds or cutting tool, such that a valuable tool for research and development of biomedical devices.

1.2.1.3 Selective Laser Sintering

A laser is used in the 3D printing process known as selective laser sintering (SLS) to fuse powdered materials like nylon or titanium one layer at a time to create the required shape, as shown in Fig. 1.3. With its high accuracy, mechanical strength, functionality, and biocompatibility, SLS makes it possible to create devices with varying degrees of porosity and the ability to combine several materials into a single object. This makes it ideal for generating functional prototypes, implants, and surgical equipment. Porous structures are a desirable alternative for creating biomedical devices because they can be utilized to promote the formation of new tissue or to offer a surface for bone ingrowth in orthopedic implants.

Giubilini et al. focused on the production and characterization of bio-based and biodegradable microspheres for 3D printing utilizing selective laser sintering (SLS) technology. The microspheres were tuned for morphological, thermal, and flowability properties, and it was discovered that PHBH has promising SLS applicability and marks the first step in widening the variety of polymeric materials for this additive manufacturing process (Giubilini et al. 2023). Jeong Hun Park et al. have successfully 3D printed a unique architected auxetic for large-volume soft tissue engineering utilizing polycaprolactone (PCL) selective laser sintering (SLS).

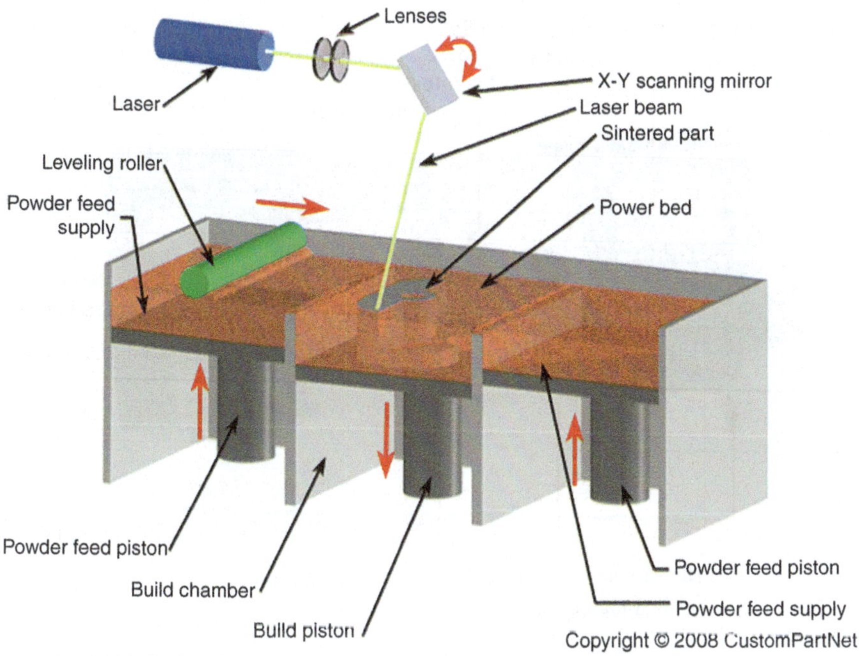

Fig. 1.3 Schematic of selective laser sintering (CustomPartNet 2023c)

Despite PCL's rather stiff and linear mechanical characteristics, the 3D auxetic design produced considerable initial flexibility and nonlinear stress–strain response to uniaxial compression using finite element simulation. The 3D auxetic also displayed significant cell survivability and cell functionality within a cell-laden hydrogel, highlighting the possibility of clinically viable 3D implants for large-volume soft tissue reconstruction (Park et al. 2023). SLS is a clean and environmentally friendly additive manufacturing process, the unused powder also be reused in the next production cycle, reducing material waste and overall production costs.

1.2.2 CNC Machining

Using computer-controlled machines to remove material from a block of material to create a part or component with exact specifications is known as CNC machining, the commercial machine is shown in Fig. 1.4. Despite being widely employed in sectors like aerospace, automotive, and electronics, CNC machining has also demonstrated promise for producing biomedical devices. In particular, the creation of biomedical equipment benefits substantially from its ability to produce high precision and complicated geometry. To ensure that the finished product fits the specified criteria, CNC machines can make parts with tolerances as small as a few microns. The creation of implants, such as dental, orthopedic, and surgical tools,

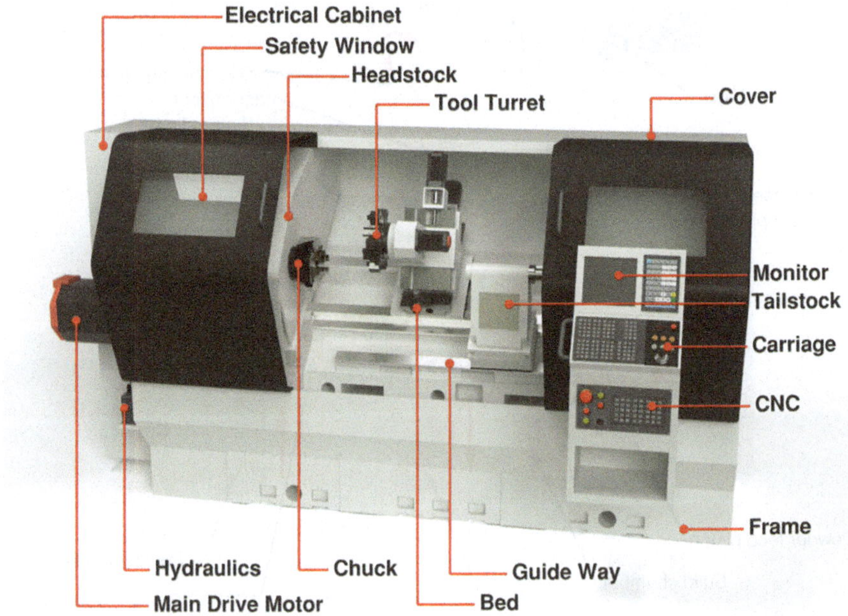

Fig. 1.4 CNC Lathe machine (CNC Masters 2023)

made of titanium or other biocompatible materials that can resist the demanding conditions of the human body, depends on this level of accuracy. Once the design is complete and the CNC program is developed, it will be simple to scale up the production to generate huge numbers of pieces. Because of this, CNC machining is one of the most effective manufacturing methods for biomedical devices that need to be produced in large quantities. In addition, it has the capacity to create intricate surface features, such as undercuts and curved surfaces, which are challenging to achieve using other production processes, especially when producing specialized surgical tools.

Mangolika Bhattacharya et al. investigated the use of an Artificial Neural Network (ANN) for real-time tool offset correction in the production of prosthetic knees using Adaptive Machining. The CNC machining cell incorporates smart sensor technology to collect force data, which is then expended to relate the functioning of a random forest classification algorithm and Bi-directional Long-Term Short Memory (LSTM) neural networks. Pre-processing modifications and a novel projection technique to turn the 2D time series data into a 3D array for the Bi-directional LSTM model results are recommended for future deployments utilizing real training data (Bhattacharya et al. 2023). The supply chain for CNC machining is well established, the technology is mature also it is economically advantageous manufacturing technology for the creation of biomedical devices because. Therefore, it is anticipated to keep playing a prominent role in the field of biomedical engineering.

1.2.3 Laser Cutting

A powerful laser is used in the subtractive manufacturing process of laser cutting to etch or cut materials like metal, plastic, or ceramic, as shown in Fig. 1.5. Compared to other conventional cutting techniques, it can generate cuts with a precision of up to 10 μm. To fabricate biomedical devices with intricate geometries, such stents or vascular grafts, a high level of precision is required. Additionally, it enables us to create devices with a variety of attributes, including biocompatibility, durability, and strength, and some instances of these materials are stainless steel, titanium, and polymers. Moreover, it may be simply incorporated into CAD and CAM systems, enabling the production of intricate and unique biological equipment. As a result, biomedical devices that are tailored to the individual demands of the patient can be quickly prototyped and produced. Scott Downen et al. covered the design and construction of a low-cost microfluidics cartridge with fluid storage and manipulation capabilities via a proprietary pressure-driven check valve. The cartridge parts

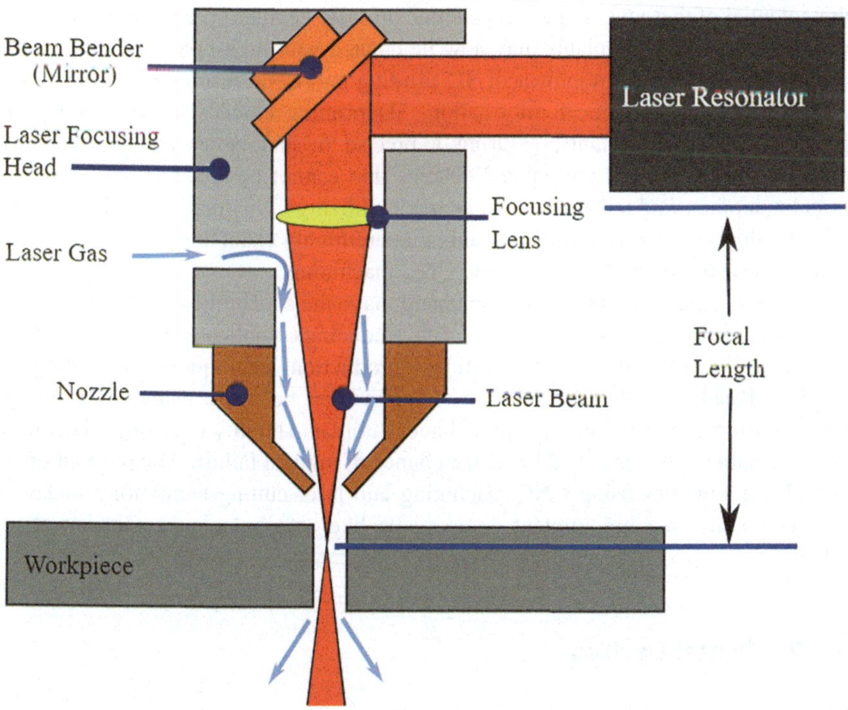

Fig. 1.5 Schematic of laser cutting (Purdue.edu 2023)

are made with a desktop CNC and laser cutter, and the check valve is made with PDMS in a bespoke acrylic mold. The cartridge was subjected to preliminary testing, which included fluid manipulation and usage for molecular diagnostics. Because of its low cost, ease of production, and fluid storage and manipulation capabilities, the design is excellent for research and high-volume testing in low-resource contexts (Downen et al. 2023).

1.3 Applications of Digital Manufacturing in Biomedical Devices

1.3.1 Orthopedic Implants

The field of orthopedics has undergone a revolution thanks to digital manufacturing technology, which offers several advantages over traditional manufacturing techniques, especially when it comes to creating orthopedic implants like knee, hip, and spinal implants. It made it possible to design highly precise, replicable implants that may be tailored to a patient's unique anatomy, enhancing patient outcomes and lowering problems.

Numerous materials, such as polyethylene, cobalt-chromium, and titanium, can be used to make knee implants using techniques like casting or forging. However, the potential of these techniques to generate intricate geometries and unique designs is constrained. Knee implants may now be created with high precision and repeatability through the development of 3D printing and CNC machining. Based on a patient's unique anatomical information, 3D printing enables the production of personalized knee implants, assuring a precise fit and better patient outcome. Complex geometry and specialized designs that cannot be created using conventional manufacturing techniques can be made utilizing CNC machining. Regardless of individuals specialties, knee implants that are highly exact and reproducible can be created using both 3D printing and CNC machining.

Hip and spinal implants, on the one hand, have the capabilities to use the similar range of materials alike knee implants. Yet, producing complicated and personalized geometries is difficult with conventional production techniques like casting or forging (Pashley et al. 2023). Porous implants can be made using 3D printing, which promotes bone ingrowth and enhances implant stability over time. This may enhance patient outcomes and lower the chance of implant failure. The production of complex geometries using CNC machining and laser cutting technology makes it perfect for creating hip implant components like acetabular cups (Tredan et al. 2023).

1.3.2 Dental Devices

The dental sector has been transformed by digital manufacturing technologies, which offer precise and effective ways to make dental equipment like crowns, bridges, aligners, and retainers. Digital technology has lowered manufacturing errors, expedited up production, and enhanced patient results.

Dental restorations including crowns and bridges are used to replace missing or damaged teeth, which were traditionally made by taking physical imprints of the patient's teeth, sending those impressions to a dental laboratory, and then waiting several days for the restoration to be finished. However, this procedure has been simplified owing to digital manufacturing technologies. An intraoral scanner can be used to take a digital impression of the patient's teeth, which can then be transferred to CAD software. A 3D model of the restoration is created by the software and delivered to a CAM machine for computer-aided fabrication. A block of ceramic or other material is milled into the restoration using the CAM machine. The duration of the patient's therapy might be cut down by placing the final restoration with cement on the same day (Yu et al. 2022a).

After receiving orthodontic treatment, aligners and retainers are used to maintain alignment and straighten teeth. Traditionally, aligners and retainers were made by physically imprinting the patient's teeth, shipping the impressions to a dental laboratory, and waiting several days for the device to be created. Digital manufacturing technologies, on the other hand, have significantly enhanced this procedure. An intraoral scanner can be used to take a digital impression of the patient's teeth, which can then be transferred to CAD software. A 3D printer is used to print the aligners or retainers after the program creates a 3D model of the patient's teeth. Patient outcomes are improved because of the shorter production time and higher precision provided by the digital fabrication process (Naeem et al. 2022).

Digital manufacturing technologies offer the potential to create dental products to match the unique demands of each patient in addition to the advantages of accuracy and efficiency. For instance, using CAD software, the size and shape of a dental replacement can be precisely customized to meet the demands of the patient. We can create intricate shapes using 3D printing technology that would be challenging to build using more conventional techniques. This personalization results in dental equipment that fits the patient more comfortably.

The use of digital manufacturing technology in the creation of dental devices is not without its restrictions, though. The expense of the tools and software needed for the fabrication process is a significant restriction. For smaller dental practices or those located in less-developed areas, this expense can be prohibitive. Additionally, the quality of the initial digital impression affects how accurate the final output will be. The finished product might not fit perfectly if the imprint is not properly taken, necessitating more time and money to make the necessary adjustments. Finally, even if the fabrication process has been greatly enhanced by digital manufacturing technology, some conventional methods, such hand-finished polishing, may still be necessary to attain the ideal level of aesthetics.

1.3.3 Prosthetics and Assistive Devices

The quality of life for those with impairments has significantly improved using prosthetics and assistive technology. The conventional production method for these devices is expensive and time-consuming. However, with improvements in digital manufacturing techniques, it is now quicker, more accurate, and more affordable to make prosthetics and other assistive equipment. It is now feasible to build prosthetics and assistive devices with better precision, tailored to the patient's specific demands, and in a shorter amount of time particularly for applications like limb prosthetics, hearing aids, and wheelchairs.

A digital model of the patient's intact leg and ear canal is built using 3D scanning technology for prosthetic and assistive equipment like hearing aids, which are frequently manufactured using digital manufacturing technology. Using additive manufacturing methods like 3D printing or selective laser sintering, a custom-fitted prosthetic socket and hearing aid shell are then designed using this model. The remaining parts of the prosthetic device, including the joints and prosthetic limb, are also 3D printed or milled using CAM. Device fit, comfort, and functionality may all be precisely customized through digital fabrication (Jia et al. 2023; Valadez Mesta 2022). The widely used biomedical implants/devices using various digital manufacturing technology is shown in Table 1.2.

Another form of assistive device that can profit from digital manufacturing is wheelchairs. Wheelchair frames are typically handcrafted from welded steel tubing; as a result of the development of digital manufacturing, wheelchair frames may now be made using CNC milling or 3D printing, allowing for greater customization and lightweight design. For instance, unique seating and support structures can be produced using 3D printing, but robust, lightweight titanium frames can be produced using CNC milling (Nace et al. 2023).

1.4 Recent Trends and Developments in Digital Manufacturing for Biomedical Devices

1.4.1 Advanced Materials

A new development and trend in digital manufacturing for biomedical devices is the use of advanced materials. These materials are made to specifically suit the functional, durable, and biocompatibility needs of biomedical equipment. Advanced materials such as shape-memory alloys, nanomaterials, and biodegradable polymers are a few examples that are employed in biomedical equipment.

The body can safely absorb and metabolize biodegradable polymers, which makes them perfect for use in implantable medical devices including sutures, screws, and plates. The need for additional procedures to remove the device can be decreased because these materials can deteriorate with time. Complex geometries with biodegradable polymers can be produced using digital manufacturing processes like

Table 1.2 Biomedical implants/devices using various digital manufacturing technology and its limitations

Sl. no.	Implant/device	Materials used	Digital manufacturing technology	Improvements	Limitations	Ref.
1.	Spinal implant for C1/C2 arthrodesis	Titanium alloy	Selective laser melting (SLM)	Customized implant, great uneventful recovery, and pain relief, reduced overall surgical time and risk	High cost, lack of standards, requirements of 3D implant modeling specific skills	Phan et al. (2016)
2.	Acetabular cup—hip implant	Titanium alloy	Electron beam melting (EBM)	100% patient satisfaction and no mechanical failure, less operative time and complication rates	More time-consuming in design and fabrication, high associated cost	Wyatt (2015)
3.	Hip stem protheses	Titanium alloy Ti6Al4V	CNC machining and EBM	35% cost reduction comparison to CNC machining, creation of open-celled net structures for bone ingrowth	Extra post processing required—hipping, yields lower fatigue strength	Torres et al. (2016)
4.	Cranial implant and bone fracture fixture plate	Stainless steel 316L with PEEK polymer	Fused filament fabrication (FFF)	Complex porous design flexibility, lower cost and lead time, patient comfort and process feasibility	Extra post processing of polymer debinding and sintering.	Chacon et al. (2022)
5.	Maxillofacial reconstruction protheses	Prime cast polymer and titanium	SLA and casting	Perfectly fit the defect during operation and reduced surgical time	Two-stage manufacturing process leads to high production time.	Singare et al. (2008)
6.	Dental model and aligners	Photocurable resin and thermoplastic polyurethane (TPU)	SLA and thermoforming	Patient-specific clear aligner for orthodontic treatment, aesthetic, compatible, and efficient appliance.	Single-layer TPU exhibits lower strength	Yu et al. (2022b)
7.	Dental implants	Polymer/metal multi-material	Hybrid AM (SLM -SLA)	Customize multi-material high strength dental crown and bridge implant with functional	High cost and limited curable biocompatible materials for dental implants	Silva et al. (2017)

(continued)

Table 1.2 (continued)

Sl. no.	Implant/device	Materials used	Digital manufacturing technology	Improvements	Limitations	Ref.
				gradients for edentulism problem		
8.	Prosthetic and surgical guide for dental implant surgery	Polyamide	Selective laser sintering (SLS)	Minimize problems related to occlusal adjustment and misfitting of prosthesis with fixed interim dental implant loading, immediate dental prosthetic fabrication	Prosthetic fractures observed after 3 month of implant delivery	Di Giacomo et al. (2016)
9.	Hearing aids	ENG hard and flexible resin mixed with ciprofloxacin–fluocinolone acetonide antibiotics	Digital light processing (DLP)	Infection free, patient specific hearing aids with antibiotic properties	Lower life span of hearing aids, i.e., 2 weeks	Vivero-Lopez et al. (2021)
10.	Kidney micro 3D scaffolds for tissue engineering	Poly-propylene fumarate (PPF) and diethyl fumarate (DEF)	Micro SLA	Biodegradable and biocompatible 3D micro-scaffolds with totally interlinked pores by 3D printing	Post processing requirement and shrinkages exhibit poor dimensional accuracy	Choi et al. (2009)
11.	Transtibial prosthetic socket	Polyamide	Fused filament fabrication (FFF)	Reduced fabrication time, high strength and patient comfort and fitting	Slightly heavy than conventionally made	Ng et al. (2002)
12.	Finger prothesis	Polylactic acid (PLA) with 1% copper nanoparticles	Fused filament fabrication (FFF)	Patient-specific finger protheses produced with antibacterial properties at low cost	Post processing after fabrication needed	Zuniga (2018)

stereolithography and 3D printing, enabling the creation of more specialized and accurate devices.

Another revolutionary material that has been applied to biomedical equipment is shape-memory alloys. These alloys are perfect for use in flexible and adaptable devices like stents and catheters because they can alter their shape in response to changes in temperature or stress. Shape-memory alloys can be formed into complex shapes using digital manufacturing processes like selective laser melting, allowing for the creation of more accurate and efficient medical devices.

Another sort of cutting-edge material that has showed promise in biomedical device applications is nanomaterials. These substances have special physical and chemical characteristics that can be tuned to medical uses, such as tissue engineering or medication delivery. With exact control over their properties and dimensions, nanomaterial-based structures and devices can be made using digital manufacturing processes like electrospinning and inkjet printing. The most common advanced materials using various digital manufacturing technology for various biomedical applications are shown in Table 1.3.

1.4.1.1 Biodegradable Materials

A new development in digital manufacturing for biomedical equipment is the use of biodegradable materials. Due to their capacity to deteriorate over time, lower the danger of long-term problems, and foster tissue regeneration, these materials have grown in favor. Implants, scaffolds, and medication delivery systems can all be made of biodegradable materials.

It is possible to create biodegradable devices with complex geometries using digital manufacturing techniques like 3D printing and stereolithography, which are difficult or impossible to do using conventional production methods. Biomedical applications frequently employ biodegradable polymers like poly (lactic acid), poly (glycolic acid), and their copolymers (PLGA). These materials can be made in a variety of forms and sizes, and the amount of lactic acid to glycolic acid in the copolymer can be changed to influence how quickly they degrade (Gharbi et al. 2023).

Devices that can administer medications directly to the site of an injury or disease have been developed; thanks to developments in biodegradable materials. For the treatment of coronary artery disease, biodegradable drug-eluting stents have been created, and biodegradable sutures have been created for the healing of wounds.

Additionally, it is possible to construct multifunctional devices with improved therapeutic qualities by combining biodegradable materials with other cutting-edge materials like hydrogels and nanoparticles.

1.4.1.2 Shape-Memory Alloys

Shape-Memory Alloys (SMAs) has the unusual ability to "remember" its original shape even after being distorted. They may be bent to fit a specific shape or position within the body and then recover to their original shape once in place, making them perfect for use in biomedical devices. SMAs can be utilized in additive manufacturing techniques like selective laser melting in digital manufacturing to

Table 1.3 Advanced materials using various digital manufacturing technology for biomedical application

Sl. no.	Advanced materials	Digital manufacturing	Implants/devices	Improvements	Ref.
1.	Titanium alloys (Ti6Al4V)	EBM	Tibial knee stems, hip stems and intermedullary rods	Geometrical array of cellular, reticular mesh, and open cell interconnected porosities has potential for unique bone compatibility and bone ingrowth	Murr et al. (2010)
2.	Titanium ELI alloy	DMLS	Facial orbital bone implant	Exact fitting of implants, improved accuracy, and reduced operation time and patient morbidity	Salmi et al. (2012)
3.	Polymethyl methacrylate (PMMA)/β-tricalcium phosphate (β-TCP)	SLS	Bone grafts and implants	SLS 3D printing has been shown to be a viable method for producing bone scaffolds and implants. Inherent process induced porosity improves bone cell ingrowth	Velu et al. (2018), Velu and Singamneni (2014)
4.	Polycaprolactone diacrylate (PCL-DA) coated by polydopamine and hydroxy apatite mineralize	DLP	Bone scaffolds	Bio inspired customized bone scaffolds, biocompatible and osteoconductive for cell proliferation	Cheng et al. (2016)
5.	Yttria-stabilized zirconia (TZ-3YS-E)	DLP	Dental implants	Tailored zirconia dental implants with adequate dimensional accuracy and flexural strength effectively proven to be printed by 3D printing	Osman et al. (2017)
6.	Carbon fibre reinforced CFR-PEEK	FFF	Orthopaedic and dental implants	Biocompatible and proper strength polymer composite proven to be potential for bone grafting and tissue engineering applications	Han et al. (2019)
7.	Strontium doped bioactive glasses	3D bioprinting	Bone scaffolds for tissue engineering and implants	Better structural control and enhanced mechanical strength, high apatite-forming capacity and stimulates osteoblast cell proliferation and differentiation	Zhang et al. (2014), Kargozar et al. (2019)

8.	Tantalum (Ta) metal	SLM	Orthopaedic bone implants	Excellent osteoconductive complex porous implant with higher fatigue strength and ductility, biocompatible and good functional bonding between implant and regenerated bone	Wauthle et al. (2015)
9.	Fibrous collagen/poly (ε-capro-lactone) (PCL)/HA composite with hydrogel	3D bioprinting	Bone scaffolds	Functional scaffold with enhanced osteogenesis to the human adipose stem cells (hASCs)	Aram et al. (2008)
10.	Polylactide (PLA)/calcium carbonet (CC)	SLS	Bone scaffolds and cranial implant	Complex interconnected pore structure, better viability for osteoblast cells, and biocompatibility.	Gayer et al. (2019)

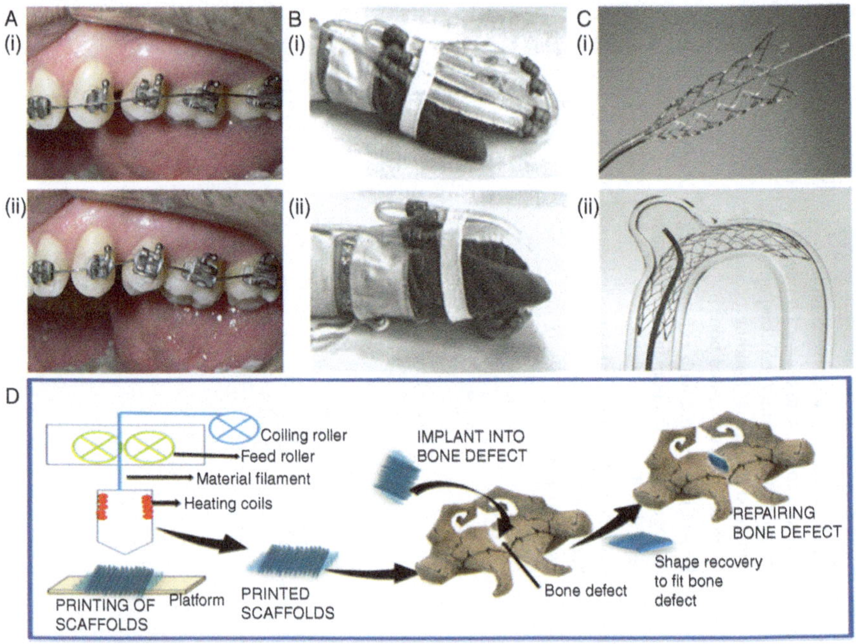

Fig. 1.6 Typical application of SMAs in biomedical; (**a**) orthodontic arch wires of super elastic NiTi (i) before and (ii) after bracket engagement (Fernandes et al. 2011); (**b**) gloves with SMA wires with position at (i) low temperature and (ii) high temperature (Petrini and Migliavacca 2011); (**c**) self-expandable neurosurgical stent of NiTi alloy (i) before and (ii) after insertion (Petrini and Migliavacca 2011) (reproduced with permission under CC BY license); (**d**) 4D printed shape memory polymer bone tissue scaffolds for repairing of bone defects (reproduced with prior permission from Subash and Kandasubramanian 2020)

build complicated shapes accurately and precisely for biomedical devices. SMAs have been employed in a wide range of biological applications such as cardiovascular devices, orthopedic implants, stents, and various applications, as shown in Fig. 1.6 (Sato and Guo 2023).

New alloys with improved qualities, such as better biocompatibility and increased endurance, have been the focus of recent developments in SMAs. In addition, new uses for SMAs have been investigated in fields like tissue engineering and medication delivery.

1.4.1.3 Nanomaterials

Due to their distinct physicochemical properties, nanomaterials have become a viable field in digital manufacturing for biological devices. Materials with diameters in the nanometer range, usually between 1 and 100 nm, are referred to as nanomaterials. Nanomaterials have been applied to biomedical devices to improve their biological and mechanical capabilities. Figure 1.7 shows the schematic for Metal-Organic Framework (MOF)–based nanomaterials for bone tissue and wound

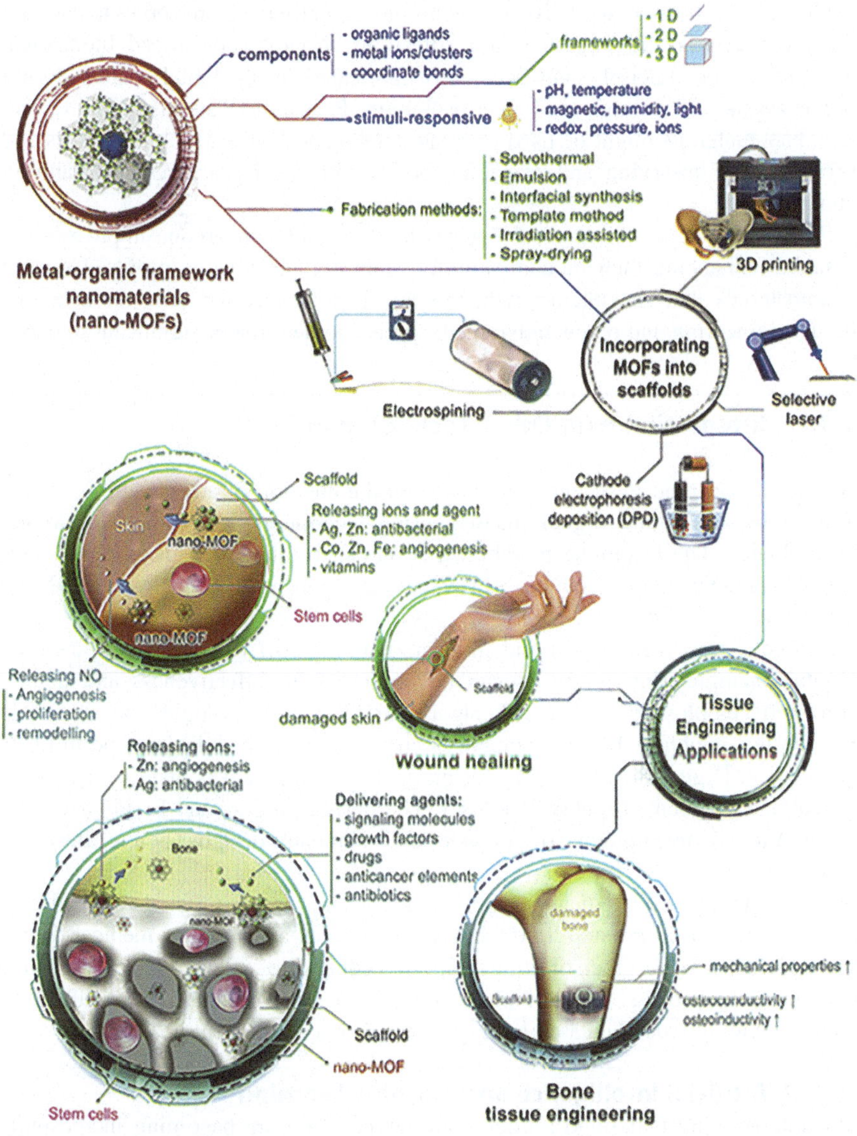

Fig. 1.7 Schematic for Metal-Organic Framework (MOF)–based nanomaterials with different components, frameworks, stimuli-responsive and scaffold fabrication methods for bone tissue engineering and wound healing applications. (Reproduced with permission from Fardjahromi et al. 2022)

healing applications. Drug delivery systems have also used nanomaterials to increase the effectiveness and targeting of medications. Nanomaterial-based biomedical devices can be precisely and accurately fabricated using digital manufacturing processes like 3D printing and electrospinning. Researchers are also looking into how nanomaterials might be used to create intelligent devices, such as sensors and actuators, for observing and managing bodily biological processes (Fardjahromi et al. 2022).

Nanomaterials for biomedical devices have recently undergone improvements aimed at enhancing their biocompatibility, stability, and toxicity profile. Creating nanomaterials that can interact with biological molecules and cells for uses like tissue engineering and regenerative medicine is another area of significant interest.

1.4.2 Integration with Other Technologies

An increasing trend in recent years has been the creation of advanced biomedical devices by combining digital manufacturing technology with other developing technologies. The discipline of robotics is one such integration. Robotic systems can help in the manufacturing process by automating inspection, quality control, and assembly.

Artificial intelligence (AI) and machine learning (ML) integration is another. Digital manufacturing processes can be improved for effectiveness and quality control by employing AI and ML algorithms. These technologies can also help with design, enabling the development of customized medical devices and intricate geometries. Digital manufacturing for biomedical equipment is also incorporating virtual and augmented reality (VR/AR). The design process can be improved by using VR/AR technology to envision and simulate designs before they are manufactured.

The Internet of Medical Things and sensors are combined with digital manufacturing as a last step. IoMT devices may track and monitor medical device performance in real time, offering helpful feedback to enhance the design and manufacturing process. Additionally, sensors can be built right into medical equipment, providing crucial data on both device function and patient health.

1.4.2.1 Artificial Intelligence and Machine Learning

Machine learning (ML) and artificial intelligence (AI) are becoming increasingly important in the design and manufacture of biomedical equipment, as well as in numerous aspects of healthcare. These technologies have transformed the sector by allowing for the analysis of vast amounts of data and the creation of personalized devices for individual patients. AI and machine learning algorithms have improved the performance and dependability of biomedical devices, making them more effective and lowering the risk of complications. Furthermore, these technologies can produce individualized implant designs that better match with each patient's anatomy by using algorithms that assess patient imaging data. This customization results in a better fit, which reduces the likelihood of complications like implant loosening or dislocation. Process optimization for digital manufacturing is another application of AI and ML in biomedical equipment; it can optimize the production process by analyzing data from sensors and other sources, increasing efficiency, decreasing waste, and ensuring consistent quality in the product also to aid with decision-making, disease prediction, and monitoring in the field of cardiovascular diseases (CVDs). These technologies have been shown to be effective in identifying arrhythmic heartbeats, forecasting irregularities, and evaluating electrocardiogram (ECG) signals. They have also been used to detect disorders such as atrial fibrillation (AF) and abdominal aortic aneurysm (AAA) (Shin et al. 2022). Artificial intelligence–assisted surgery has emerged as a prominent use of AI in healthcare. AI technologies, for example, can help surgeons evaluate massive volumes of data, anticipate risks, direct surgical procedures, and improve postoperative care, among other things. Machine learning algorithms, for example, have been created to predict difficulties in spine procedures and postoperative fatalities in cardiac patients, allowing surgeons to take preemptive measures to increase patient safety. Clinical accuracy can be enhanced, and real-time glucose levels can be delivered by merging AI-based techniques with glucose-monitoring equipment. Machine learning algorithms trained on numerous input features can detect human glucose levels correctly, assisting in the prediction of diabetes patterns, diagnosing diabetes risk, and tailoring nutrition/diet plans based on individual parameters. CGMs (continuous glucose monitors) improve diabetes control and management by delivering real-time glucose readings. AI and machine learning advancements have also had a substantial impact on cancer identification and therapy. These technologies have shown promise in the early diagnosis, screening, categorization, and prediction of outcomes in several forms of cancer. Cancer stages and outcomes can be accurately predicted using computational models constructed by analyzing clinical data, pathological data, and genetic polymorphisms. Figure 1.8a depicts the role of AI-based approaches in various themes of biomedical healthcare applications. Machine learning techniques aid in pattern detection and the extraction of useful characteristics from large datasets. Figure 1.8b shows the 3D bioprinting process optimization based on machine learning algorithms for printing human organs using biomaterials. AI used in conjunction with immunohistochemical approaches has demonstrated great sensitivity and selectivity in diagnosing certain forms of cancer, such as HER2-overexpressed breast cancer (Shah et al. 2019).

1.4.2.2 Augmented Reality and Virtual Reality

Emerging technologies like augmented reality (AR) and virtual reality (VR) have the potential to completely alter how medical devices are created. Before constructing actual prototypes, designers and engineers may use AR and VR to test and visualize their ideas in a virtual environment, which can save time and costs.

Additionally, surgical planning and training can make use of AR and VR. AR and VR can be used by surgeons to model operations, practice difficult procedures, and more precisely plan operations. By offering a more engaging and immersive experience, augmented reality and virtual reality can also aid in patient education and rehabilitation.

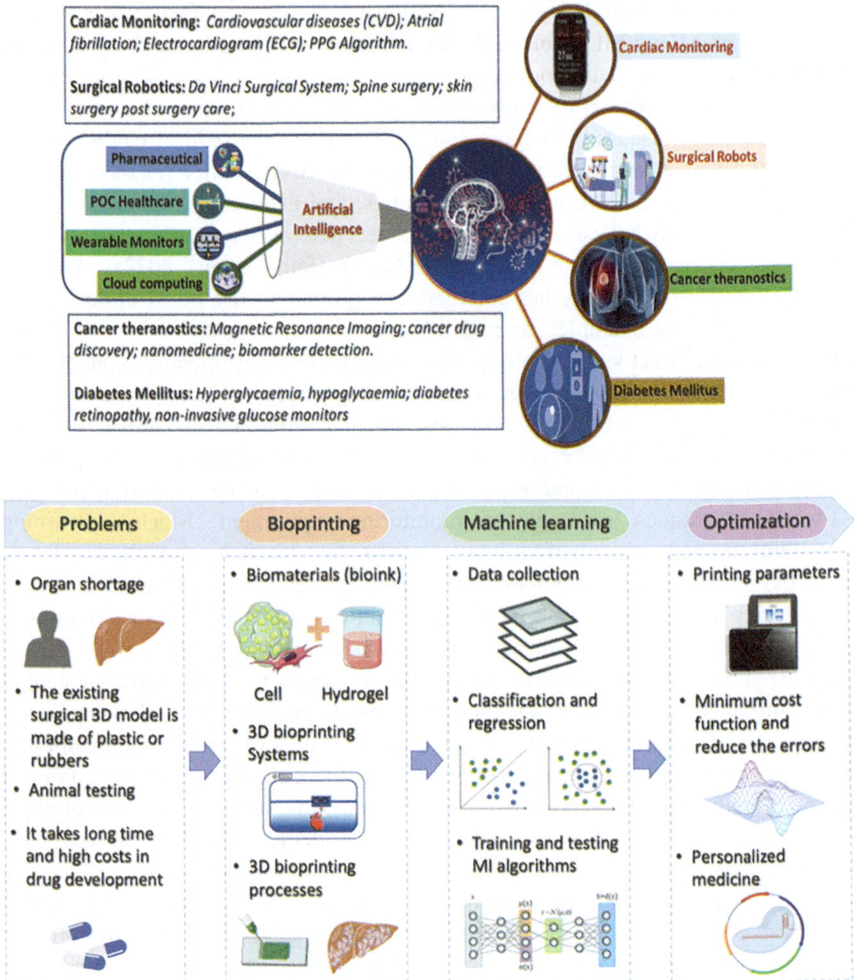

Fig. 1.8 (**a**) Role of AI-based approaches in various themes of biomedical healthcare, including cardiac monitoring, surgery, cancer theragnostic, and diabetes mellitus management (reproduced with permission under CC BY license from Manickam et al. 2022). (**b**) 3D bioprinting of human organ using biomaterials and process optimization based on machine learning algorithms (reproduced with permission under CC BY license from Shin et al. 2022)

AR and VR can be used to increase the accuracy and precision of manufacturing processes in the context of digital manufacturing. For instance, AR can be used to directly show virtual pictures of quality control standards and manufacturing instructions onto the actual parts being created. By doing so, errors can be decreased, and the overall quality of the manufactured parts can be raised (Balani and Tümler 2021).

1.4.2.3 Internet of Medical Things

The Internet of Medical Things (IoMT) is a technology that bridges the gap between digital manufacturing and the healthcare business. Connecting various devices and sensors to the Internet allows them to gather and transmit data in real time, allowing healthcare practitioners to remotely monitor and operate medical devices. This connectedness enables efficient patient health tracking, quicker intervention, and improved healthcare outcomes. Insulin pumps can be linked to sensors that continually monitor blood sugar levels and may be communicated to healthcare practitioners, who can subsequently make educated judgments regarding altering insulin levels. This real-time feedback loop ensures that patients receive appropriate treatment as soon as possible, resulting in better illness control and quality of life.

IoMT is also useful in the production of biomedical devices, manufacturers may monitor their operations in real time by connecting their industrial gear and equipment to the internet. This enables proactive maintenance and quality control, lowering the chance of mistakes and enhancing total manufacturing efficiency. As a result, biomedical equipment may be manufactured with greater consistency and quality. When paired with IoMT systems, AI algorithms enable the collection, processing, and analysis of massive volumes of data generated by various sensors. This information may be utilized to uncover patterns, trends, and possible markers of chronic illnesses, enabling early identification and intervention. Furthermore, combining AI analysis with IoT sensors has proven useful in handling healthcare emergencies like as the COVID-19 pandemic. IoT devices with sensors may collect crucial health data, which AI systems can subsequently evaluate to deliver significant insights to healthcare staff. This technology allows for remote monitoring of patients, early detection of symptoms, and effective allocation of healthcare resources (Manickam et al. 2022; Dinesh Kumar et al. 2021).

Other areas where IoMT is having a big influence include point-of-care sensing devices, wearable devices, and e-diagnosis via IoT platforms. These AI-enabled gadgets, such as smart textiles, smartwatches, and wristbands, can continually measure vital indications such as blood pressure, heart rate, and body temperature. The acquired data may be examined in real time, giving useful information for individualized healthcare management. E-diagnostic using IoT systems enables remote diagnosis, which is especially useful in locations with limited healthcare resources. It lowers the need for patients to attend healthcare institutions in person and allows them to obtain rapid and accurate diagnoses at a lesser cost. This strategy has the potential to enhance healthcare access and outcomes, particularly in underserved or distant communities.

1.5 Challenges and Prospects

The use of digital manufacturing in biological equipment raises several regulatory and ethical issues. These include regulatory compliance, intellectual property protection, privacy and security, quality control procedures, ethical considerations, and limiting environmental effect. Adoption of digital manufacturing must include cost-effectiveness and scalability while giving universal access to healthcare technologies. Despite the early costs, digital manufacturing can save money in the long run by decreasing waste and increasing efficiency. It also provides the ability to produce gadgets in response to the needs of the healthcare system. To fully realize the promise of digital manufacturing, it is critical to optimize resources and manufacturing processes, capitalize on economies of scale, and investigate collaborations between healthcare providers and manufacturers. Digital manufacturing has the potential to enhance patient outcomes, hasten the development of treatments and technologies, and promote healthcare sustainability. Machine learning (ML) is critical in optimizing 3D bioprinting techniques for the generation of tissues and organs. ML can find data trends to improve the quality of printed results and detect abnormalities, saving time and resources. However, due to the difficulties connected with gathering large amounts of biomedical data, there are fewer investigations using ML in bioprinting than in other domains. The future of data collecting is likely to be facilitated by the expansion of open-source platforms and more data sharing. Personalized treatment is possible by utilizing patient-specific data from computed tomography and magnetic resonance imaging. The transferability of AI models is one difficulty, which can be addressed by data selection optimization and transfer learning to improve adaptability across domains. It is possible to overcome these problems and improve manufacturing processes by integrating advanced AI/ML approaches with physics models, which duplicates real-world experiments in virtual models. Big data can be used to facilitate in silico trials and boost efficiency, resulting in more digitized and automated bioprinting products. ML has the potential to transform 3D bioprinting, and its future trends will be driven by technological advancement and optimization.

AI/ML has several applications in healthcare, including enhanced monitoring, diagnosis, and therapy. ML can interpret complex sensor data and improve decision-making abilities. It may extract analytical insights from low-resolution or noisy datasets, ultimately increasing biosensor system performance. However, there are obstacles to overcome to commercialize and adapt AI/ML in healthcare. These difficulties include collecting accurate and substantial patient data, managing data heterogeneity, and assuring data security and privacy. Technological improvements and powerful ML algorithms can help with these difficulties. Connectivity is an important feature of Internet of Medical Things (IoMT) devices, with communication protocols such as Wi-Fi and Bluetooth playing an important role in linking sensors to portable devices and central hubs. To sustain network persistence in noisy RF environments, Wi-Fi modules must provide efficient scanning methods. Traditional medical devices frequently rely on complicated and heavy electronic components, but the development of single integrated circuit (IC) solutions, such as Analog Front Ends (AFEs), allows for the miniaturization of IoMT devices. To connect with diverse sensors, future IoMT devices should include multifunctional AFEs with multiple channels. Mobile health technologies have improved IoMT capabilities by providing telecommunication, low-cost online consultations, and control via mobile apps. However, it is critical that these applications handle security and privacy concerns. AI in healthcare confronts hurdles in managing large amounts of data, maintaining scalability, and dealing with data privacy concerns. Although AI's multitasking capabilities are restricted, comprehensive computer replacement of a physician's diagnostic job remains a long-term aim. AI/ML integration with IoMT devices has enormous promise in the healthcare sector. Nanotechnology and microelectronics advancements will contribute to the development of AI-based IoMT devices with improved functionality, sensitivity, downsizing, and low power consumption, ultimately boosting access to high-quality healthcare. Material science breakthroughs, interaction with other technologies, scalability and cost-effectiveness, and customization and personalization of biomedical devices are all potential future research fields. The continued advancement of digital manufacturing in the biomedical industry has the potential to change the design, manufacturing, and delivery of medical devices, hence improving the healthcare system.

1.6 Conclusion

The integration of digital manufacturing and modern technology has changed biomedical device creation. Three-dimensional printing and other digital manufacturing techniques have enabled the faster and more cost-effective fabrication of patient-specific implants, prosthetic limbs, surgical equipment, tissue engineering scaffolds, and medication delivery systems. Shape-memory alloys, nanomaterials, artificial intelligence, machine learning, augmented reality, virtual reality, and the Internet of Medical Things have all been used to improve the manufacturing process, resulting in increased productivity, lower costs, and higher product quality. Despite obstacles such as the expense of tools and software and the quality of initial digital impressions, the potential of these technologies is enormous. Artificial intelligence and machine learning have the potential to improve healthcare through improving biomedical equipment design and production, as well as improving diagnosis, therapy, and monitoring in a variety of medical sectors. These technologies enable the analysis of enormous datasets, device personalization, and process optimization, resulting in better patient care, cost savings, and potentially the saving of lives. The combination of the Internet of Medical Things with nanomaterials, artificial intelligence, and IoT platforms has important implications for healthcare. This integration has had a favorable impact on real-time patient health monitoring, enhanced manufacturing processes, early disease prediction, and remote healthcare management, to name a few. These developments have the potential to alter healthcare delivery, enhance patient outcomes, and reshape how healthcare is delivered. Finally, advances in digital manufacturing and the incorporation of novel technology in the healthcare industry show significant potential for transforming patient care, improving medical device production, and improving overall healthcare results. We can unlock new potential in healthcare and pave the road for a more efficient, tailored, and accessible healthcare system by properly harnessing these technologies and tackling the associated obstacles.

References

Aram MR, Czaderski C, Motavalli M (2008) Debonding failure modes of flexural FRP-strengthened RC beams. Compos Part B 39(5):826–841

Balani MS, Tümler J (2021) Usability and user experience of interactions on VR-PC, HoloLens 2, VR cardboard and AR smartphone in a biomedical application. In: Virtual, augmented and mixed reality: 13th international conference, VAMR 2021, held as part of the 23rd HCI international conference, HCII 2021, virtual event, July 24–29, 2021, proceedings. Springer International Publishing, Cham, pp 275–287

Bandyopadhyay A, Traxel KD, Bose S (2021) Nature-inspired materials and structures using 3D printing. Mater Sci Eng R Rep 145:100609

Bhattacharya M, O'Neill P, Southern M, Hayes M (2023) Training and tuning of neuro-fuzzy control laws for the machining of prosthetics. Proc Comput Sci 217:1057–1065

Chacon JM, Nunez PJ, Caminero MA, Garcia-Plaza E, Vallejo J, Blanco M (2022) 3D printing of patient-specific 316L–stainless–steel medical implants using fused filament fabrication technology: two veterinary case studies. Biodesign Manuf 5(4):808–815

Cheng YL, Chen YW, Wang K, Shie MY (2016) Enhanced adhesion and differentiation of human mesenchymal stem cell inside apatite-mineralized/poly (dopamine)-coated poly (-ε-caprolactone) scaffolds by stereolithography. J Mater Chem B 4(38):6307–6315

Choi JW, Wicker R, Lee SH, Choi KH, Ha CS, Chung I (2009) Fabrication of 3D biocompatible/biodegradable micro-scaffolds using dynamic mask projection microstereolithography. J Mater Process Technol 209(15–16):5494–5503

CNC Masters (2023) CNC mills and milling machines for sale. https://www.cncmasters.com/. Accessed 21 Apr 2023

CustomPartNet (2023a) Rapid prototyping—stereolithography (SLA). https://www.custompartnet.com/wu/stereolithography. Accessed 21 Apr 2023

CustomPartNet (2023b) Fused deposition modeling (FDM). https://www.custompartnet.com/wu/fused-deposition-modeling. Accessed 21 Apr 2023

CustomPartNet (2023c) Rapid prototyping—selective laser sintering (SLS). https://www.custompartnet.com/wu/selective-laser-sintering. Accessed 21 Apr 2023

Di Giacomo GDA, Cury PR, da Silva AM, da Silva JV, Ajzen SA (2016) A selective laser sintering prototype guide used to fabricate immediate interim fixed complete arch prostheses in flapless dental implant surgery: technique description and clinical results. J Prosthet Dent 116(6):874–879

Dinesh Kumar JR, Ganesh Babu C, Balaji VR, Priyadharsini K, Karthi SP (2021) Performance investigation of various SRAM cells for IoMT based wearable biomedical devices. In: Inventive communication and computational technologies: proceedings of ICICCT 2020. Springer, Singapore, pp 573–588

Downen RS, Dong Q, Chen JL, Li Z (2023) Design and fabrication of a low-cost microfluidic cartridge with integrated pressure-driven check valve for molecular diagnostics platforms. bioRxiv. https://doi.org/10.1101/2022.12.29.522222

Ertugrul I, Ulkir O, Ersoy S, Ragulskis M (2023) Additive manufactured strain sensor using stereolithography method with photopolymer material. Polymers 15(4):991

Fardjahromi MA, Nazari H, Tafti SA, Razmjou A, Mukhopadhyay S, Warkiani ME (2022) Metal-organic framework-based nanomaterials for bone tissue engineering and wound healing. Mater Today Chem 23:100670

Fernandes DJ, Peres RV, Mendes AM, Elias CN (2011) Understanding the shape-memory alloys used in orthodontics. ISRN Dent 2011:1–6. https://doi.org/10.5402/2011/132408

Gayer C, Ritter J, Bullemer M, Grom S, Jauer L, Meiners W et al (2019) Development of a solvent-free polylactide/calcium carbonate composite for selective laser sintering of bone tissue engineering scaffolds. Mater Sci Eng C 101:660–673

Gharbi A, Kallel AY, Kanoun O, Cheikhrouhou-Koubaa W, Contag CH, Antoniac I et al (2023) A biodegradable bioactive glass-based hydration sensor for biomedical applications. Micromachines 14(1):226

Giubilini A, Colucci G, De Trane G, Lupone F, Badini C, Minetola P et al (2023) Novel 3D printable bio-based and biodegradable poly (3-hydroxybutyrate-co-3-hydroxyhexanoate) microspheres for selective laser sintering applications. Mater Today Sustain 22:100379

Gummaluri VS, Vadakke Matham M (2023) Stereolithography assisted controllable random lasing device for tunable threshold, linewidth, and wavelength. Adv Eng Mater 25(3):2200474

Han X, Yang D, Yang C, Spintzyk S, Scheideler L, Li P et al (2019) Carbon fiber reinforced PEEK composites based on 3D-printing technology for orthopedic and dental applications. J Clin Med 8(2):240

Jia X, Zhang K, Qiang M, Han Q, Zhao G, Wu Y, Chen Y (2023) Design of well-matched end-structure of anatomical proximal femoral locking plate based on computer-assisted imaging combined with 3d printing technology: a quality improvement study. Int J Surg 109:10–1097

Kargozar S, Montazerian M, Fiume E, Baino F (2019) Multiple and promising applications of strontium (Sr)-containing bioactive glasses in bone tissue engineering. Front Bioeng Biotechnol 7:161

Manickam P, Mariappan SA, Murugesan SM, Hansda S, Kaushik A, Shinde R, Thipperudraswamy SP (2022) Artificial intelligence (AI) and internet of medical things (IoMT) assisted biomedical systems for intelligent healthcare. Biosensors 12(8):562. https://doi.org/10.3390/bios12080562

Murr LE, Gaytan SM, Medina F, Lopez H, Martinez E, Machado BI et al (2010) Next-generation biomedical implants using additive manufacturing of complex, cellular and functional mesh arrays. Philos Trans R Soc A Math Phys Eng Sci 368(1917):1999–2032

Nace S, Tiernan J, Ní Annaidh A, Holland D (2023) Development and evaluation of a facile mesh-to-surface tool for customised wheelchair cushions. 3D Print Med 9(1):3

Naeem OA, Bencharit S, Yang IH, Stilianoudakis SC, Carrico C, Tüfekçi E (2022) Comparison of 3-dimensional printing technologies on the precision, trueness, and accuracy of printed retainers. Am J Orthod Dentofac Orthop 161(4):582–591

Ng P, Lee PSV, Goh JCH (2002) Prosthetic sockets fabrication using rapid prototyping technology. Rapid Prototyp J 8:53

Osman RB, van der Veen AJ, Huiberts D, Wismeijer D, Alharbi N (2017) 3D-printing zirconia implants; a dream or a reality? An in-vitro study evaluating the dimensional accuracy, surface topography and mechanical properties of printed zirconia implant and discs. J Mech Behav Biomed Mater 75:521–528

Park JH, Park HJ, Tucker SJ, Rutledge SR, Wang L, Davis ME, Hollister SJ (2023) 3D printing of poly-ε-caprolactone (PCL) Auxetic implants with advanced performance for large volume soft tissue engineering. Adv Funct Mater 33:2215220

Pashley J, Blunt LA, Bills PJ, Racasan R (2023) Development of fused metrology methods for the analysis of hip implant tribology. Surf Topogr Metrol Prop 11:024003

Pertusio R, Roatta S (2023) 3D-printed encapsulation of thin-film transducers for reliable force measurement in biomedical applications. Biomechanics 3(1):115–123

Petrini L, Migliavacca F (2011, Figure 1) Biomedical applications of shape memory alloys. J Metall 2011:1–15. https://doi.org/10.1155/2011/501483

Phan K, Sgro A, Maharaj MM, D'Urso P, Mobbs RJ (2016) Application of a 3D custom printed patient specific spinal implant for C1/2 arthrodesis. J Spine Surg 2(4):314

Purdue.edu (2023) Laser cutting. Bechtel Innovation Design Center. https://www.purdue.edu/bidc/resources/printing-and-prototyping/laser-engraving-and-cutting/. Accessed 21 Apr 2023

Rajkumar V, Nahaad V, Krishnan RM, Felix R (2020) Correction to: Experimental investigation of robotic 3D printing of high-performance thermoplastics (PEEK): a critical perspective to support automated fibre placement process. Int J Adv Manuf Technol 108(4):1027–1027

Rajzer I, Kurowska A, Frankova J, Sklenářová R, Nikodem A, Dziadek M et al (2023) 3D-printed polycaprolactone implants modified with bioglass and Zn-doped bioglass. Materials 16(3):1061

Salmi M et al (2012) Patient-specific reconstruction with 3D modeling and DMLS additive manufacturing. Rapid Prototyp J 18(3):209–214. https://doi.org/10.1108/13552541211218126

Sato Y, Guo Y (2023) Shape-memory-alloys enabled actuatable fiber sensors via the preform-to-fiber fabrication. ACS Appl Eng Mater 1(2):822–831

Shah P, Kendall F, Khozin S, Goosen R, Hu J, Laramie J et al (2019) Artificial intelligence and machine learning in clinical development: a translational perspective. NPJ Digit Med 2(1):69

Shilov SY, Rozhkova YA, Markova LN, Tashkinov MA, Vindokurov IV, Silberschmidt VV (2022) Biocompatibility of 3D-printed PLA, PEEK and PETG: adhesion of bone marrow and peritoneal lavage cells. Polymers 14(19):3958

Shin J, Lee Y, Li Z, Hu J, Park SS, Kim K (2022) Optimized 3D bioprinting technology based on machine learning: a review of recent trends and advances. Micromachines 13(3):363. https://doi.org/10.3390/mi13030363

Silva M, Felismina R, Mateus A, Parreira P, Malça C (2017) Application of a hybrid additive manufacturing methodology to produce a metal/polymer customized dental implant. Proc Manuf 12:150–155

Singare S, Liu Y, Li D, Lu B, He S (2008) Individually prefabricated prosthesis for maxilla reconstruction. J Prosthodont 17(2):135–140

Song Q, Chen Y, Hou P, Zhu P, Helmer D, Kotz-Helmer F, Rapp BE (2023) Fabrication of multi-material pneumatic actuators and microactuators using stereolithography. Micromachines 14(2):244

Subash A, Kandasubramanian B (2020) 4D printing of shape memory polymers. Eur Polym J 134:109771. https://doi.org/10.1016/j.eurpolymj.2020.109771

Torres J, Cole M, Owji A, DeMastry Z, Gordon AP (2016) An approach for mechanical property optimization of fused deposition modeling with polylactic acid via design of experiments. Rapid Prototyp J 22:387

Tredan DA, Mobbs RJ, Maharaj M, Parr WC (2023) Combining virtual surgical planning and patient-specific 3D-printing as a solution to complex spinal revision surgery. J Pers Med 13(1):19

Valadez Mesta BL (2022) Development of a custom, 3D-printed, multi-microphone, noise-cancelling, hearing protection device with a magnetically attached printed ear canal for sound localization preservation

Velu R, Singamneni S (2014) Selective laser sintering of polymer biocomposites based on polymethyl methacrylate. J Mater Res 29(17):1883–1892

Velu R, Kamarajan BP, Ananthasubramanian M, Ngo T, Singamneni S (2018) Post-process composition and biological responses of laser sintered PMMA and β-TCP composites. J Mater Res 33(14):1987–1998

Velu R, Vaheed NM, Venkatesan C, Raspall F, Krishnan M (2019) Experimental investigation on fabrication of thermoset prepreg composites using automated fibre placement process and 3D printed substrate. Proc CIRP 85:296–301

Velu R, Ramachandran MK, Anand Kumar S (2023a) State-of-the-art overview and recent trends in additive manufacturing: opportunities, limitations, and current market. In: Nanotechnology-based additive manufacturing: product design, properties and applications, vol 1. Wiley, pp 1–25

Velu R, Tulasi R, Ramachandran MK (2023b) Environmental impact, challenges for industrial applications and future perspectives of additive manufacturing. In: Nanotechnology-based additive manufacturing: product design, properties and applications, vol 2. Wiley, pp 691–709

Vivero-Lopez M, Xu X, Muras A, Otero A, Concheiro A, Gaisford S et al (2021) Anti-biofilm multi drug loaded 3D printed hearing aids. Mater Sci Eng C 119:111606

Wauthle R, Van Der Stok J, Yavari SA, Van Humbeeck J, Kruth JP, Zadpoor AA et al (2015) Additively manufactured porous tantalum implants. Acta Biomater 14:217–225

Wyatt MC (2015) Custom 3D-printed acetabular implants in hip surgery–innovative breakthrough or expensive bespoke upgrade? Hip Int 25(4):375–379

Yu J, Chen Y, Liu X, Islam R, Alam MK (2022a) A novel method of 3D printing locating guide for abutment screw removal in cement-retained implant-supported prostheses. J Dent Sci 17(4): 1665–1668

Yu X, Li G, Zheng Y, Gao J, Fu Y, Wang Q et al (2022b) 'Invisible' orthodontics by polymeric 'clear' aligners molded on 3D-printed personalized dental models. Regen Biomater 9:rbac007

Zaeri A, Cao K, Zhang F, Zgeib R, Chang RC (2022) A review of the structural and physical properties that govern cell interactions with structured biomaterials enabled by additive manufacturing. Bioprinting 26:e00201

Zhang J, Zhao S, Zhu Y, Huang Y, Zhu M, Tao C, Zhang C (2014) Three-dimensional printing of strontium-containing mesoporous bioactive glass scaffolds for bone regeneration. Acta Biomater 10(5):2269–2281

Zuniga JM (2018) 3D printed antibacterial prostheses. Appl Sci 8(9):1651

Futuristic Biomaterials for 3D Printed Healthcare Devices

2

Pauline John, Arun Karthick Selvam, Mannat Uppal, and S. Mohammed Adhil

Contents

P. John (✉)
Division of Engineering, New York University Abu Dhabi, Abu Dhabi, UAE
e-mail: pj2266@nyu.edu

A. K. Selvam
Department of Biomedical Engineering, Sri Sivasubramaniya Nadar College of Engineering, Kalavakkam, Tamil Nadu, India

M. Uppal
HealthCubed India Private Limited, Bengaluru, Karnataka, India

S. Mohammed Adhil
Amrita Hospital, Faridabad, Haryana, India

R. Velu et al. (eds.), *Digital Design and Manufacturing of Medical Devices and Systems*, https://doi.org/10.1007/978-981-99-7100-8_2

Abstract

3D printing is revolutionizing and extending the frontiers in the medical field from rapid manufacturing of healthcare devices and medical implants, to the bioprinting of human organs and tissues. A wide variety of biomaterials, both natural and synthetic, are used in 3D printing of biomedical devices, which is described comprehensively in this chapter. Firstly, this chapter provides an overview of the evolution and different processes of 3D printing technology. Secondly, this chapter provides insights on the various futuristic biomaterials, including biopolymers and bio-nano materials, and their suitable characteristics for fabricating 3D-printed medical devices. Thirdly, this chapter discusses the vital applications of biomaterials in tissue engineering, pharmaceutical, medical and healthcare industries. Finally, this chapter highlights the future challenges and solutions of 3D printing and also underscores the role of artificial intelligence in 3D printing.

Keywords

3D printing · Medical devices · Biomaterials · Biometals · Biopolymers · Bioprinting · Tissue engineering · Biomedical applications

2.1 Introduction

3D printing technology is revolutionizing the medical field in various ways. The virtues of 3D printing technology, which include rapid manufacturing process, low cost, high precision, fabrication of complex structures, and customized designs, are the main reasons for this technology to be chosen over conventional manufacturing technology for designing and developing medical devices (Yadav et al. 2020; Sharafeldin et al. 2018). This technology is a boon to the clinical and medical field in not only manufacturing medical devices which can be implanted into human bodies but also aiding in the design and development of biological human organs and parts of the body, such as bone, heart, liver, and cornea, with the advancements in tissue engineering (Fetah et al. 2019; Gu et al. 2020; Mahdavi et al. 2020). This will certainly improve the life expectancy of people who have lost hope of getting organ transplantation due to the lack of donors, unfavorable host response, and organ rejection. The integration of microfluidic technology and 3D cell printing technology has led to an improvement in the vascularization of engineered tissues, which serves as a test platform in drug discovery (Sharafeldin et al. 2018; Jang et al. 2018).

In addition to the applications to manufacturing and development of medical devices and human organs, 3D printing technology is also used in disease modeling, which is widely used in precision medicine (Jang et al. 2018). Metallic biomaterials

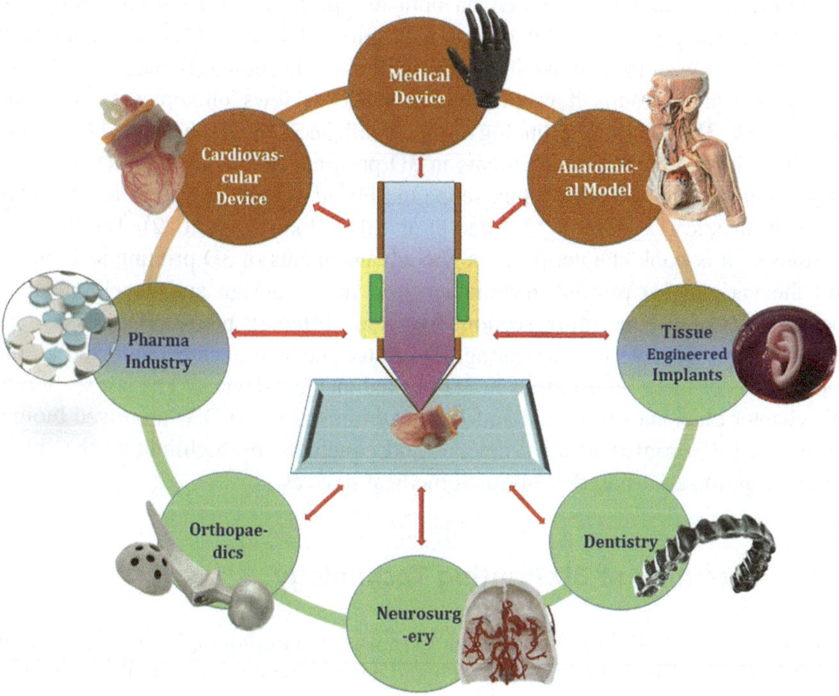

Fig. 2.1 Architecture of a 3D-printed healthcare device

such as stainless steel, cobalt, titanium, and magnesium alloys are commonly preferred for orthopedic implants and long bones (Tapscott and Wottowa 2022). However, bioresorbable biomaterials such as ceramics and polymers are generally used in orthopedics for soft bones (Yadav et al. 2020; Jammalamadaka and Tappa 2018). Bioresorbable materials find their way toward circular economy and sustainability. Several other materials such as polymers, alloys, composites, ceramics, and functionally graded materials are used for various medical applications such as dental implants, corneal implants, and cochlear implants (Yadav et al. 2020; Rokkanen et al. 2000; Salinas et al. 2013). Biomaterial-based approaches are generally applicable in tissue regeneration. Advancements in both biomaterial use and 3D printing technologies have resulted in the development of lab-on-paper, lab-on-chip, and organ-on-chip systems (Fetah et al. 2019; Xu et al. 2016; Tai et al. 2021). Bioinks and polymers are widely used biomaterials for fabricating tissues and organs such as vasculature, skin, bone, brain, cardiac tissues, liver, gut, and kidney (Wang et al. 2022; Derakhshanfar et al. 2018). Furthermore, hydrogel, which is a type of polymer, is used in manufacturing cell-encapsulated tissue, scaffolds, and drug delivery systems (Derakhshanfar et al. 2018). Figure 2.1 shows the architecture of the enormous applications of 3D-printed medical devices in various medical fields.

3D printing technologies based on optical approaches utilizing ultraviolet and infrared light sources along with digital micromirror devices (DMD) incorporated in the system are used to facilitate dynamic maskless 3D printing (Soman et al. 2013). Several research groups have provided detailed reviews on topics such as the progress of 3D printing technology, its significance in the field of healthcare, non-optical and optical advancements in 3D printing, the unique characteristics of smart biomaterials, and their future scope in 3D and 4D printing applications in the biomedical field (Li et al. 2022; Miao et al. 2017; John et al. 2022). The first two sections of this book chapter describe the advancements of 3D printing technology and the various 3D printing techniques used in the design and development of medical devices. The third section lists the different biomaterials and their characteristics suitable for fabricating 3D-printed medical devices, followed by the applications of these biomaterials in 3D-printed medical devices. The last section of this chapter elucidates the Food and Drug Administration (FDA)-approved biomaterial-based 3D-printed medical devices and concludes by highlighting the future scope of biomaterial-based 3D-printed medical devices.

2.2 Evolution of 3D Printing Technology

The first invention of 3D printing technology was stereolithography by Charles Hull in 1984, which underwent much research and development for a valuable application process. Different inventions in 3D printing have made rapid prototyping and additive manufacturing (AM) a topic of interest in various fields. As we know, 3D printing is the study of combining manufactured layers into a single product. Figure 2.2 shows the general development of 3D bioprinting.

3D-printed medical devices create more impact nowadays as they help in avoiding the scarcity of artificial organs, prosthesis, bionic arms, robotics, and so on. 3D bioprinting of medical devices emerged in the 1990s, and it reached milestones in 2009. Figure 2.3 describes the brief timeline of 3D printing technology that helps us understand its evolution from technology to data.

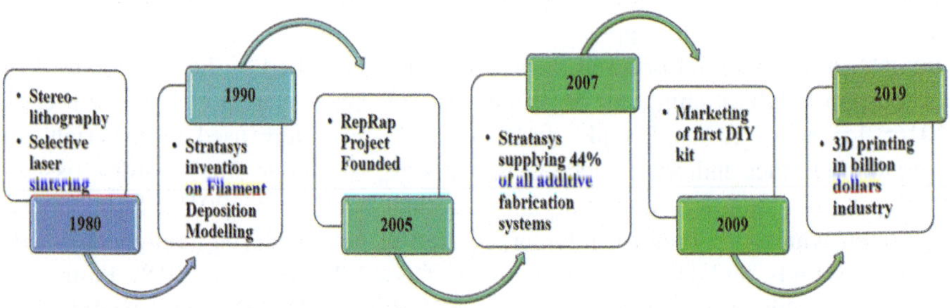

Fig. 2.2 Evolution of 3D printing technology (Panda et al. 2016)

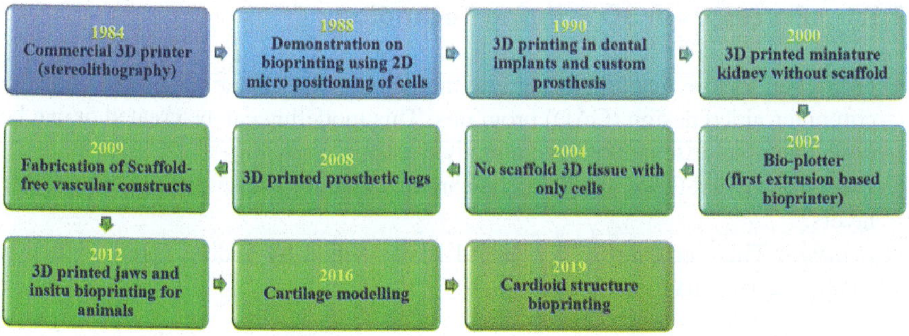

Fig. 2.3 Brief timeline of 3D printing in biomedical applications (Yan et al. 2018)

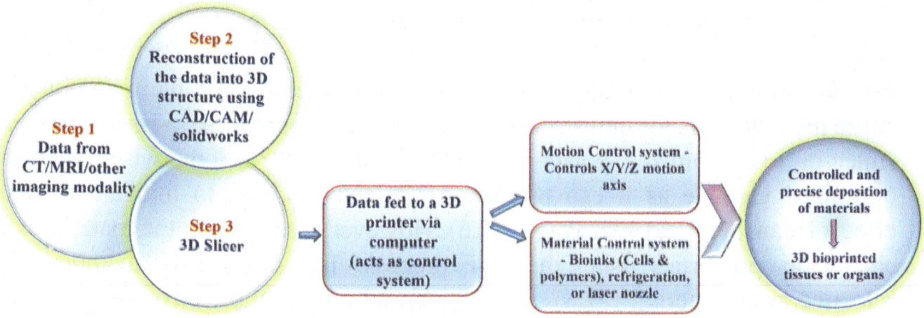

Fig. 2.4 Processes in 3D printing technology

2.3 Various 3D Printing Techniques for Designing Medical Devices

By utilizing AM, more layers can be added to the 3D-printed object using CAD software to create the object's physical components (Bozkurt and Karayel 2021), owing to its intricate components, efficiency in use of time, and rapid manufacture (Murr 2016; Squelch 2018). These technologies are employed in the biomedical sector of the medical device industry in addition to the development of artificial organs. Tissue engineering, stem cell research, prosthetics, and implants are the various applications of it in addition to dental imaging (Bücking et al. 2017) and medical imaging (Shahrubudin et al. 2019). Figure 2.4 shows the various processes in 3D printing technology.

2.3.1 Processes in 3D Printing Technology

- *Modeling*: Before manufacturing, the modeling of the material is prepared using computer-aided design (CAD) programs. This modeling can be created or can be downloadable or scannable if it already exists.
- *Printable layers*: Once modeled, they are obtained into several slices of printable layers.
- *Printing*: Thus, printing of a material is performed by adding layers, which is called additive manufacturing.

According to the primary material's physical state—solid, liquid, or powder—3D printing techniques may be categorized. For various types of materials, several processes are employed. Figure 2.5 shows the classification of various 3D bioprinting techniques in terms of materials and material type.

1. **Powder Bed Fusion (PBF)**: It is a 3D printing method capable of producing entire metallic parts for industrial applications using sources like a laser. They can sinter or fuse atomized powder particles jointly. PBF is otherwise called an optimized variable as it can produce optimized products to mitigate thermal effects (Stansbury and Idacavage 2016). However, overheating the material will change its properties using the PBF process. The major PBF methods like selective laser sintering (SLS), stereolithography (SLA), selective laser melting (SLM), and material extrusion are discussed below.
   - **Selective laser sintering (SLS)**: A laser source is used to fuse the powder layer into solid parts in the powder bed surface. The solid parts are produced

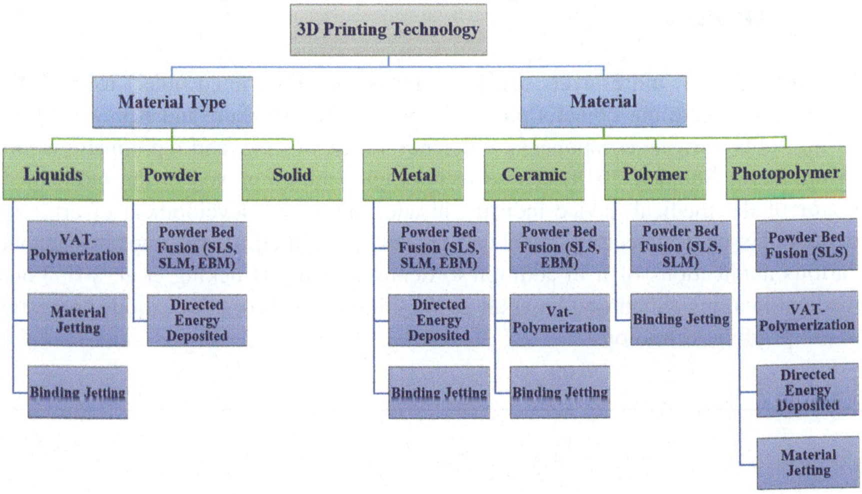

Fig. 2.5 Classification of 3D printing technologies based on materials and material type (Bozkurt and Karayel 2021)

by heating powder with a laser source, and they are arranged one over the other to form a solid part (Shirazi et al. 2015). Parameters like laser scanning speed, its energy density, a strategy of scanning, bed-time temperature and the distance between the layers are important for manufacturing (Shuai et al. 2014; Senthilkumar et al. 2020). It can be used to produce polymers, metals, ceramics, and composites.

- **Selective laser melting (SLM)**: It is like the SLS technique, but the major difference is that the addition of powder materials is done after the complete melting of materials rather than sintering. Like SLS, a laser source is used for PBF. The liquid starts to harden when the temperature drops. The unmelted powder element of the mixture supports the structure, while the molten material produces the item. The leftover material (the dust) when the process is finished and the part is built will be eliminated (Meier and Haberland 2008). This method involves the powder layer being laser scanned and used to build the product as a result of laser energy (Antonini et al. 2021). The SLM process is mostly ideal for metallic materials, compared to the SLS method. Like other AM processes, SLM offers nearly limitless geometry and flexibility through the tuning of variables, including the material of the powder, size of the powder, input energy of the laser, morphology, scan strategy, and speed.
- **Stereolithography (SLA)**: It is the most important method in AM as it uses photopolymers or resins, which are used for producing complex parts in many applications. Since it uses photopolymers, these materials have a greater impact on mechanical properties and chemical properties when exposed to light. Due to their good surface quality, they are used in wide applications.
- **Material extrusion**: Fusion deposition modelling (FDM) and electron beam modelling are two examples of material extrusion. It uses thermoplastic in the form of filament as the main material. Layer thickness and extrusion tip diameter are some of the crucial processing parameters of the approach. In the beginning, heating of the used polymer takes place above the transition temperature of glass and then feeding into the extruder in semi-melt filament form takes place, followed by forcing through a nozzle (Shashi et al. 2017; Park et al. 2014). As the extrusion head moves, the filament drops to the ground and solidifies as it cools. The process is repeated while the platform descends in the interim. Layered production takes place as a result of the filament being placed on top of the hardened filament layer. Preprinted and cooled filaments that are placed on top of the hot filament are heated up as well. Thus, the layer of solidified filament is melted once more and combined with the most recent layer to be added. This allows for the provision of the tiered structure. Postprocessing was typically needed after operations were complete, and when the part was printed, layers were visible on the surface (Pranzo et al. 2018; Low et al. 2017). Figure 2.6 shows the material extrusion process.

2. **Vat polymerization**: In 3D printing, vat polymerization is sometimes referred to as curing photo-reactive polymers with lasers, and ultraviolet (photo polymerization) light sources. Using resin and liquid photopolymer, the sculpture is built up

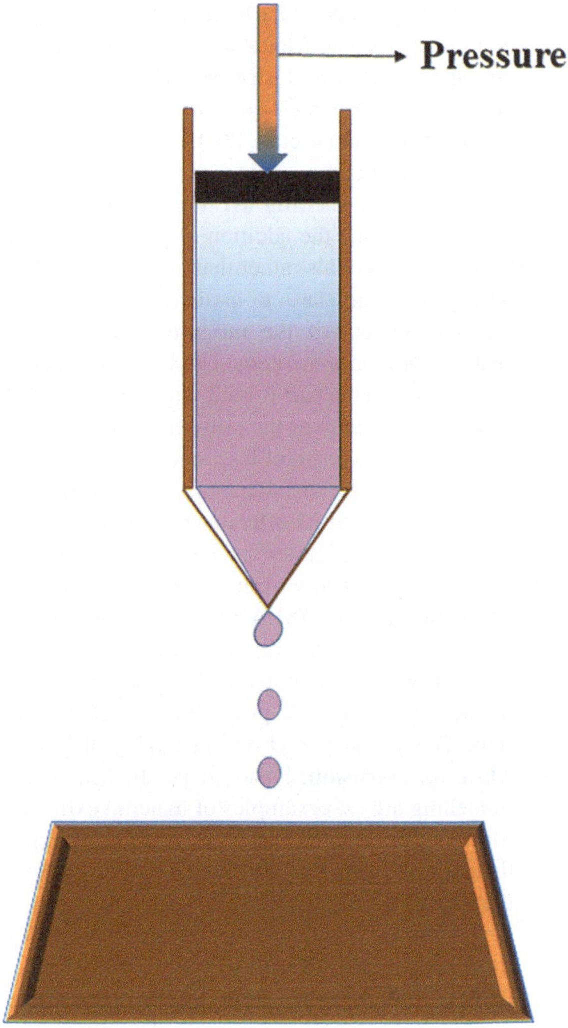

Fig. 2.6 Material extrusion process

layer by layer. Materials are employed in a liquid state, and after exposure to UV light, they become hard. SLA and digital light processing (DLP) are two examples (Hitzler et al. 2018). They are found to be similar in process, but major differences are based on the light sources used (Tofail et al. 2018). The procedure for photopolymerization is as follows:

- The layer thickness causes the construction platform to descend from the resin vat's top.
- The resin is gradually cured with a UV lamp. Additional layers are added on top of the earlier ones as the platform descends farther.

- To create a smooth resin foundation for the next layer to be built on, some machines use a blade that moves between the layers.
- The resin is then emptied from the vat when the piece is finished.

3. **Directed energy deposition (DED)**: It is a 3D printing method that can produce complete metallic parts for industrial applications like PBF (Yap et al. 2017). In this approach, powder material or wire is fed into the substrate using an electron beam, laser beam plasma, or electric arc, thus finally forming a small-size melt pool by continuously passing layer by layer. They are used for depositing in highly performative materials like ceramics, composites, Ti-based alloys, Co-based alloys, shape memory alloys (SMA), high-entropy alloys, and functionally graded materials (FGM). The process of DED is as follows:
   - Solidification of substrate as heating sources move forward, thus forming the metal track
   - Overlapping of the metal track on the predefined hatch space
   - Once one layer is completed, the feedstock delivery system, along with the deposition head, moves upward by a slice thickness to form the next layer
4. **Materials jetting**: Like VAT polymerization, material jetting uses a UV light source for curing photopolymers. Using a method called material jetting, which uses light to cure photopolymers, multiple materials can be printed simultaneously. Sometimes, wax is also utilized. This process produces supporting structures from a variety of materials that are necessary for some applications (Nichetti and Manas-Zloczower 1999). Material jetting selectively deposits construction material drop by drop; thus, viscosity is found to be an important parameter. Products with a good dimensional precision and a very smooth surface finish are produced using material jetting (Nahmias et al. 2005). The process of material jetting is as follows:
   - Curing of photopolymers and creating droplets
   - Solidifying the layers
   - Fixing it layer by layer
   - Final printing and coloring are done based on application needs.

   Figure 2.7 shows the process of material jetting.
5. **Binding jetting**: In this approach, the binder is employed during the binder jetting procedure in the powder bed. The binder is used to make sure that the powder particles are linked. The structures that connect to one another to form layers are topped with new layers. In this way, layered manufacturing is realized. The advantages of the PBF method discussed earlier are present in this procedure. Due to the physical support provided by the powder, the pieces made in the powder bed do not need supporting structures. As a result, the supporting structures are not required in this manner. Additionally, powders that are unused can be recycled, as in PBF techniques. Gypsum-based powder and water-based binders can be employed, as they were when they were initially used. Additionally, various materials and binders can be employed. Like material jetting, colored parts can be produced. Table 2.1 enlists the applications of several 3D printing technologies in the biomedical domain.

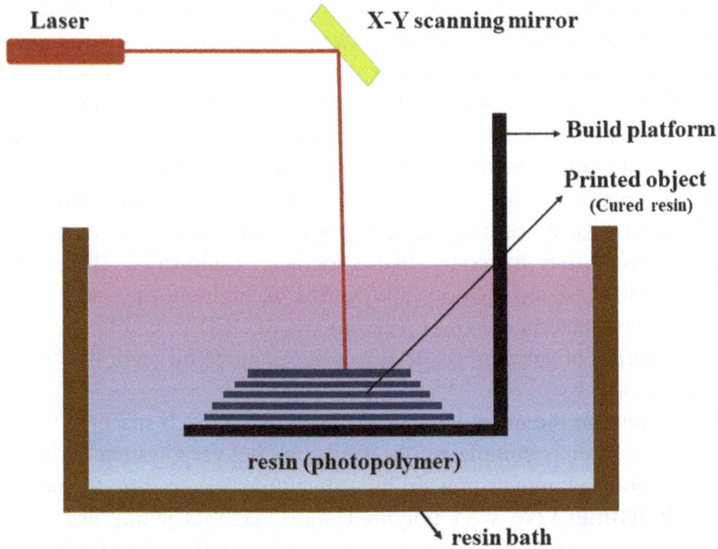

Fig. 2.7 Material jetting process

Table 2.1 Biomedical applications of several 3D printing technologies (Stansbury and Idacavage 2016; Shirazi et al. 2015; Shuai et al. 2014; Senthilkumar et al. 2020; Meier and Haberland 2008; Antonini et al. 2021; Shashi et al. 2017; Park et al. 2014; Pranzo et al. 2018; Low et al. 2017; Hitzler et al. 2018; Tofail et al. 2018; Yap et al. 2017; Nichetti and Manas-Zloczower 1999; Nahmias et al. 2005)

Technology	Applications
Powder bed fusion	
Selective laser sintering (SLS)	Prosthesis and implants
Selective laser melting (SLM)	
Stereolithography (SLA)	Orthodontics, oral surgery
Material extrusion	Bone models, vascular models, and soft tissue models
Vat polymerization	Drug delivery, cardiovascular stents, dental splint, microarray, scaffolds, implants, etc.
Directed energy deposition	Surgical planning models, bioreactors, tissue repair, implants, etc.
Material jetting	Anatomical models for presurgical planning and educational purposes
Binding jetting	Computerized tomography (CT) analysis, low-dose tablets and its microstructure, drug delivery system

6. **Droplet-based bioprinting**: Other than the aforementioned 3D printing methods, there is also droplet-based bioprinting, which uses droplets as the basic units and produces materials with high resolution compared to extrusion-based bioprinting. These can be classified based on their principles, as shown in Fig. 2.8.

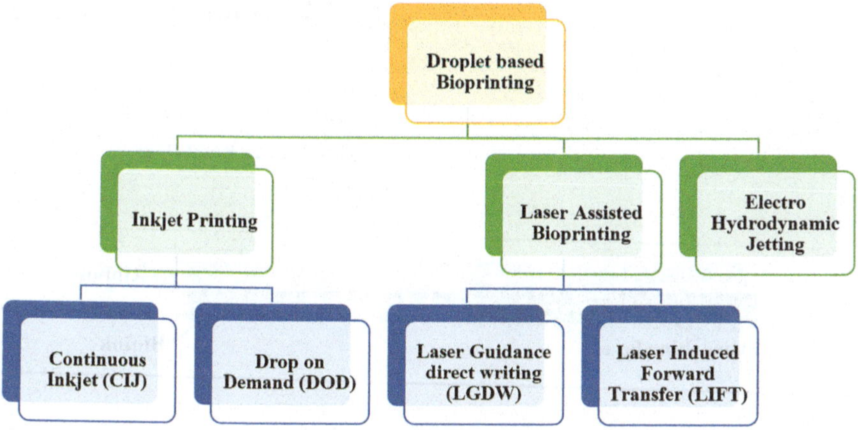

Fig. 2.8 Classification of droplet-based bioprinting (Gu et al. 2020)

The method uses different actuators, like electrodes, piezoelectric transducers, thick film resistors, and so on, for producing layers. Continuous inkjet printing is electrically conductive, and thus they need an electric and magnetic field to drive the bioink that can produce high-frequency droplets. Drop-on-Demand (DOD) printing produces low-frequency droplets when required with higher resolutions by moving nozzles at the desired location. Laser-assisted bioprinting uses a laser source for producing the required droplets. Laser guided direct writing (LGDW) uses weak laser pulses for producing substrates, but it is not a topic of research currently (Kiran and Ramakrishna 2021). Laser-induced forward transfer (LIFT) uses an absorbing layer where the laser beam gets focused and produces high-pressure bubbles in the substrate for driving material with the cell. Its process is shown in Fig. 2.9. Electrohydrodynamic drives the bioink with the electric field produced in between the nozzle and substrate. Figure 2.10 shows the different DOD processes.

2.4 Biomaterials and Their Characteristics Suitable for Fabricating 3D-Printed Medical Devices

Biomaterials are classified into two major types of inorganic and organic materials. Metals and ceramics are examples of inorganic materials, whereas polymers are examples of organic materials. These classifications are based on the chemical bonding of each material. The desired properties of biomaterials that can be used for 3D fabrication include biocompatibility, non-toxicity, host response, tear and wear corrosion, and some mechanical properties like hardness, toughness, and melting temperature. On top of all the other characteristics, the cost-effectiveness

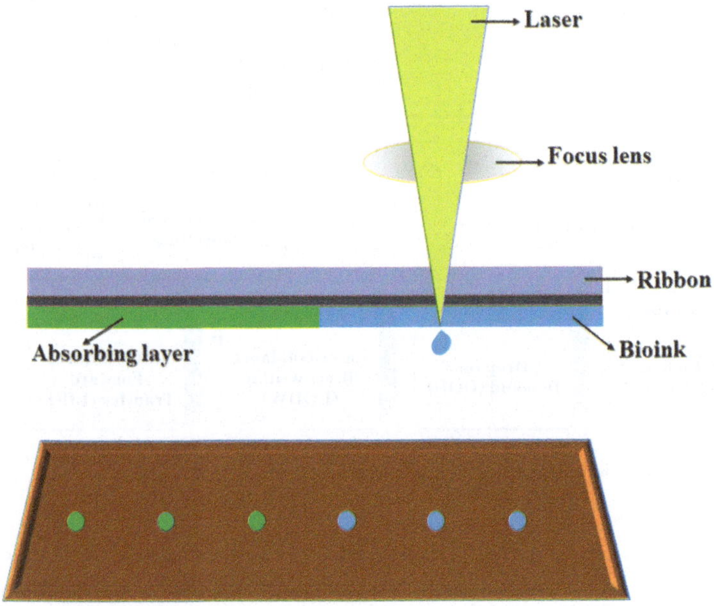

Fig. 2.9 Process of laser-induced forward transfer

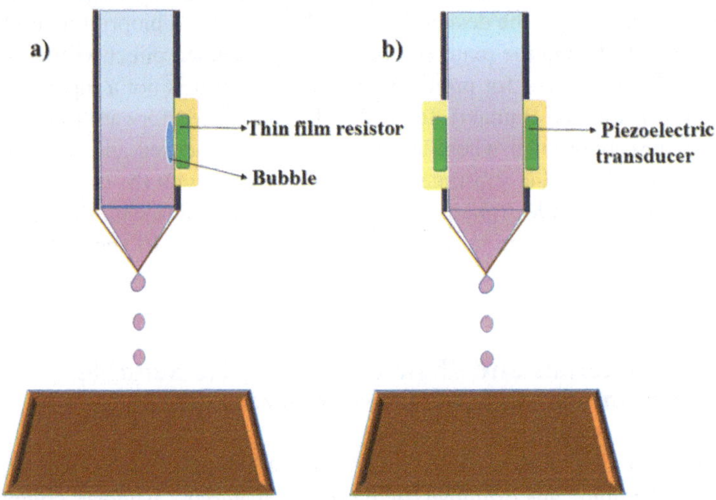

Fig. 2.10 Drop on demand (DOD) process of (**a**) thin film resistor DOD printing and (**b**) piezoelectric transducer DOD printing

of the biomaterials and biological response and reactions of tissue/organs toward the biomaterials are the main concerns.

Figure 2.11 shows the primary requirement of designing biomaterials.

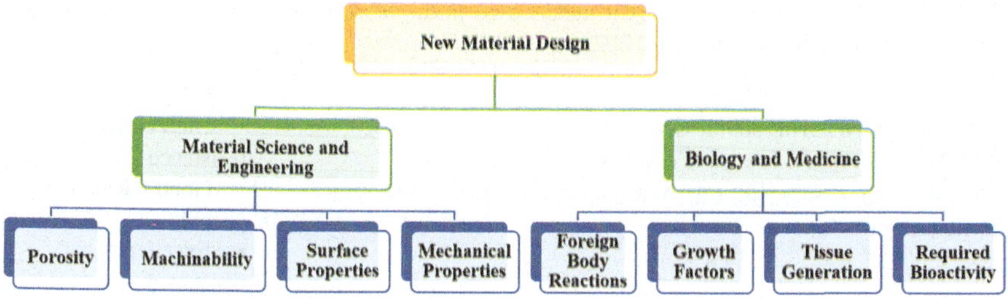

Fig. 2.11 Primary requirements for designing new biomaterials (dos Santos 2015)

2.4.1 Bio-metals

In contrast to ceramics and polymers, metals' characteristics may be changed throughout the production process. Because of their superior heat conductivity and mechanical qualities, metals are employed in medicinal applications. These metals can be divided into ferrous (steel and cast iron) and non-ferrous (pure metals and alloys of aluminum, copper, nickel, silver, titanium, zinc, and cobalt) categories (Groover 2013). Ferrous metals include steel and cast iron. Metals are susceptible to corrosion-induced degradation, which might release byproducts that could cause negative biological interactions. Corrosion resistance is a critical quality to consider for a surgically implanted alloy, since metal alloys are exposed to an especially hostile medium mainly chloride ions and proteins present in body fluids. Dissolved oxygen is changed into hydroxide ions, and the alloy's metallic components are oxidized to take on their ionic forms during the corrosion process. Stainless steel 316L in particular is still the most common type of metallic material utilized in medical applications (Jani et al. 2014).

SMA, which can memorize the shape and deform back to its original shape, is temperature dependent and magnetic field dependent. Nitinol, which is a combination of nickel and titanium, is an example of SMA (Obeidi et al. 2021). Their ability to memorize is due to high fatigue strength. These are used in applications where the materials can change their shape and regain their original shape by heating at a certain temperature or responding to external stimuli (Duerig et al. 1999). In 3D printing-based medical device applications, they are used due to their high corrosion resistance and non-magnetic and biocompatible nature, along with their physical characteristics that suit superelastic behavior. This behavior correlates with the stress–strain relationship of tendons in human bones, making SMA the best material for stents in cardiology; they are also used for eyeglass frames, orthodontic applications, bone implants, aneurysm treatments, pneumatic valves, myocardial assist devices, and so on (Santos 2017). Table 2.2 lists the characteristics of metallic materials used in the fabrication of medical devices.

Table 2.2 Characteristics of different metals used in the fabrication of medical devices (Santos 2017; Pina et al. 2018; Obeidi et al. 2021)

Materials	Characteristics
Titanium-based: 316L stainless steel, Ti (commercially pure), Ti-6Al-4V, Ti-5Al-2.5Fe, and Ti-Al-Nb	• High corrosion resistance • Good mechanical properties • Excellent wear resistance • Osseointegration
Cobalt-based: Co-Cr-Mo, Cast Wrought Co, Nickel-Cr-Mo, and Nickel-Cr-W	
Shape memory alloy: Nitinol	• High corrosion resistance • Non-magnetic • Biocompatible • High fatigue strength

2.4.2 Bioceramics

Bioceramics are designed as a replacement for metallic implants due to their good hardness, strength, and chemical inertness. They are natural or synthetic and possess the ability to bond with bone (Subedi 2013). These bioceramics are the forms of carbides, oxides, nitrides, sulfides of metals, and metalloids (Kargozar et al. 2020) and can be used in soft tissue repair and regeneration (Punj et al. 2021). Even though biomaterials are more useful than metals in terms of density, porosity, elastic modulus, and hardness, its demerits involve poor machinability, ductility, and sinterability (Guzzi and Tibbitt 2020). The synthetic bioceramics are subclassified as bioinert, bioresorbable, and bioactive. Table 2.3 enumerates the synthetic bioceramics and their characteristics for developing 3D-printed medical devices.

2.4.3 Biopolymers

Biopolymers are synthetic materials made by living organisms. Starch polymers are typically what they are. These have monomeric building blocks. Polynucleotides, polypeptides, and polysaccharides are the three primary categories of biopolymers, which are further divided based on the monomers employed and the final biopolymer structure. Polymers are favorable and widely used in 3D printing due to their availability in different forms as filaments, powders, solutions, and gels to be used in FDM, SLS, SLA, and direct ink writing (DIW), respectively (Pugliese et al. 2021; Festas et al. 2020). They may also be dissolved in fast-evaporating organic solvents like dichloromethane, tetrahydrofuran, or dimethyl sulfoxide, and they have biocompatibility, adjustable mechanical characteristics, and degradation rates. Chitosan-based biopolymers, which are a form of hydrogel-based polymers widely used in organ/cell 3D printing, provide promising results in tissue engineering and organ replacement (Jayashankar et al. 2022). A tensile strength of 60 MPa and

Table 2.3 Characteristics of bioceramics used in the fabrication of medical devices (Ligon et al. 2017)

Bioceramics	Classification	Materials	Characteristics
	(a) Bioinert	Alumina	• Y: 380 GPa • CS: 4500 MPa • TS: 380 MPa • Physically stable • Density: 3.94 g/cm^3 • Grain size: $<$4 μm
		Zirconia	• Y: 200 GPa • CS: 2000 MPa • TS: 200 MPa • Density: 3.94 g/cm^3 • Porosity: $<$1.0 vol% • Grain size: 0.2–0.4 μm
		Titania	• Y: 110 GPa • CS: 485 MPa • TS: 760 MPa • Density: 4.23 g/cm^3
		Carbon/CNT	• Y: 28 GPa • CS: 517 MPa • TS: 560 MPa • Density: 2.26 g/cm^3 • Grain size: 3.4 nm
	(b) Bioresorbable	Porous BCP	• CS: 100 MPa • TS: 3 MPa • Osteoconductive
		Tri CAP	• Y: 117 GPa • CS: 896 MPa • TS: 193 MPa • Insoluble in water • Soluble in dilute HCl and nitric acid
		Calcium carbonate and gypsum	• Y: 69.9 GPa • CS: 6 MPa • TS: 23.3 MPa • Strength is high • Poor soluble in water
	(c) Bioactive	Glass/glass ceramics	• Y: 35 GPa • CS: 500 MPa • TS: 83 MPa • Hard and brittle • Density of glass: 2.5 g/cm^3 • Density of glass ceramic: 2.8 g/cm^3
		Hydroxy-apatite	• Y: 120 GPa • CS: 1000 MPa • TS: 300 MPa • Bone mimic

CAP calcium phosphate, *BCP* biphasic calcium phosphate, *MPa* mega Pascal, *GPa* giga Pascal, *CNT* carbon nanotube, *HCl* hydrochloric acid, *Y* Young's modulus, *CS* compressive strength, *TS* tensile strength

Table 2.4 Characteristics of different polymers used in 3D printing technologies (Dos Santos et al. 2017)

Form of polymers	Different polymers	Characteristics
Solid polymers-based ink	Acrylonitrile butadiene styrene (ABS)	• Good strength and flexibility • Temperatures of 20–80 °C • Melting point of 105 °C
	Poly lactic acid (PLA)	• Low cost • Easy processability • Bio-compatible • Biodegradable • Melting temperature: 175 °C
	Poly D,L lactide (PDLLA)	• Bio-compatible • High mechanical strength • Highly resorbable • Biodegradable
	Polycaprolactone (PCL)	• Biodegradable • Bio-compatible • High porosity • Extended stiffness and degradation (3 years)
	Polypropylene fumarate (PPF)	• Osteoconductivity • Amenability • Resorbability • Molecular mass range of 700–3000 Da
	Polyamides	• Tensile strength of 10 MPa • High load-bearing capacity • Good stability, rigidity, flexibility, and shock resistance
	Thermoplastic polyurethane (TPU)	• High durability • Flexible • Abrasion-resistant thermoplastic
Polymeric hydrogel-based inks	Collagen, fibrin, chitosan, matrigel, gelatin methylacrylamide, alginate, spider silk, agarose, self-assembling peptide	• Biocompatibility • Viscoelasticity • Softness • A range of storage moduli, from 259–3552 Pa

biological properties such as biocompatibility, non-toxicity, and biodegradability are their unique attributes to be used in medical applications of AM (Jayashankar et al. 2022). Table 2.4 shows the characteristics of different polymers used in 3D printing technologies.

2.4.4 Bio-nano Materials

Nano-technology is used in the synthetization of nano materials like ceramics, polymers, composites, metals, and some self-assembled materials that are used in biomedical applications like medical diagnostics and surgery, dentistry, tissue engineering, and drug delivery (Velu et al. 2019). These bio-nano materials and their composites are found to be more compatible with modern techniques like AM for the fabrication of medical implants, customized prosthetics, functional implantable devices, and so on (Dutra et al. 2020). The nano-based fillers are a matrix that is used along with these materials to provide electrical, mechanical, and physical properties. Several nano-based fillers, like metallic fillers (gold and silver nanoparticles), ceramic fillers, carbon fillers, and cellulose fillers, are used for several biomedical applications, which have been enlisted in Table 2.5. These nano-based biomaterials seek more attention from specific communities due to their robustness, chemical stability, biocompatibility, and good physical and mechanical properties. There are certain protocols and guidelines provided for the fabrication of these by the International Standard Organization (ISO) and the Food and Drug Administration (FDA). The protocols involved (1) the development of material and its characterization, (2) in vitro testing, (3) in vivo implantation, and (4) human study trial (Narayan 2017).

Table 2.5 Different nano-based fillers and their biomedical applications (Rahmani et al. 2022)

S. no.	Nano-based fillers	Applications
1.	Metallic nano fillers	Antimicrobial activity, antibiotic drug, wound dressing, avoiding inflammation for musculoskeletal tissue engineering
2.	Ceramic nano fillers	Artificial bone tissue scaffolds, surgeon gloves, warm water bags, titanium implants
3.	Carbon nano fillers	Collagen, chitosan, carbon nanotubes (CNT), implant coating
4.	Cellulose nano fillers	Bone and cartilage regeneration, dental grafting, soft tissue replacement, heart valve tissue, wound dressing, vascular grafting

2.5 FDA-Approved Biomaterial-Based 3D-Printed Healthcare Devices

3D objects are manufactured using 3D printing technology by fabricating successive layers of raw materials. Designers may simply have to adjust the necessary control parameters, thanks to 3D printing's versatility, without having to set up extra tools or equipment. Additionally, it enables manufacturers to design devices with extremely complicated internal structures or devices that are anatomically tailored for a patient. The growth of 3D-printed healthcare devices, including prostheses, medical implants, and human organs, has seen a significant surge in attention as a result of these properties, in addition to the technology's numerous uses in the food, industrial, and sociocultural sectors. Table 2.6 provides a list of biomaterials used in 3D printing technology for various medical applications, such as the fabrication of scaffolds, drug delivery devices, surgical guides, and implants.

FDA approval for 3D-printed biomaterials is based on how the human body reacts to the materials in terms of biocompatibility, biological responses, and immunological responses. These tests are performed prior to approval for medical applications such as tissue engineering, organ replacement, and fixation. The mechanical properties of the material are also evaluated with biological responses to determine its stability, usability, and durability. The research efforts by the FDA open new scopes in IVD tests, biomarkers, and several other screening tools. Table 2.7 provides a list of FDA-approved materials along with their medical applications.

2.6 Various Applications of Biomaterial-Based 3D Printing

This section provides details of various applications of biomaterial-based 3D printing in developing tissues and organs, tools and models for surgery, tissue engineering, medical device, and pharmaceutical industry, which is shown in Fig. 2.12.

2.6.1 Bioprinting of Tissues and Organs

With the help of 3D bioprinters that make use of guided pipettes via computers to print tissues and organs by layering the bioinks, transplantation of bone, cartilage, vascular grafts, skin, and even heart tissues is possible. These bioprinted tissues and organs exactly mimic the native structure and functionality and are highly economical for organ transplantation (Kumar et al. 2021). Plant-derived bioinks (nanocellulose, pectin, green algae, brown algae, and red algae) are used in 3D printing of tissues and organs. Due to its easy availability, biocompatibility, and natural rigidity, it has a wide range of applications in biomedical engineering, drug targeting, and medical prosthetics (Mahendiran et al. 2021). The fibrous morphology exhibited by nanocellulose, with an interconnected porous network supporting cellular activity, makes it a suitable mimic for the extracellular matrix of tissues.

Table 2.6 List of biomaterials used in 3D printing technology for fabricating medical devices

S. no.	Technology	Material used/applications	Ref.
1.	Fused deposition modeling (FDM) or free form fabrication (FFF)	• *Scaffolds for tissue engineering and regeneration*: Biodegradable calcium phosphate glass combined with PCL (polycaprolactone) + chitosan, PCL + β-TCP, and PLA (poly lactic acid) • *Drug delivery*: PLA, PCL, oleo-gum-resins (Myrrha, olibanum, and benzoin,) doped with metal oxide nanoparticles (TiO_2, Cu_2O, MoO_3, and P25), PVA (poly vinyl alcohol) • *Surgical guides and implants*: Acrylonitrile butadiene styrene (ABS), TPU—Thermoplastic urethane	Dong et al. (2017), Shim et al. (2017), Almeida et al. (2014)
2.	Extrusion based bioprinting	Methacrylate hyaluronic acid (MHA), PVA, and phytagel (1:1), crosslinked gelatin, nano-fibrillated cellulose (NFC), alginate, calcium silicate, calcium sulfate hydrate, mesoporous bio glass, polyethyleneimine, and biphasic calcium phosphate (HA/-TCP = 60:40) *Applications*: Cartilage fabrication, tissue engineering in cartilage, construction of chondral, modeling of disease, tissue transplantation, toxicity analysis, drug development	Laronda et al. (2017), Tan et al. (2017)
3.	Material sintering	*Stereolithography*: Epoxy resins, glass-filled polycarbonate, ABS, polypropylene, polyurethane, Bakelite, etc. *Applications*: Patient-specific models, implantable device production (biodegradable implants), tissue engineering (repairable scaffolds), and hydrogel-coated cells	Sun et al. (2016)
4.	Inkjet or binder jet printing	• *Substrate*: 2-pyrrolidone (zb63), hydroxyapatite, Gantrez AN 169 BF (poly (methyl vinyl ether-co-maleic anhydride)) microneedles, vinyl polymer, and carbohydrate mesoporous silica nanoparticles, polyethyleneimine, furosemide, and propylene glycol,	Wang et al. (2017), Sandler et al. (2011), Strobel et al. (2014)

(continued)

Table 2.6 (continued)

S. no.	Technology	Material used/applications	Ref.
		are all present in aqueous solutions • *Powders*: α-TCP + hydroxyapatite + dextrin; α-TCP, 8.75 wt% phosphoric acid + 0.25 wt% Tween 80 • *Binding liquid*: Concentrated solution of paracetamol, theophylline, and caffeine water + glycerol, Soluplus (co-polymer of PVC-PVA-PEG) *Applications*: Tissue regeneration, cancer research, stem cell research, microarray design, anti-microbial tests, delivery of biological materials, genomics, biosensors, and drug development	
5.	Polyjet printing	The FullCure 930 TangoPlus from Stratasys, the elastic photopolymer Japanese Agilista-3200 3D printer, the rigid acrylic resin (AR-M2) photopolymer resin, the multiple photopolymer resins printed on Connex 3 polyjet, the multiple photopolymer resins printed on Connex 350, the multiple photopolymer resins printed on Objet 500 Connex, the multiple photopolymer RGD525 and Connex 500 *Applications*: Rapid prototyping of rigid and soft tissue materials	Zein et al. (2013), Waran et al. (2014)

Poor mechanical features and the requirement of physical and chemical modifications for improving stability and shape fidelity are the challenges of plant-derived bioinks (Mahendiran et al. 2021). Osmotic swelling triggered by nanofibrillated cellulose (NFC) has led to the controlled structure and geometry of bioink, which helps in tissue engineering of complex shapes (Jang et al. 2018). The self-transformation behavior of 3D-printed objects in terms of function and form using a predetermined stimulus that includes heat, light, current, osmotic pressure, or other energy sources has led to the advancement from 3D bioprinting to 4D bioprinting (Yang et al. 2017). Hybrid biomaterials based on silk fibroin exhibit intrinsic molecular and mechanical properties, which can be used for shape-morphing.

Cell-laden bioinks in combination with drug substances are found to be effective in the treatment and management of wound healing and burns. Both natural (chitin, cellulose, chitosan, alginate, hyaluronic acid, thrombin, and collagen) and synthetic biopolymers, because of their biocompatibility and biodegradability, are suitable for

Table 2.7 List of FDA-approved biomaterials and their applications (Bharadwaj 2021)

S. no.	Materials	Applications
1.	CoCrMo, tantalum, platinum, nitinol, Ti6Al4V, nickel, titanium, stainless steel	• Orthopedic • Orthodontic • Cardiovascular
2.	Zirconia, hydroxyapatite, pyrolytic carbon, alumina, beta tricalcium phosphate	• Orthopedic • Orthodontic • Cardiovascular
3.	Nylon, polymethyl methacrylate (PMMA), polyethylene, polylactic acid (PLA), celluloid, polycaprolactone (PCL), cellophane, polyglycolic acid (PGA), polyurethane, poly-lactic-co-glycolic acid (PLGA), poly (ethers) including polyethylene glycol (PEG), polyvinyl alcohol (PVA), and polyurethanes (PUS), poly tetrafluoroethylene (PTFE)	• Drug delivery systems • Medical equipment • Cancer treatments • Biological applications for hydrogels • Nanotechnology • Bioartificial organs • Tissue engineering

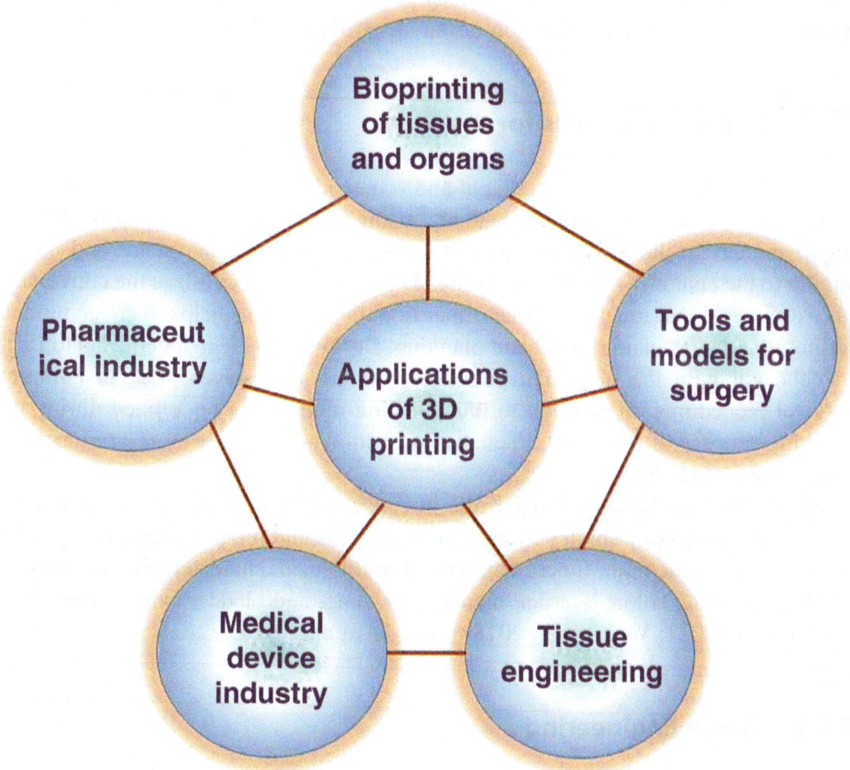

Fig. 2.12 Applications of biomaterial-based 3D printing

these applications (Chakraborty et al. 2022). Bioinks incorporated with fibroblasts and keratinocytes are also used in skin regeneration and wound healing (Tabriz and Douroumis 2022). Lignin, possessing antioxidant properties, is also used for wound healing applications (Wang et al. 2018a). Besides antioxidant properties, 3D printing of flexible wound dressing materials with antibacterial properties is demonstrated with Ag-, Zn-, and Cu-incorporated polycaprolactone filaments (Muwaffak et al. 2017). Wound dressing is prepared using 3D-printed multicomponent hydrogel loaded with silver nanoparticles and other vascular endothelial growth factors (Alizadehgiashi et al. 2021). Temporary or permanent coverage of wounds, burns, or flaps is possible using skin substitutes. Apligraf® is one such example of a skin substitute that is available on the market (Linares-Gonzalez et al. 2021). One of the novel works related to skin substitutes is the development of i-skin, which incorporates microfluidics and built-in electronics. These microfluidic channels integrated with photonic crystals provide multifunctional benefits of sensitivity toward sensing motion and multiple biomarkers (Desanlis et al. 2021). Several reviews are reported on the advancements in organ-on-chip technology, which includes 3D organs such as the heart, lung, liver, skin, gut, and vasculature (Kratz et al. 2019; Fetah et al. 2019). A biosensor system is incorporated into the organ-on-a-chip to study the health condition of the in vitro model (Shin et al. 2016).

2.6.2 Tools and Models for Surgery

Distinct tools for application in dental and orthopedics (including supporting bone plates and braces) are prepared today using a 3D printing process. Recent improvements in the field have led to the development of bone plates and braces similar to the anatomy of patients. As the 3D printing process utilizes the conversion of two-dimensional images to three-dimensional images, this helps to create models for improved physician training and planning. Designing patient-specific anatomical models will help the physician perform and train themselves prior to complex surgical procedures. In addition to this, creating models can be applied during the planning process of treatment, diagnosis, and implant engineering (Gargiulo et al. 2017; Wake et al. 2019).

3D printing is playing a crucial role in cancer research, pharmaceutical testing, and immune oncology studies by creating organoids and reliable tumor models that represent the structural, functional, and physiological characteristics of in vivo cervical, prostate, colon, ovarian, breast, liver, lung, and bladder cancers (Sánchez-Salazar et al. 2021; Wang et al. 2018b; Skardal et al. 2016).

2.6.3 Tissue Engineering

Accidents lead to tissue damage and bone injuries, which might lead to the loss of joint and organ functions. Application of tissue-engineered scaffolds is a known technique used to restore the functional activity of damaged bones and organs.

Various traditional methods used to manufacture scaffolds include freeze drying, electrospinning, solution casting, gas foaming, and emulsification methods (Derakhshanfar et al. 2018; Turnbull et al. 2018). Fibrillar collagen from bovine Achilles tendon is used in creating 3D-printed scaffolds without using strategies such as electrospinning, crosslinking, low temperature, or hybrid ink (Nocera et al. 2018). Studies using bioresorptive cellulose-incorporated collagen scaffolds are reported, wherein the mechanical properties and the interaction of the cell material are suggested to be achieved by varying the concentration of cellulose and the degree of oxidation (Kacvinská et al. 2022). An efficient fabrication of scaffolds based on multiscale porous bioactive (MPB) inorganic nanoparticle with a shape-memory polymer matrix of poly(D,L-lactide-co-trimethylene carbonate) is reported for bone tissue engineering applications (Wang et al. 2021a). Another work suggests the use of 3D-printed fabrication of cobalt-doped bioceramic and magnesium-doped β-TCP tissue engineering scaffolds for enhancement of osteogenic and angiogenic properties for bone repair (Li et al. 2021; Gu et al. 2019). Manufacturing of scaffolds for tissue engineering application by the 3D printing process is a recent advancement as it offers advantages like minimal cost, personalized design customization, and fabrication (Tofail et al. 2018). Applications of 2D nanomaterials as a replacement for metals, polymers, and ceramics are found in the repair and regeneration of cartilage tissue, osseointegration, neural regeneration, and the treatment of osteosarcoma (Das et al. 2021).

2.6.4 Pharmaceutical Industry

3D printing methods like inkjet, laser-assisted, and pressure-assisted methods are used in the pharmaceutical industry (Murphy and Atala 2014). Tablets manufactured using the 3D printing process are categorized into two classes: (1) single active pharmaceutical ingredient (API) tablets and (2) multiple API tablets. Among all the methods mentioned above, the inkjet printing process is the commonly adopted process in the pharma industry (Goyanes et al. 2016; Ozbolat and Yu 2013). 3D printed tablets offer many benefits like personal customization, increased production rate with higher resolution, highly reliable with lesser production cost. Recently, Fabrication of transdermal skin patches for drug delivery using microneedles are manufactured using a 3D printing process (Goyanes et al. 2015).

2.6.5 Medical Device Industry

Medical devices are classified into three groups (1) instrumentation, (2) implants, and (3) prosthesis. 3D printing plays a major role in year-on-year updation and is broadly accepted by the medical device industry. Surgical tools like retractors, clips, staples, and hemostats are easily manufactured using the 3D printing process. In recent years, tools and instruments of superior accuracy are mainly chosen in dentistry. Medical devices by 3D printing find its applications in various medical fields such as cardiology, gastro-enterology, maxillofacial and oral implants, neurosurgery, plastic and vascular surgery, otolaryngology, oncology, and orthopedic surgery (Wu et al. 2015).

2.7 Future Challenges

Despite all the progress made over these years in 3D printing, many challenges remain unanswered. In 3D bioprinting, the challenges can be classified into three areas: (1) printing section, (2) structural integrity, and (3) cell incorporation problems. To overcome problems in the printing section and structural integrity, the feed solution needs to have a constant stable printing streamline. For cell incorporation problems, the bioink should maintain the viability of the cells and cytocompatibility (Kim et al. 2018; Derakhshanfar et al. 2018). In the case of 4D printing, two requirements are essential: first, the feed solution needs to be stimuli-reactive and, second, there should be an external stimulus for triggering. Moreover, producing a programmable and stimuli-reactive 3D-printed object that undergoes modification against time due to ambient conditions such as heat, humidity, light, ultrasound, magnetic field, pH, and osmotic pressure is critical (Lee et al. 2017). In addition to this, the common difficulties include maintaining the temperature at 37°C and sterilizing the production environment, which is the most realistic hurdle in this process. It is noteworthy that there is no approved sterilization method for the bioprinting process. Also, during the extraction process, the effect of shear stress on the living cells needs to be kept to a minimum (Jakus 2018).

Though different biomaterials are used by 3D printing techniques, the research has changed from fabricating different smart materials to smart structures. The smart structures can be triggered by external stimuli or by ambient physiological changes. With the introduction of smart structures using smart bioinks, the future direction of tissue engineering and regenerative medicine involves the expansion of the limited choice of printable smart biomaterials for scaffolds and other implantable goods. In addition, the development of novel bioinks shows a vibrant role in attaining higher resolution capability for organ 3D printing. There are a limited number of feed solutions appropriate to carry the cell with adequate mechanical strength and cytotoxicity. Moreover, the printing time is an important concern that leads to a decrease in the functionality of the feed solution and indemnifies the partially printed area as printing time increases. Utilizing multi-head parallel printing will help address the timing problem. Manufacturing organs by 3D printing is the future direction that involves development of novel bioinks and advanced 3D printing manufacturing processes.

Artificial intelligence (AI), which is a superset of machine learning and deep learning, is a game-changer in today's modern industrial era. These AI-based technologies substitute the need for manual requirements and enhance the automation of the process. Researchers in the current medical industry use AI technologies in disease prediction, non-invasive diagnostic technologies, production and packaging processes in the pharmaceutical industry, 3D printing of desired organs, and also laser surgery. AI-based 3D printing approaches played a vital role in drug production during the Covid-19 outbreak (Banerjee et al. 2022). In situ AI-based 3D printing of medical devices provides the remedy for ex situ-based 3D printing, which leads to the problem of dynamic and geometrical mismatching of the interface between printed materials and target surface (Zhu et al. 2021). AI incorporated in the Internet of Things (IoT), cloud computing, and blockchain are used in 3D printing in the pharmaceutical industry for medicine delivery navigation, prediction purposes, and mass production based on the needs of patients (Elbadawi et al. 2021). In Rojek et al. (2023), the production of the upper limb exoskeleton has been discussed based on the Medical Devices Regulation (MDR) and the ISO 13485 and ISO 10993 standards, where AI optimization plays a major role. AI also aids in the simulation of 3D-printed computation-modeled heart (Wang et al. 2021b).

2.8 Conclusion

The evolution of 3D printing technology has led to the immense growth and development of biomaterial-based devices in the medical field. In this industrial revolution 4.0 era, AI, which includes machine learning and deep learning approaches, plays a significant role in AM in several aspects, such as designing, processing, tuning, predicting, and optimizing various features and also assessing the functionality of 3D-printed products even prior to manufacturing (Zhu et al. 2021). The various 3D printing techniques used for designing such biomedical devices, which include PBF, directed energy deposition, material jetting, binding jetting, and droplet-based bioprinting, are discussed in this chapter. The futuristic biomaterials and their beneficial properties in developing biomedical devices are also mentioned. The vast applications of biomaterial-based medical devices, not only in fabricating medical implants and prosthetic devices, disease modeling, and pharmaceutical industry, but also in developing patient-specific 3D hard and soft tissue scaffolds, vasculatures, and organs, are described in this chapter.

References

Alizadehgiashi M, Nemr CR, Chekini M, Pinto Ramos D, Mittal N, Ahmed SU, Khuu N, Kelley SO, Kumacheva E (2021) Multifunctional 3D-printed wound dressings. ACS Nano 15(7): 12375–12387

Almeida CR, Serra T, Oliveira MI, Planell JA, Barbosa MA, Navarro M (2014) Impact of 3-D printed PLA- and chitosan-based scaffolds on human monocyte/macrophage responses: unraveling the effect of 3-D structures on inflammation. Acta Biomater 10(2):613–622

Antonini E, Kaya FE, Palermo M, Pretelli M (2021) Applications of additive manufacturing in construction and historic building restoration/rehabilitation

Banerjee A, Haridas HK, SenGupta A, Jabalia N (2022) Artificial intelligence in 3D printing: a revolution in health care. In: Emerging applications of 3D printing during CoVID 19 pandemic. Springer, pp 57–79

Bharadwaj A (2021) An overview on biomaterials and its applications in medical science. In: IOP conference series: materials science and engineering, vol 1116(1). IOP Publishing, p 012178

Bozkurt Y, Karayel E (2021) 3D printing technology; methods, biomedical applications, future opportunities and trends. J Mater Res Technol 14:1430–1450
Bücking TM, Hill ER, Robertson JL, Maneas E, Plumb AA, Nikitichev DI (2017) From medical imaging data to 3D printed anatomical models. PLoS One 12(5):e0178540
Chakraborty J, Mu X, Pramanick A, Kaplan DL, Ghosh S (2022) Recent advances in bioprinting using silk protein-based bioinks. Biomaterials 287:121672
Das M, Ambekar RS, Panda SK, Chakraborty S, Tiwary CS (2021) 2D nanomaterials in 3D/4D-printed biomedical devices. J Mater Res 36(19):4024–4050
Derakhshanfar S, Mbeleck R, Xu K, Zhang X, Zhong W, Xing M (2018) 3D bioprinting for biomedical devices and tissue engineering: a review of recent trends and advances. Bioactive Mater 3(2):144–156
Desanlis A, Albouy M, Rousselle P, Thépot A, Santos MD, Auxenfans C, Marquette C (2021) Validation of an implantable bioink using mechanical extraction of human skin cells: first steps to a 3D bioprinting treatment of deep second degree burn. J Tissue Eng Regen Med 15(1):37–48
Dong L, Wang SJ, Zhao XR, Zhu YF, Yu JK (2017) 3D-printed poly (ε-caprolactone) scaffold integrated with cell-laden chitosan hydrogels for bone tissue engineering. Sci Rep 7(1):1–9
dos Santos GA (2015) Tecnologia dos Materiais Metálicos: Propriedades, Estruturas e Processos de Obtenção. Saraiva Educação SA
Dos Santos V, Brandalise RN, Savaris M (2017) Engineering of biomaterials. Springer, Berlin, pp 1–86
Duerig T, Pelton A, Stöckel DJMS (1999) An overview of nitinol medical applications. Mater Sci Eng A 273:149–160
Dutra GVS, Neto WS, Dutra JPS, Machado F (2020) Implantable medical devices and tissue engineering: an overview of manufacturing processes and the use of polymeric matrices for manufacturing and coating their surfaces. Curr Med Chem 27(10):1580–1599
Elbadawi M, McCoubrey LE, Gavins FK, Ong JJ, Goyanes A, Gaisford S, Basit AW (2021) Harnessing artificial intelligence for the next generation of 3D printed medicines. Adv Drug Deliv Rev 175:113805
Festas AJ, Ramos A, Davim JP (2020) Medical devices biomaterials—a review. Proc Inst Mech Eng L J Mater Des Appl 234(1):218–228
Fetah K, Tebon P, Goudie MJ, Eichenbaum J, Ren L, Barros N, Nasiri R, Ahadian S, Ashammakhi N, Dokmeci MR, Khademhosseini A (2019) The emergence of 3D bioprinting in organ-on-chip systems. Progress Biomed Eng 1(1):012001
Gargiulo P, Árnadóttir Í, Gíslason M, Edmunds K, Ólafsson I (2017) New directions in 3D medical modeling: 3D-printing anatomy and functions in neurosurgical planning. J Healthcare Eng 2017:1
Goyanes A, Buanz AB, Hatton GB, Gaisford S, Basit AW (2015) 3D printing of modified-release aminosalicylate (4-ASA and 5-ASA) tablets. Eur J Pharm Biopharm 89:157–162
Goyanes A, Det-Amornrat U, Wang J, Basit AW, Gaisford S (2016) 3D scanning and 3D printing as innovative technologies for fabricating personalized topical drug delivery systems. J Control Release 234:41–48
Groover MP (2013) Principles of modern manufacturing, 5th edn. John Wiley, Sons Inc, New York, 1024 p
Gu Y, Zhang J, Zhang X, Liang G, Xu T, Niu W (2019) Three-dimensional printed Mg-doped β-TCP bone tissue engineering scaffolds: effects of magnesium ion concentration on osteogenesis and angiogenesis in vitro. Tissue Eng Regen Med 16(4):415–429
Gu Z, Fu J, Lin H, He Y (2020) Development of 3D bioprinting: from printing methods to biomedical applications. Asian J Pharm Sci 15(5):529–557
Guzzi EA, Tibbitt MW (2020) Additive manufacturing of precision biomaterials. Adv Mater 32(13):1901994
Hitzler L, Alifui-Segbaya F, Williams P, Heine B, Heitzmann M, Hall W, Merkel M, Öchsner A (2018) Additive manufacturing of cobalt-based dental alloys: analysis of microstructure and physicomechanical properties. Adv Mater Sci Eng 2018:8213023

Jakus A (2018) An introduction to 3D printing: past, present, and future promise. In: 3D printing in orthopaedic surgery. Elsevier, p 1

Jammalamadaka U, Tappa K (2018) Recent advances in biomaterials for 3D printing and tissue engineering. J Funct Biomater 9(1):22

Jang J, Park JY, Gao G, Cho DW (2018) Biomaterials-based 3D cell printing for next-generation therapeutics and diagnostics. Biomaterials 156:88–106

Jani JM, Leary M, Subic A, Gibson MA (2014) A review of shape memory alloy research, applications and opportunities. Mater Des (1980–2015) 56:1078–1113

Jayashankar DK, Gupta SS, Velu R, Jayakumar A (2022) Chitosan biopolymer for 3D printing: a comprehensive review. In: Natural polymers: perspectives and applications for a green approach. CRC Press, pp 91–116

John P, Antony IR, Whenish R, Jinoop AN (2022) A review on fabrication of 3D printed biomaterials using optical methodologies for tissue engineering applications. Proc Inst Mech Eng H J Eng Med 236(11):1583–1594

Kacvinská K, Trávníčková M, Vojtová L, Poláček P, Dorazilová J, Kohoutek M, Hlináková K, Pajorová J, Tirpáková M, Bačáková L (2022) Porous cellulose-collagen scaffolds for soft tissue regeneration: influence of cellulose derivatives on mechanical properties and compatibility with adipose-derived stem cells. Cellulose 29(15):8329–8351

Kargozar S, Singh RK, Kim HW, Baino F (2020) "Hard" ceramics for "soft" tissue engineering: paradox or opportunity? Acta Biomater 115:1–28

Kim SH, Yeon YK, Lee JM, Chao JR, Lee YJ, Seo YB, Sultan M, Lee OJ, Lee JS, Yoon SI, Hong IS (2018) Precisely printable and biocompatible silk fibroin bioink for digital light processing 3D printing. Nat Commun 9(1):1–14

Kiran ASK, Ramakrishna S (2021). www.worldscientific.com/doi/pdf/10.1142/9789811228186_0004#:~:text=The%20tensile%20strength%2C%20yield%20strength,properties%20are%20of%20top%20priority

Kratz SRA, Höll G, Schuller P, Ertl P, Rothbauer M (2019) Latest trends in biosensing for microphysiological organs-on-a-chip and body-on-a-chip systems. Biosensors 9(3):110

Kumar R, Kumar M, Chohan JS (2021) The role of additive manufacturing for biomedical applications: a critical review. J Manuf Process 64:828–850

Laronda MM, Rutz AL, Xiao S, Whelan KA, Duncan FE, Roth EW, Woodruff TK, Shah RN (2017) A bioprosthetic ovary created using 3D printed microporous scaffolds restores ovarian function in sterilized mice. Nat Commun 8(1):1–10

Lee JY, An J, Chua CK (2017) Fundamentals and applications of 3D printing for novel materials. Appl Mater Today 7:120–133

Li J, Zhao C, Liu C, Wang Z, Ling Z, Lin B, Tan B, Zhou L, Chen Y, Liu D, Zou X (2021) Cobalt-doped bioceramic scaffolds fabricated by 3D printing show enhanced osteogenic and angiogenic properties for bone repair. Biomed Eng Online 20(1):1–24

Li X, Lu W, Xu X, Wang Y, Chen SC (2022) Advanced optical methods and materials for fabricating 3D tissue scaffolds. Light Adv Manuf 3(2):1–32

Ligon SC, Liska R, Stampfl J, Gurr M, Mülhaupt R (2017) Polymers for 3D printing and customized additive manufacturing. Chem Rev 117(15):10212–10290

Linares-Gonzalez L, Rodenas-Herranz T, Campos F, Ruiz-Villaverde R, Carriel V (2021) Basic quality controls used in skin tissue engineering. Life 11(10):1033

Low ZX, Chua YT, Ray BM, Mattia D, Metcalfe IS, Patterson DA (2017) Perspective on 3D printing of separation membranes and comparison to related unconventional fabrication techniques. J Membr Sci 523:596–613

Mahdavi SS, Abdekhodaie MJ, Kumar H, Mashayekhan S, Baradaran-Rafii A, Kim K (2020) Stereolithography 3D bioprinting method for fabrication of human corneal stroma equivalent. Ann Biomed Eng 48(7):1955–1970

Mahendiran B, Muthusamy S, Sampath S, Jaisankar SN, Popat KC, Selvakumar R, Krishnakumar GS (2021) Recent trends in natural polysaccharide based bioinks for multiscale 3D printing in tissue regeneration: a review. Int J Biol Macromol 183:564–588

Meier H, Haberland C (2008) Experimental studies on selective laser melting of metallic parts. Mater Werkst 39(9):665–670

Miao S, Castro N, Nowicki M, Xia L, Cui H, Zhou X, Zhu W, Lee SJ, Sarkar K, Vozzi G, Tabata Y (2017) 4D printing of polymeric materials for tissue and organ regeneration. Mater Today 20(10):577–591

Murphy SV, Atala A (2014) 3D bioprinting of tissues and organs. Nat Biotechnol 32(8):773–785

Murr LE (2016) Frontiers of 3D printing/additive manufacturing: from human organs to aircraft fabrication. J Mater Sci Technol 32(10):987–995

Muwaffak Z, Goyanes A, Clark V, Basit AW, Hilton ST, Gaisford S (2017) Patient-specific 3D scanned and 3D printed antimicrobial polycaprolactone wound dressings. Int J Pharm 527(1–2): 161–170

Nahmias Y, Schwartz RE, Verfaillie CM, Odde DJ (2005) Laser-guided direct writing for three-dimensional tissue engineering. Biotechnol Bioeng 92(2):129–136

Narayan R (2017). https://www.sciencedirect.com/book/9780081007167/nanobiomaterials#book-description

Nichetti D, Manas-Zloczower I (1999) Influence of molecular parameters on material processability in extrusion processes. Polym Eng Sci 39(5):887–895

Nocera AD, Comín R, Salvatierra NA, Cid MP (2018) Development of 3D printed fibrillar collagen scaffold for tissue engineering. Biomed Microdevices 20(2):1–13

Obeidi MA, Monu M, Hughes C, Bourke D, Dogu MN, Francis J, Zhang M, Ahad IU, Brabazon D (2021) Laser beam powder bed fusion of nitinol shape memory alloy (SMA). J Mater Res Technol 14:2554–2570

Ozbolat IT, Yu Y (2013) Bioprinting toward organ fabrication: challenges and future trends. IEEE Trans Biomed Eng 60(3):691–699

Panda B, Tan MJ, Gibson I, Chua CK (2016) The disruptive evolution of 3D printing. In: Second international conference on progress in additive manufacturing, pp 152–157

Park SI, Rosen DW, Choi SK, Duty CE (2014) Effective mechanical properties of lattice material fabricated by material extrusion additive manufacturing. Addit Manuf 1:12–23

Pina S, Rebelo R, Correlo VM, Oliveira JM, Reis RL (2018) Bioceramics for osteochondral tissue engineering and regeneration. Adv Exp Med Biol 1058:53–75

Pranzo D, Larizza P, Filippini D, Percoco G (2018) Extrusion-based 3D printing of microfluidic devices for chemical and biomedical applications: a topical review. Micromachines 9(8):374

Pugliese R, Beltrami B, Regondi S, Lunetta C (2021) Polymeric biomaterials for 3D printing in medicine: an overview. Ann 3D Print Med 2:100011

Punj S, Singh J, Singh K (2021) Ceramic biomaterials: properties, state of the art and future prospectives. Ceram Int 47(20):28059–28074

Rahmani S, Maroufkhani M, Mohammadzadeh-Komuleh S, Khoubi-Arani Z (2022) Polymer nanocomposites for biomedical applications. In: Fundamentals of bionanomaterials. Elsevier, pp 175–215

Rojek I, Mikołajewski D, Dostatni E, Kopowski J (2023) Specificity of 3D printing and AI-based optimization of medical devices using the example of a group of exoskeletons. Appl Sci 13(2): 1060

Rokkanen PU, Böstman O, Hirvensalo E, Mäkelä EA, Partio EK, Pätiälä H, Vainionpää S, Vihtonen K, Törmälä P (2000) Bioabsorbable fixation in orthopaedic surgery and traumatology. Biomaterials 21(24):2607–2613

Salinas AJ, Esbrit P, Vallet-Regí M (2013) A tissue engineering approach based on the use of bioceramics for bone repair. Biomater Sci 1(1):40–51

Sánchez-Salazar MG, Álvarez MM, Trujillo-de Santiago G (2021) Advances in 3D bioprinting for the biofabrication of tumor models. Bioprinting 21:e00120

Sandler N, Määttänen A, Ihalainen P, Kronberg L, Meierjohann A, Viitala T, Peltonen J (2011) Inkjet printing of drug substances and use of porous substrates-towards individualized dosing. J Pharm Sci 100(8):3386–3395

Santos G (2017) The importance of metallic materials as biomaterials. Adv Tissue Eng Regen Med Open Access 3(1):300–302

Senthilkumar V, Velmurugan C, Balasubramanian KR, Kumaran M (2020) Additive manufacturing of multi-material and composite parts. In: Additive manufacturing applications for metals and composites. IGI Global, pp 127–146

Shahrubudin N, Lee TC, Ramlan R (2019) An overview on 3D printing technology: technological, materials, and applications. Proc Manuf 35:1286–1296

Sharafeldin M, Jones A, Rusling JF (2018) 3D-printed biosensor arrays for medical diagnostics. Micromachines 9(8):394

Shashi GM, Laskar MAR, Biswas H, Saha AK (2017) A brief review of additive manufacturing with applications. In: Proceedings of 14th global engineering and technology conference, Dec 2017

Shim JH, Won JY, Park JH, Bae JH, Ahn G, Kim CH, Lim DH, Cho DW, Yun WS, Bae EB, Jeong CM (2017) Effects of 3D-printed polycaprolactone/β-tricalcium phosphate membranes on guided bone regeneration. Int J Mol Sci 18(5):899

Shin SR, Zhang YS, Kim DJ, Manbohi A, Avci H, Silvestri A, Aleman J, Hu N, Kilic T, Keung W, Righi M (2016) Aptamer-based microfluidic electrochemical biosensor for monitoring cell-secreted trace cardiac biomarkers. Anal Chem 88(20):10019–10027

Shirazi SFS, Gharehkhani S, Mehrali M, Yarmand H, Metselaar HSC, Kadri NA, Osman NAA (2015) A review on powder-based additive manufacturing for tissue engineering: selective laser sintering and inkjet 3D printing. Sci Technol Adv Mater 16(3):033502

Shuai C, Zhuang J, Peng S, Wen X (2014) Inhibition of phase transformation from β-to α-tricalcium phosphate with addition of poly (L-lactic acid) in selective laser sintering. Rapid Prototyp J 20(5):369–376

Skardal A, Devarasetty M, Forsythe S, Atala A, Soker S (2016) A reductionist metastasis-on-a-chip platform for in vitro tumor progression modeling and drug screening. Biotechnol Bioeng 113(9):2020–2032

Soman P, Chung PH, Zhang AP, Chen S (2013) Digital microfabrication of user-defined 3D microstructures in cell-laden hydrogels. Biotechnol Bioeng 110(11):3038–3047

Squelch A (2018) 3D printing and medical imaging. J Med Radiat Sci 65(3):171–172

Stansbury JW, Idacavage MJ (2016) 3D printing with polymers: challenges among expanding options and opportunities. Dent Mater 32(1):54–64

Strobel LA, Rath SN, Maier AK, Beier JP, Arkudas A, Greil P, Horch RE, Kneser U (2014) Induction of bone formation in biphasic calcium phosphate scaffolds by bone morphogenetic protein-2 and primary osteoblasts. J Tissue Eng Regen Med 8(3):176–185

Subedi MM (2013) Ceramics and its importance. Himal Geol 4:80–82

Sun M, Liu A, Shao H, Yang X, Ma C, Yan S, Liu Y, He Y, Gou Z (2016) Systematical evaluation of mechanically strong 3D printed diluted magnesium doping wollastonite scaffolds on osteogenic capacity in rabbit calvarial defects. Sci Rep 6(1):1–14

Tabriz AG, Douroumis D (2022) Recent advances in 3D printing for wound healing: a systematic review. J Drug Deliv Sci Technol 74:103564

Tai WC, Chang YC, Chou D, Fu LM (2021) Lab-on-paper devices for diagnosis of human diseases using urine samples—a review. Biosensors 11(8):260

Tan Z, Parisi C, Di Silvio L, Dini D, Forte AE (2017) Cryogenic 3D printing of super soft hydrogels. Sci Rep 7(1):1–11

Tapscott DC, Wottowa C (2022) Orthopedic implant materials. In: StatPearls. StatPearls Publishing, Treasure Island, FL

Tofail SA, Koumoulos EP, Bandyopadhyay A, Bose S, O'Donoghue L, Charitidis C (2018) Additive manufacturing: scientific and technological challenges, market uptake and opportunities. Mater Today 21(1):22–37

Turnbull G, Clarke J, Picard F, Riches P, Jia L, Han F, Li B, Shu W (2018) 3D bioactive composite scaffolds for bone tissue engineering. Bioactive Mater 3(3):278–314

Velu R, Calais T, Jayakumar A, Raspall F (2019) A comprehensive review on bio-nanomaterials for medical implants and feasibility studies on fabrication of such implants by additive manufacturing technique. Materials 13(1):92

Wake N, Alexander AE, Christensen AM, Liacouras PC, Schickel M, Pietila T, Matsumoto J (2019) Creating patient-specific anatomical models for 3D printing and AR/VR: a supplement for the 2018 Radiological Society of North America (RSNA) hands-on course. 3D Print Med 5(1):1–10

Wang Y, Wang K, Li X, Wei Q, Chai W, Wang S, Che Y, Lu T, Zhang B (2017) 3D fabrication and characterization of phosphoric acid scaffold with a HA/β-TCP weight ratio of 60: 40 for bone tissue engineering applications. PLoS One 12(4):e0174870

Wang J, Tian L, Luo B, Ramakrishna S, Kai D, Loh XJ, Yang IH, Deen GR, Mo X (2018a) Engineering PCL/lignin nanofibers as an antioxidant scaffold for the growth of neuron and Schwann cell. Colloids Surf B Biointerfaces 169:356–365

Wang X, Zhang X, Dai X, Wang X, Li X, Diao J, Xu T (2018b) Tumor-like lung cancer model based on 3D bioprinting. 3 Biotech 8(12):1–9

Wang J, Gao H, Hu Y, Zhang N, Zhou W, Wang C, Binks BP, Yang Z (2021a) 3D printing of pickering emulsion inks to construct poly (D, L-lactide-co-trimethylene carbonate)-based porous bioactive scaffolds with shape memory effect. J Mater Sci 56(1):731–745

Wang DD, Qian Z, Vukicevic M, Engelhardt S, Kheradvar A, Zhang C, Little SH, Verjans J, Comaniciu D, O'Neill WW, Vannan MA (2021b) 3D printing, computational modeling, and artificial intelligence for structural heart disease. Cardiovasc Imaging 14(1):41–60

Wang M, Li W, Hao J, Gonzales A, Zhao Z, Flores RS, Kuang X, Mu X, Ching T, Tang G, Luo Z (2022) Molecularly cleavable bioinks facilitate high-performance digital light processing-based bioprinting of functional volumetric soft tissues. Nat Commun 13(1):1–18

Waran V, Narayanan V, Karuppiah R, Owen SL, Aziz T (2014) Utility of multimaterial 3D printers in creating models with pathological entities to enhance the training experience of neurosurgeons. J Neurosurg 120(2):489–492

Wu D, Rosen DW, Wang L, Schaefer D (2015) Cloud-based design and manufacturing: a new paradigm in digital manufacturing and design innovation. Comput Aided Des 59:1–14

Xu Y, Liu M, Kong N, Liu J (2016) Lab-on-paper micro-and nano-analytical devices: fabrication, modification, detection and emerging applications. Microchim Acta 183(5):1521–1542

Yadav D, Garg RK, Ahlawat A, Chhabra D (2020) 3D printable biomaterials for orthopedic implants: solution for sustainable and circular economy. Resour Policy 68:101767

Yan Q, Dong H, Su J, Han J, Song B, Wei Q, Shi Y (2018) A review of 3D printing technology for medical applications. Engineering 4(5):729–742

Yang H, Leow WR, Wang T, Wang J, Yu J, He K, Qi D, Wan C, Chen X (2017) 3D printed photoresponsive devices based on shape memory composites. Adv Mater 29(33):1701627

Yap YL, Wang C, Sing SL, Dikshit V, Yeong WY, Wei J (2017) Material jetting additive manufacturing: an experimental study using designed metrological benchmarks. Precis Eng 50:275–285

Zein NN, Hanouneh IA, Bishop PD, Samaan M, Eghtesad B, Quintini C, Miller C, Yerian L, Klatte R (2013) Three-dimensional print of a liver for preoperative planning in living donor liver transplantation. Liver Transpl 19(12):1304–1310

Zhu Z, Ng DWH, Park HS, McAlpine MC (2021) 3D-printed multifunctional materials enabled by artificial-intelligence-assisted fabrication technologies. Nat Rev Mater 6(1):27–47

Design and Manufacturing of 3D Printed Sensors for Biomedical Applications

3

Sridhar Chandrasekaran, Arunkumar Jayakumar, Rajkumar Velu, and S. Stella Mary

Contents

Abstract

Recently, three-dimensional (3D) printing technology has been evolving rapidly in the healthcare sector, specifically for the development of small-scale medical implants. 3D printing technology is a precise and easy-to-deployable technology

S. Chandrasekaran (✉)
School of Electronics Engineering, Vellore Institute of Technology, Chennai, Tamil Nadu, India
e-mail: sridhar.c@vit.ac.in

A. Jayakumar
Department of Electrical and Electronics Engineering, St. Peter's Institute of Higher Education and Research, Chennai, Tamil Nadu, India

R. Velu
Additive Manufacturing Research Laboratory, Mechanical Engineering, Indian Institute of Technology Jammu, Jammu, Jammu and Kashmir, India

S. S. Mary
Department of Physics, St. Peter's Institute of Higher Education and Research, Chennai, Tamil Nadu, India

R. Velu et al. (eds.), *Digital Design and Manufacturing of Medical Devices and Systems*, https://doi.org/10.1007/978-981-99-7100-8_3

that is a low-cost fabrication technique with minimal waste during the manufacturing process. Biomedical sensors are generally used to analyze the human body fluid or surface nature through which the analysis of human health is obtained. In this chapter, we will discuss in detail the various printing methods used for the manufacturing of biomedical sensors and access those sensors that could be rapidly manufactured using 3D printing technology. Also, we provide the future perspective of printable sensors in various cutting-edge applications.

Keywords

Biomedical sensors · Additive manufacturing · Implantable sensors · Electrochemical sensors · Textile-embedded sensors · Wearable sensors · Haptic sensors · Microfluidic sensors

3.1 Introduction

Additive manufacturing (AM) technology is revolutionizing the present industrial world by providing rapid and sustainable solutions to many complex real-time problems faced by humanity. In addition, AM technology offers precise and rapid solutions to complex manufacturing issues with minimal waste generation during the process. These advantages of AM technology have allowed vast penetration of this technology across interdisciplinary fields such as mechanical devices, electronic devices, and biomedical devices (Al Rashid et al. 2020). The emergence of Industry 4.0 and the incorporation of AM technology are extremely promising for biomedical applications due to their potential to achieve complex and compact adaptable structures (Dilberoglu et al. 2017). The biomedical field is facing a huge revolution due to the emergence of artificial intelligence–assisted smart hospitals, which have significantly increased the number of sensory and actuating units in the healthcare ecosystem (Haleem et al. 2022, 2023). Biomedical sensors play a prominent role in the next-generation healthcare infrastructure, as these sensors have the potential for real-time monitoring of vital organs of the human body (Chen et al. 2023; Wang et al. 2022; Hua et al. 2022). Figure 3.1 depicts the recently emerged biomedical sensors that interact and interface with the human body, such as brain implants, organs on chips, haptic sensors, and smart fabric sensors. Additionally, the emergence of brain–computer interfacing in the recent past has broadened the scope of implantable and haptic sensors in the healthcare ecosystem (Hochberg and Donoghue 2006; Faisal et al. 2023; George et al. 2012; Fleury et al. 2020). These sensing technologies are predicted to dominate the next generation of the biomedical industry, which is strongly expected to have artificial intelligence and machine learning as driving forces for futuristic applications. Thus, even the sensors and sensory circuits need upgrading to rapidly evolve to the growing needs of the industry. Biomedical sensors can be classified based on their sensing operations across various parts of the human body. These sophisticated biomedical sensors can offer various solutions, such as brain implants, heart-on-chip devices, E-textile-

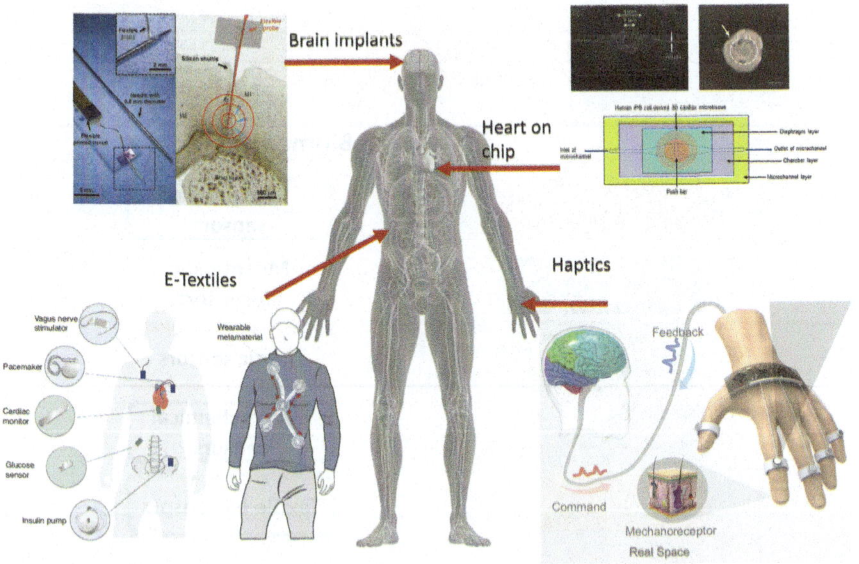

Fig. 3.1 Human–machine interface of various sensors and supporting systems connecting various forms of the human body. (Reprinted with permission Guo et al. 2022; Sun et al. 2022; Tian et al. 2023; Abulaiti et al. 2020)

based monitoring, and haptic sensing, as depicted in Fig. 3.2. In a study, the authors developed micro-fluidic-based heart-on-chip devices that are capable of monitoring acute hypoxia (Liu et al. 2020). Similarly, heart-on-chip devices are found to be effective in testing the drug efficacy analysis (Zhang et al. 2021). Specifically, implants for the human brain are a rapidly growing field, and it requires sophisticated analysis on the choice of electrode materials, which determine the brain signal detection efficacy (Cho et al. 2021). The future of augmented reality is based on the haptic sensors in feedback, which could evolve the futuristic applications in various industries, ranging from medical to commercial gaming applications (Xiong et al. 2021). These broad and dynamic futuristic applications are the key factors that motivate researchers to develop sensors based on printable technology (Hua et al. 2022; Hochberg and Donoghue 2006; Faisal et al. 2023).

As depicted in Fig. 3.2, the entire class of the biomedical sensing elements can be classified as implantable or biocompatible sensors, microfluidic sensors, skin-surface-contact-based haptic sensors, electrochemical sensors, and textile-based wearable sensors (Ali et al. 2022). The integral challenge faced by the researchers is to convert these sophisticated sensors into printable sensors without losing their key properties, such as biocompatibility, sensitivity, adaptability, and electrical efficiency (Dahiya et al. 2019). Additionally, on converting them into rapid prototyping technology, these sensors offer users the higher degree of freedom to obtain rapid customization across various application spaces, including futuristic biomedical applications.

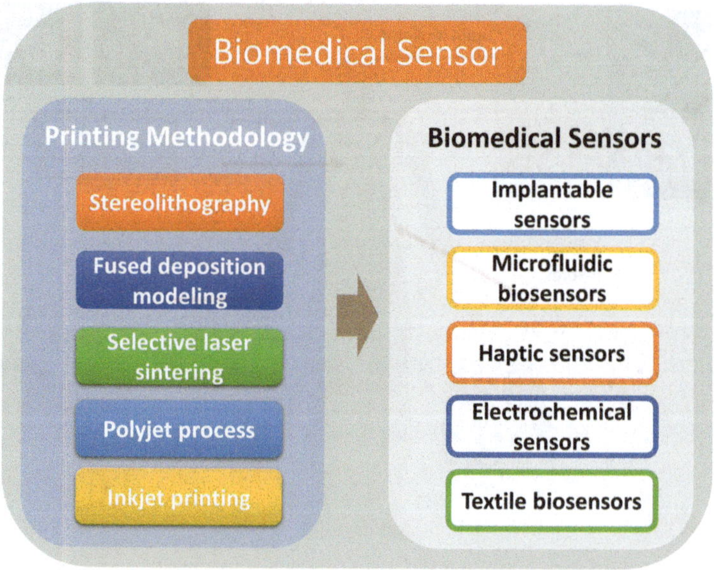

Fig. 3.2 Block diagram of the various biomedical sensors and their printing methodology used for fabrication

The biomedical sensors can be effectively printed by using various printing technologies such as stereolithography, fuse deposition modelling (FDM), selective laser sintering, polyjet processing, and inkjet printing, as depicted in Fig. 3.3. Sensors are 3D printed in general by either directly printing the sensors on the substrates or by integrating the sensors into a complete sensing system. Thus, the 3D-printed sensors can be effectively classified based on the method of fabrication into directly printed sensors and integrated sensors. Both the integrated sensor and directly printed sensor can be effectively used for the development of next-generation bio-medical sensors and supporting systems. The next generation of healthcare ecosystem is moving toward interconnected artificial intelligence–assisted technology, and the integrated biomedical sensors have a promising future in the next-generation healthcare ecosystem (Bozkurt and Karayel 2021). In near future, the additive manufacturing technology is going to evolve by integrating with intelligent systems, which will further enhance the reliability of the additive manufacturing technology (Heiden et al. 2021). Similarly, the standalone direct-printed sensor is practically used in direct sensing applications such as blood glucose sensing, temperature sensing, pressure sensing, virus detection, and other micro detection can be effectively obtained by using direct implantable sensors. These sensors are cost-effective with minimal resources required for analyzing the sensing patch or supporting system.

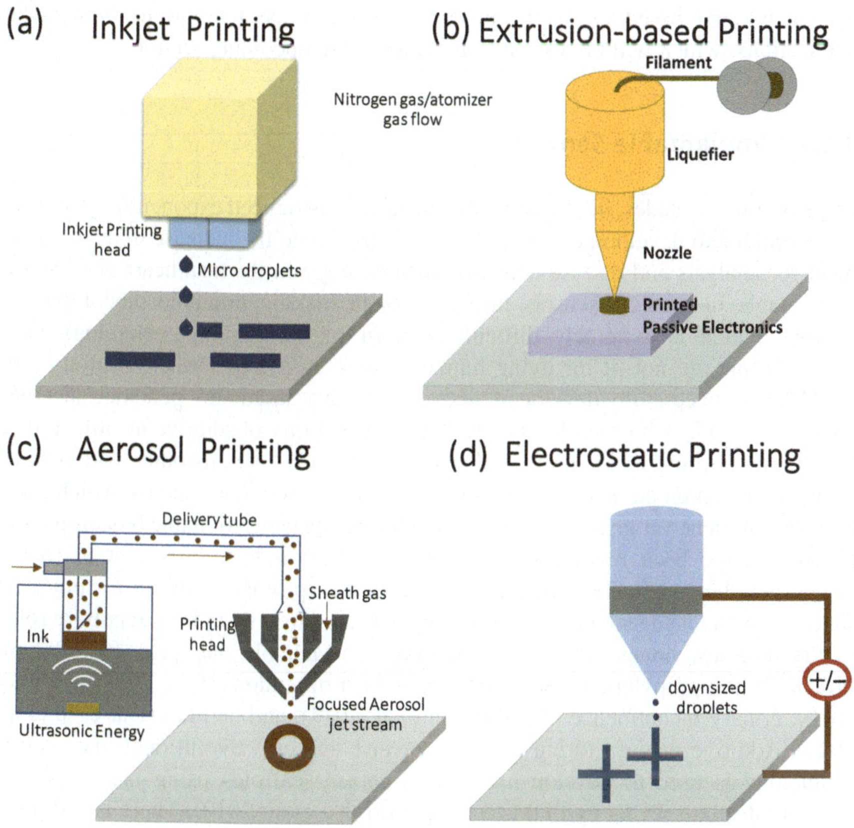

Fig. 3.3 Various printing methods such as (**a**) inkjet printing, (**b**) extrusion-based fused deposition modeling, (**c**) aerosol printing, (**d**) electrostatic printing. (Reprinted from Chandrasekaran et al. 2022)

3.2 Biomedical Sensors

Ever since the commencement of the industry 4.0 revolution, additive manufacturing technology has been penetrating all sectors of the industry; among them, the healthcare sector is never limited. Recently, artificial intelligence–assisted technology has been penetrating large-scale healthcare applications to achieve an intelligent healthcare ecosystem and subsequently highly effective sensors, thus combating rapid industrial growth. It is essential to develop adaptive technology to develop rapid, manufacturable sensors for biomedical applications. Ever since the surge of COVID-19, humankind experienced the worst-ever catastrophic effect on the healthcare ecosystem, and the demand for rapidly manufacturable biomedical sensors has been exponentially increasing due to their precise and effective manufacturing process during the catastrophic condition. The biomedical sensors are categorized based on their functionality and scope for various biomedical applications, which will be discussed in detail in the upcoming section.

3.2.1 Implantable Sensors

In the past few decades, implantable sensors have experienced exponential growth in the research and development space, prominently due to the increase in the requirement for analysis and disease detection methodology in the healthcare ecosystem. Implantable biomedical sensors face hurdles in making printable biocompatible sensors, which is extremely difficult as most of the printing technology uses materials that are not fit for living human tissues. In a leap further, Britton et al. (2021) have successfully developed biocompatible ink based on x-pentadecalactone-co-e-decalactone, which further increases the adaptability of additive manufacturing technology into printable biomedical sensors. Similarly, various other studies have been conducted on passive biocompatible materials rather than sensors, which open pathways for a newer generation of implantable ecosystems. Meltable biocompatible polymers have been revolutionizing the biomedical industry for over a decade because of their meltable property, which acts as a promising future for practical surgery. As the name suggests, passive implants are those that play supportive roles to the muscles, bones, and other vital organs. Meltable and printable Ethicon Prolene™ polypropylene is used for the treatment of tendons (Pike and Gelberman 2010), urinary incontinence (Zyczkowski et al. 2014), and hernia (Tanasescu et al. 2021). Additive manufacturing is highly precise and effective in dentistry, as this technology is used to develop highly customized scaffolds using biocompatible polycabrolactone (PCL) by FDM technique (Probst et al. 2010). There is a significant leap in printable passive implantable, which offers various possible biocompatible materials in developing next-generation biocompatible sensors using these materials. In an interesting leap toward implantable sensors, the printable bionic ears are attracting attention as they could effectively transmit the audio signal via radio frequency transmission, which is based on conductive silver nanoparticle ink with biological cells (Mannoor et al. 2013). In another significant breakthrough for the future of printable implants, Huo et al. (2023) have successfully developed soft ionotronics, which is a game changer because of its ability to adapt to the human body both electrically and mechanically. In this study, they explored the ionic diodes, transistors, rectifiers, and touchpads, which lead to a prosperous future for printable implantable sensors. Also, in another study, printed microgel was used for the development of implantable strain sensors based on carbopol and deep eutectic solvents, which act as the future of wearable and implantable technologies (Vo et al. 2023). Organ on chip is also increasingly popular among the printable implantable biomedical systems, with its attractive application, which could revolutionize the way drug delivery systems work, on-chip heart with cardiac functionality, and glioblastoma-on-a-chip, which is especially useful for analyzing the patient response to chemotherapy (Yi et al. 2019; Lind et al. 2017; Ma et al. 2021).

3.2.2 Microfluidic Biosensors

In the traditional microfluidic biosensors, the fabrication system components such as microchannels, microvalves, and others often require highly expensive cleanroom fabrication, which makes them a capital-intensive research space. In recent days, after the emergence of additive manufacturing, even microfluidic sensor manufacturing has driven to such smart and lean manufacturing of sensors. A study reported by Michael J. Beauchamp et al. has developed a microfluidic bio-marker that can determine the risk for preterm birth, and it is effectively printed using stereolithographic 3D printing (Beauchamp et al. 2019). Colorimetric Analysis is widely used in point-of-care settings, and a 3D-printed microfluidic component composed of valves and pumps is seemingly advanced in conducting such an intensive point-of-care application (Chan et al. 2016). The microfluidic biosensor offers a wide variety of biomedical sensing applications such as Pathogen Detection, Lung Disease, Bioanalysis, Diagnostics, and other microfluidic devices (Kumar et al. 2022; Ding et al. 2021; Berlanda et al. 2021). Brain research is seemingly popular in recent years because of its extraordinary cognitive functionality and understanding of the physicality of the extraordinary features of the human brain. In future, printed microfluidic devices will be an effective tool for understanding the function of the brain, and future pathways for brain research will be poised around the microfluidic manipulation and chip (Wan et al. 2022). Another important finding by Daehoon Han et al. is the printable bio-inspired needle array, which has the potential to replace the traditional drug delivery needles (Han et al. 2020).

3.2.3 Haptic Sensors

Ever since the induction of wearable electronic devices into the commercial market space, the demand for biomedical haptic sensors is increasing at an exponential rate, leading to ground-breaking innovations (Ali et al. 2022; Wan et al. 2017). In this section, the various haptic printable sensors that could be part of future clinical wearable medical devices have been discussed in detail. As the haptic sensor comes into the picture, most efforts are toward the development of a flexible printable capacitive tactile sensor, attracting attention because of their broad support for the future of wearable and printable biomedical devices (El-Molla et al. 2016; Salim and Lim 2017; Gaspar et al. 2017). The future of wearables is also progressing toward triboelectric tactile sensors, which can effectively sense human touch (Wang et al. 2020). In another study, highly mechanically stable cantilever-based flexible strain sensors and pressure sensors for the e-skin application are also promising in the field of e-skin-based wearable electronic devices (Kanao et al. 2015). Highly stretchable and printable e-skin with outstanding sensitivity of 150 kPa^{-1} to touch and load has been reported by Roy et al. (2022). Thiyagarajan et al. have reported a low-cost flexible and printable multi-wall carbon nanotube-based temperature sensor for clinical monitoring of sensory patches (Thiyagarajan et al. 2022). In another study, biomimicking soft haptic devices are found to be effective in force sensing for brain–

computer interface applications (Mutlu et al. 2023). Even the haptic microgripper is efficient for physical rehabilitation purposes, where the motion tissue is monitored on a real-time basis (Mutlu et al. 2023). In a study, the authors developed fully flexible and printable actuators that are highly desired for the future of augmented reality and virtual reality applications, as the future of the medical industry is also expected to adopt advanced technologies offered by artificial intelligence, which plays a pivot role in the healthcare industry (Grasso et al. 2023).

3.2.4 Electrochemical Sensors

Electrochemical sensors are widely used in the biomedical industry because of their promising nature to detect pathogens or abnormalities through the electrochemical reaction that happens between the electrodes and solution (Yamanaka et al. 2016). The adaptation of printing technology into biosensors will open a new horizon of low-cost mass production initiatives (Richter et al. 2019; Cardoso et al. 2020; Hamzah et al. 2018). The electrode of the electrochemical sensors is often expensive because of their requirement to be inert in nature (Pt, Au, boron diamond, and glassy carbon), which leads to higher manufacturing costs for fabricating industrial standard electrochemical sensors (Bakker and Telting-Diaz 2002). AM technology is a low-cost alternative to the highly expensive electrochemical sensors based on the traditional manufacturing process. Additionally, AM technology could offer conductive thermoplastics such as graphene, graphite, metallic nanoparticles, and carbon nanotubes. FDM, inkjet, and screen printing are the widely adapted manufacturing technology for the fabrication of electrochemical sensors (Stefano et al. 2022a; Taleat et al. 2014; Li et al. 2015). Cheng Yang et al. reported the use of printable microelectrode for the detection of dopamine, which could crucially be a game changer for the neurotransmitter study (Yang et al. 2018). Gold-plated printed stainless-steel electrodes are effective in sensing the DNA with the targeted DNA, which offers additional scope for the scalable DNA sensors (Loo et al. 2017). In a study, carbon black/polylactic acid-based electrochemical biosensors were used for detecting muscle contraction for the measurement in the anorectum (Hamzah et al. 2019). Jéssica Santos Stefano et al. have developed a lab-made filament that is effective in fabricating printable biosensors that can detect SARS-CoV-2 (Stefano et al. 2022b). In another innovative attempt, the researcher has successfully developed a printed cell-on-chip device that is effective in determining caffeine and paracetamol (Katseli et al. 2020). In this study, the authors used the extrusion-based printing technology for developing this cell-on-chip device using polylactic acid non-conductive filament and acrylonitrile butadiene styrene conductive filament (Katseli et al. 2020).

3.2.5 Textile-Based Biosensors

Textile-based electronics and sensory system are attracting increased attention among researchers as the future of continuous and real-time monitoring system will be poised around this theme, which is clearly evidenced by the recent trend in publication data of the researcher around the globe. The textile-based sensors in the biomedical domain can be realized by using two methods—namely, directly printable on textiles and by stitching/embroidering the conductive fabric on the textile surface. Printing technology is seemingly effective in terms of fabrication cost and easy process flow but has lesser advantages with the lesser wash cycle. Conversely, the yarn-based sensory system can sustain multiple wash cycles with minimal damage to the conductive line at higher manufacturing costs. One of the major advantages of textile-based sensors is the continuous skin or body contact with the user, which makes them a promising technology for wearable electronics applications. In a recent review, authors discussed the use of textile-based sensors for biological signal (ECG & EMG) monitoring and detection, which gives a detailed discussion of the future of printable technology on textile-based wearable monitoring systems for biomedical applications (Blachowicz et al. 2021). Jose et al. (2022) developed printable pH sensors on fabric surfaces using organic and polymeric materials such as PEDOT:PSS, carbon-alizarin, and graphene/polyaniline. Electrical bioimpedance tomography is a highly effective technology with the ability to conduct non-invasive biomedical imaging for accurate determination of bone fracture and lung function. In this study, the authors have developed a highly stretchable and flexible bioimpedance sensor on the textile substrate (Jose et al. 2021). In a detailed review, Ikra Iftekhar Shuvo et al. discussed the various biological vital sign monitoring by using various textile-based biomedical sensors (Shuvo et al. 2022). This review provides a strong message to the reader that the dominant role of electronic textile-based biomedical sensors is going to revolutionize the healthcare industry in the future (Shuvo et al. 2022). Human–machine interaction on wearables is going to revolutionize the world of the electronic manufacturing sector by introducing textile-based printable sensors. In this study, the authors fabricated washable textile-based electronic Touch/Gesture Tribo-Sensors, which play a prominent role in human–machine interactions (Cao et al. 2018).

3.3 Outlook

The future of the healthcare ecosystem will be strongly driven by the penetration of artificial intelligence-controlled sensory systems, thus introducing additive manufacturing technology into the edge sensing application, which will provide a higher degree of flexibility in providing an easy and controlled manufacturing ecosystem. Additionally, futuristic applications such as augmented reality and virtual reality systems require a highly reliable strain and haptic sensor for the proper functionality of such a system. Brain–computer interfacing is also one of the promising areas to research, as this sophisticated interfacing system requires smart and reliable biomedical sensors to transceiver the brain signals. Fabrication of implantable medical device such as orthopedic implants and hearing aids is highly attractive because of the potential of AM to match the complex form and mechanics of individual human bodies. Externally worn and implantable tissue-support devices, such as ankle or knee braces and hernia repair mesh, offer a new opportunity for AM to mimic tissue-like mechanics and improve both patient outcomes and comfort.

3.4 Conclusion

The various manufacturing and biomedical sensors based on the ease of operation across the healthcare industry have been elaborately discussed. A holistic assessment of various AM-based printing technologies, which could play a significant role in the future of large-scale manufacturing sectors and is believed to play a commanding role in biomedical sensor manufacturing and fabrication, has been discussed in detail.

Initially, the various kinds of printable manufacturing technology, such FDM, inkjet printing, aerosol jet printing, and electrostatic printing, were discussed. Even the future of manufacturing is going to revolutionize by incorporating artificial intelligence into rapid manufacturing technology.

Additionally, an elaborate discussion on the various biomedical sensors such as implantable sensors, microfluidic sensors, haptic sensors, electrochemical sensors, and textile-based sensors for various applications from medical grade usage to wearable applications in the healthcare ecosystem was made in order to emphasize on the importance of wearable sensors. Thus, the emergence of such smart and rapidly manufacturable sensors will further open the pathways for the highly customizable biomedical monitoring and control system. Also, the value addition of this printable sensor will further improve the intrusion of artificial intelligence–based technology into the healthcare ecosystem.

Also, the 3D-printed lattice structures provide an effective surface for osseointegration, and the addition of coatings will further enhance bone in-growth and improve functionality, including enhanced durability and antimicrobial properties. The pivotal role of printable technologies for futuristic applications such as AR/VR, organ on chip, and implantable brain sensors was also holistically discussed.

References

Abulaiti M et al (2020) Establishment of a heart-on-a-chip microdevice based on human iPS cells for the evaluation of human heart tissue function. Sci Rep 10(1):19201. https://doi.org/10.1038/s41598-020-76062-w

Al Rashid A, Khan SA, Al-Ghamdi SG, Koç M (2020) Additive manufacturing: technology, applications, markets, and opportunities for the built environment. Autom Constr 118:103268. https://doi.org/10.1016/j.autcon.2020.103268

Ali MA, Hu C, Yttri EA, Panat R (2022) Recent advances in 3D printing of biomedical sensing devices. Adv Funct Mater 32(9). https://doi.org/10.1002/adfm.202107671

Bakker E, Telting-Diaz M (2002) Electrochemical sensors. Anal Chem 74(12):2781–2800. https://doi.org/10.1021/ac0202278

Beauchamp MJ, Nielsen AV, Gong H, Nordin GP, Woolley AT (2019) 3D printed microfluidic devices for microchip electrophoresis of preterm birth biomarkers. Anal Chem 91(11): 7418–7425. https://doi.org/10.1021/acs.analchem.9b01395

Berlanda SF, Breitfeld M, Dietsche CL, Dittrich PS (2021) Recent advances in microfluidic technology for bioanalysis and diagnostics. Anal Chem 93(1):311–331. https://doi.org/10.1021/acs.analchem.0c04366

Blachowicz T, Ehrmann G, Ehrmann A (2021) Textile-based sensors for biosignal detection and monitoring. Sensors 21(18):6042. https://doi.org/10.3390/s21186042

Bozkurt Y, Karayel E (2021) 3D printing technology; methods, biomedical applications, future opportunities and trends. J Mater Res Technol 14:1430–1450. https://doi.org/10.1016/j.jmrt.2021.07.050

Britton J et al (2021) A flexible strain-responsive sensor fabricated from a biocompatible electronic ink via an additive-manufacturing process. Mater Des 206:109700. https://doi.org/10.1016/j.matdes.2021.109700

Cao R et al (2018) Screen-printed washable electronic textiles as self-powered touch/gesture tribo-sensors for intelligent human–machine interaction. ACS Nano 12(6):5190–5196. https://doi.org/10.1021/acsnano.8b02477

Cardoso RM et al (2020) Additive-manufactured (3D-printed) electrochemical sensors: a critical review. Anal Chim Acta 1118:73–91. https://doi.org/10.1016/j.aca.2020.03.028

Chan HN et al (2016) Simple, cost-effective 3D printed microfluidic components for disposable, point-of-care colorimetric analysis. ACS Sensors 1(3):227–234. https://doi.org/10.1021/acssensors.5b00100

Chandrasekaran S, Jayakumar A, Velu R (2022) A comprehensive review on printed electronics: a technology drift towards a sustainable future. Nanomaterials 12:23. https://doi.org/10.3390/nano12234251

Chen H, Luo Z, Lin X, Zhu Y, Zhao Y (2023) Sensors-integrated organ-on-a-chip for biomedical applications. Nano Res 16(7):10072–10099. https://doi.org/10.1007/s12274-023-5651-9

Cho Y, Park S, Lee J, Yu KJ (2021) Emerging materials and technologies with applications in flexible neural implants: a comprehensive review of current issues with neural devices. Adv Mater 33(47):2005786. https://doi.org/10.1002/adma.202005786

Dahiya R et al (2019) Large-area soft e-skin: the challenges beyond sensor designs. Proc IEEE 107(10):2016–2033. https://doi.org/10.1109/JPROC.2019.2941366

Dilberoglu UM, Gharehpapagh B, Yaman U, Dolen M (2017) The role of additive manufacturing in the era of industry 4.0. Proc Manuf 11:545–554. https://doi.org/10.1016/j.promfg.2017.07.148

Ding S, Zhang H, Wang X (2021) Microfluidic-chip-integrated biosensors for lung disease models. Biosensors (Basel) 11(11):456. https://doi.org/10.3390/bios11110456

El-Molla S et al (2016) Integration of a thin film PDMS-based capacitive sensor for tactile sensing in an electronic skin. J Sensors 2016:1–7. https://doi.org/10.1155/2016/1736169

Faisal SN et al (2023) Noninvasive sensors for brain–machine interfaces based on micropatterned epitaxial graphene. ACS Appl Nano Mater 6(7):5440–5447. https://doi.org/10.1021/acsanm.2c05546

Fleury M, Lioi G, Barillot C, Lécuyer A (2020) A survey on the use of haptic feedback for brain-computer interfaces and neurofeedback. Front Neurosci 14. https://doi.org/10.3389/fnins.2020.00528

Gaspar C, Olkkonen J, Passoja S, Smolander M (2017) Paper as active layer in inkjet-printed capacitive humidity sensors. Sensors 17(7):1464. https://doi.org/10.3390/s17071464

George L, Marchal M, Glondu L, Lécuyer A. Combining brain-computer interfaces and haptics: detecting mental workload to adapt haptic assistance. 2012. p. 124–35. https://doi.org/10.1007/978-3-642-31401-8_12.

Grasso G, Rosset S, Shea H (2023) Fully 3D-printed, stretchable, and conformable haptic interfaces. Adv Funct Mater 33(20). https://doi.org/10.1002/adfm.202213821

Guo Z et al (2022) A flexible neural implant with ultrathin substrate for low-invasive brain–computer interface applications. Microsyst Nanoeng 8(1):133. https://doi.org/10.1038/s41378-022-00464-1

Haleem A, Javaid M, Pratap Singh R, Suman R (2022) Medical 4.0 technologies for healthcare: features, capabilities, and applications. Internet Things Cyber Phys Syst 2:12–30. https://doi.org/10.1016/j.iotcps.2022.04.001

Haleem A, Javaid M, Pratap Singh R, Suman R (2023) Exploring the revolution in healthcare systems through the applications of digital twin technology. Biomed Technol 4:28–38. https://doi.org/10.1016/j.bmt.2023.02.001

Hamzah HH, Shafiee SA, Abdalla A, Patel BA (2018) 3D printable conductive materials for the fabrication of electrochemical sensors: a mini review. Electrochem Commun 96:27–31. https://doi.org/10.1016/j.elecom.2018.09.006

Hamzah HH, Keattch O, Yeoman MS, Covill D, Patel BA (2019) Three-dimensional-printed electrochemical sensor for simultaneous dual monitoring of serotonin overflow and circular muscle contraction. Anal Chem 91(18):12014–12020. https://doi.org/10.1021/acs.analchem.9b02958

Han D et al (2020) 4D Printing of a bioinspired microneedle array with backward-facing barbs for enhanced tissue adhesion. Adv Funct Mater 30(11):1909197. https://doi.org/10.1002/adfm.201909197

Heiden B, Alieksieiev V, Volk M, Tonino-Heiden B (2021) Framing artificial intelligence (AI) additive manufacturing (AM). Proc Comput Sci 186:387–394. https://doi.org/10.1016/j.procs.2021.04.161

Hochberg LR, Donoghue JP (2006) Sensors for brain-computer interfaces. IEEE Eng Med Biol Mag 25(5):32–38. https://doi.org/10.1109/MEMB.2006.1705745

Hua J, Li J, Jiang Y, Xie S, Shi Y, Pan L (2022) Skin-attachable sensors for biomedical applications. Biomed Mater Devices. https://doi.org/10.1007/s44174-022-00018-z

Huo R et al (2023) Tough transient ionic junctions printed with ionic microgels. Adv Funct Mater 33(20). https://doi.org/10.1002/adfm.202213677

Jose M, Lemmens M, Bormans S, Thoelen R, Deferme W (2021) Fully printed, stretchable and wearable bioimpedance sensor on textiles for tomography. Flexible Printed Electron 6(1):015010. https://doi.org/10.1088/2058-8585/abe51b

Jose M et al (2022) Printed pH sensors for textile-based wearables: a conceptual and experimental study on materials, deposition technology, and sensing principles. Adv Eng Mater 24(5):2101087. https://doi.org/10.1002/adem.202101087

Kanao K et al (2015) Printable flexible tactile pressure and temperature sensors with high selectivity against bending. In: 2015 28th IEEE international conference on micro electro mechanical systems (MEMS). IEEE, pp 756–759. https://doi.org/10.1109/MEMSYS.2015.7051068

Katseli V, Economou A, Kokkinos C (2020) A novel all-3D-printed cell-on-a-chip device as a useful electroanalytical tool: application to the simultaneous voltammetric determination of caffeine and paracetamol. Talanta 208:120388. https://doi.org/10.1016/j.talanta.2019.120388

Kumar N, Kumari M, Arun RK (2022) Development and implementation of portable biosensors in microfluidic point-of-care devices for pathogen detection. In: Miniaturized biosensing devices. Springer Nature, Singapore, pp 99–122. https://doi.org/10.1007/978-981-16-9897-2_5

Li J, Rossignol F, Macdonald J (2015) Inkjet printing for biosensor fabrication: combining chemistry and technology for advanced manufacturing. Lab Chip 15(12):2538–2558. https://doi.org/10.1039/C5LC00235D

Lind JU et al (2017) Instrumented cardiac microphysiological devices via multimaterial three-dimensional printing. Nat Mater 16(3):303–308. https://doi.org/10.1038/nmat4782

Liu H et al (2020) Heart-on-a-chip model with integrated extra- and intracellular bioelectronics for monitoring cardiac electrophysiology under acute hypoxia. Nano Lett 20(4):2585–2593. https://doi.org/10.1021/acs.nanolett.0c00076

Loo AH, Chua CK, Pumera M (2017) DNA biosensing with 3D printing technology. Analyst 142(2):279–283. https://doi.org/10.1039/C6AN02038K

Ma C, Peng Y, Li H, Chen W (2021) Organ-on-a-chip: a new paradigm for drug development. Trends Pharmacol Sci 42(2):119–133. https://doi.org/10.1016/j.tips.2020.11.009

Mannoor MS et al (2013) 3D Printed bionic ears. Nano Lett 13(6):2634–2639. https://doi.org/10.1021/nl4007744

Mutlu R, Singh D, Tawk C, Sariyildiz E (2023) A 3D-printed soft haptic device with built-in force sensing delivering bio-mimicked feedback. Biomimetics 8(1):127. https://doi.org/10.3390/biomimetics8010127

Pike JM, Gelberman RH (2010) Zone II combined flexor digitorum superficialis and flexor digitorum profundus repair distal to the A2 pulley. J Hand Surg Am 35(9):1523–1527. https://doi.org/10.1016/j.jhsa.2010.06.024

Probst FA, Hutmacher DW, Müller DF, Machens H-G, Schantz J-T (2010) Rekonstruktion der Kalvaria durch ein präfabriziertes bioaktives Implantat. Handchirurgie Mikrochirurgie Plastische Chirurgie 42(06):369–373. https://doi.org/10.1055/s-0030-1248310

Richter EM et al (2019) Complete additively manufactured (3D-printed) electrochemical sensing platform. Anal Chem 91(20):12844–12851. https://doi.org/10.1021/acs.analchem.9b02573

Roy AC et al (2022) Large-area 3D printable soft electronic skin for biomedical applications. ACS Biomater Sci Eng 8(12):5319–5328. https://doi.org/10.1021/acsbiomaterials.2c00241

Salim A, Lim S (2017) Review of recent inkjet-printed capacitive tactile sensors. Sensors 17(11): 2593. https://doi.org/10.3390/s17112593

Shuvo II, Shah A, Dagdeviren C (2022) Electronic textile sensors for decoding vital body signals: state-of-the-art review on characterizations and recommendations. Adv Intell Syst 4(4): 2100223. https://doi.org/10.1002/aisy.202100223

Stefano JS et al (2022a) Electrochemical (bio)sensors enabled by fused deposition modeling-based 3D printing: a guide to selecting designs, printing parameters, and post-treatment protocols. Anal Chem 94(17):6417–6429. https://doi.org/10.1021/acs.analchem.1c05523

Stefano JS et al (2022b) New conductive filament ready-to-use for 3D-printing electrochemical (bio)sensors: towards the detection of SARS-CoV-2. Anal Chim Acta 1191:339372. https://doi.org/10.1016/j.aca.2021.339372

Sun Z, Zhu M, Shan X, Lee C (2022) Augmented tactile-perception and haptic-feedback rings as human-machine interfaces aiming for immersive interactions. Nat Commun 13(1):5224. https://doi.org/10.1038/s41467-022-32745-8

Taleat Z, Khoshroo A, Mazloum-Ardakani M (2014) Screen-printed electrodes for biosensing: a review (2008–2013). Microchim Acta 181(9–10):865–891. https://doi.org/10.1007/s00604-014-1181-1

Tanasescu C, Moisin A, Mihetiu A, Serban D, Costache A, Bratu D (2021) The use of polypropylene mesh in inguinal hernia surgery: a retrospective study. Exp Ther Med 22(4):1193. https://doi.org/10.3892/etm.2021.10627

Thiyagarajan K, Rajini GK, Maji D (2022) Cost-effective, disposable, flexible, and printable MWCNT-based wearable sensor for human body temperature monitoring. IEEE Sensors J 22(17):16756–16763. https://doi.org/10.1109/JSEN.2021.3088466

Tian X et al (2023) Implant-to-implant wireless networking with metamaterial textiles. Nat Commun 14(1):4335. https://doi.org/10.1038/s41467-023-39850-2

Vo TH, Lam PK, Sheng Y-J, Tsao H-K (2023) Jammed microgels in deep eutectic solvents as a green and low-cost ink for 3D printing of reliable auxetic strain sensors. ACS Appl Mater Interfaces 15:33109. https://doi.org/10.1021/acsami.3c05209

Wan Y, Wang Y, Guo CF (2017) Recent progresses on flexible tactile sensors. Mater Today Phys 1: 61–73. https://doi.org/10.1016/j.mtphys.2017.06.002

Wan J, Zhou S, Mea HJ, Guo Y, Ku H, Urbina BM (2022) Emerging roles of microfluidics in brain research: from cerebral fluids manipulation to brain-on-a-chip and neuroelectronic devices engineering. Chem Rev 122(7):7142–7181. https://doi.org/10.1021/acs.chemrev.1c00480

Wang L et al (2020) A metal-electrode-free, fully integrated, soft triboelectric sensor array for self-powered tactile sensing. Microsyst Nanoeng 6(1):59. https://doi.org/10.1038/s41378-020-0154-2

Wang M et al (2022) A wearable electrochemical biosensor for the monitoring of metabolites and nutrients. Nat Biomed Eng 6(11):1225–1235. https://doi.org/10.1038/s41551-022-00916-z

Xiong J, Hsiang E-L, He Z, Zhan T, Wu S-T (2021) Augmented reality and virtual reality displays: emerging technologies and future perspectives. Light Sci Appl 10(1):216. https://doi.org/10.1038/s41377-021-00658-8

Yamanaka K, Vestergaard M, Tamiya E (2016) Printable electrochemical biosensors: a focus on screen-printed electrodes and their application. Sensors 16(10):1761. https://doi.org/10.3390/s16101761

Yang C et al (2018) 3D-printed carbon electrodes for neurotransmitter detection. Angew Chem Int Ed 57(43):14255–14259. https://doi.org/10.1002/anie.201809992

Yi H-G et al (2019) A bioprinted human-glioblastoma-on-a-chip for the identification of patient-specific responses to chemoradiotherapy. Nat Biomed Eng 3(7):509–519. https://doi.org/10.1038/s41551-019-0363-x

Zhang F et al (2021) Design and fabrication of an integrated heart-on-a-chip platform for construction of cardiac tissue from human iPSC-derived cardiomyocytes and in situ evaluation of physiological function. Biosens Bioelectron 179:113080. https://doi.org/10.1016/j.bios.2021.113080

Zyczkowski M et al (2014) Tension-free vaginal tape, transobturator tape, and own modification of transobturator tape in the treatment of female stress urinary incontinence: comparative analysis. Biomed Res Int 2014:1–6. https://doi.org/10.1155/2014/347856

Role of Sensing Integrated Prosthetic Socket in Comfort

4

L. Lebea, H. M. Ngwangwa, and Anand Kumar Subramaniyan

Contents

Abstract

A number of people undergo amputation of one or both of their lower limbs, which has an immediate negative influence on their quality of life. This chapter

L. Lebea (✉)
Department of Mechanical and Mechatronic Engineering, Central University of Technology, Free State, Bloemfontein, South Africa
e-mail: llebea@cut.ac.za

H. M. Ngwangwa
Department of Mechanical Engineering, University of South Africa, Johannesburg, South Africa

A. K. Subramaniyan
Additive Manufacturing Research Laboratory, Mechanical Engineering, Indian Institute of Technology Jammu, Jammu, Jammu and Kashmir, India

R. Velu et al. (eds.), *Digital Design and Manufacturing of Medical Devices and Systems*, https://doi.org/10.1007/978-981-99-7100-8_4

demonstrates the function of prosthetic sockets in comfort. Amputees require outlets connected to the residual limbs in addition to artificial joints. A socket, which is a bucket-shaped casing that houses the limb, is where a knee prosthesis is attached. Prosthesis sockets can also be designed to be less comfortable and more functional, for example, due to rigid ischial restrictions that limit relative motion between the prosthesis and the stump. Sensing and monitoring technologies therefore offer great potential to improve the quality of care for individuals who have lost lower extremities. Overall, the results of previous studies and the current case study demonstrate that 3D-printed prostheses outperform standard prostheses in functional activities involving compound grasps, individual finger movements, and differential grasp patterns and that they are not functional in activities that require a strong grasp. Meanwhile, large companies are starting to use additive manufacturing by purchasing machines and hiring dedicated technicians to operate those machines. However, experts also point out that 3D-printed prosthetic parts have limited material options and limited structural strength of the printed parts.

Keywords

Prosthesis sockets · 3D printed · Amputees · Sensor

4.1 Introduction

This chapter illustrates the role of prosthetic sockets in comfort in people who undergo amputation of one or both of their lower limbs, which has an immediate impact on their quality of life. War, the prevalence of diabetes, vascular disorders (Ngwangwa and Nemavhola 2021), and cancer are a few factors that might cause these disabilities to rapidly increase in number (Hassan and Abdul Ameer 2022). A multidisciplinary clinical team of doctors, therapists, and prosthetists is needed to provide the care and expertise necessary for recovery following significant limb loss, which is a lifelong, individual struggle. People who have lost a lower limb (Zapen 2021) (as shown in Fig. 4.1) are more likely to develop obesity, depression, osteoarthritis, cardiovascular disorders (Nemavhola 2017, 2021), and low-back pain.

A possible avenue for promoting science and innovation is through bionic designing. The bioinspired technique is also beneficial for developing distinct next-generation mechanosensors that can accurately detect four separate mechanical signals, including sound, vibration, air/water stream, and material. Upper appendage prosthetic innovation and utility have advanced dramatically, notably in terms of control of the device as well as overt criticism. The vital importance of prosthesis comfort and fit to patients is one of the main causes of the generally high abandonment rates of upper appendage prostheses (estimated at 23% in 2007). Development begins with electrical movement delivered inside the nervous system. The cortex produces this activity, which is then sent via the spinal column to the peripheral nerves and, finally, to the muscles, where it prompts muscular contractions and,

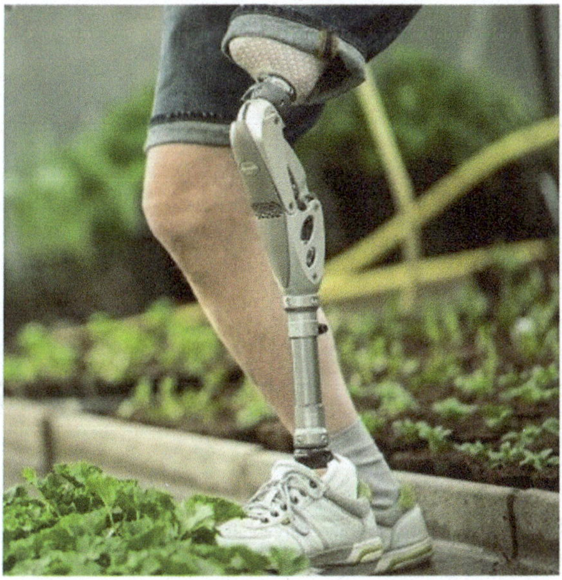

Fig. 4.1 A mechanical knee prosthetic (Zapen 2021)

eventually, the growth of appendages. The electrical movement that results from volitional development in a prosthetic hand is recorded and supplied to a controller, which classifies the desired action and generates the appropriate commands to the prosthesis to drive development. The straightforward extraction of orders from electrical impulses within the brain, particularly the sensorimotor and parietal districts of cerebral cortex, has attracted a lot of attention recently.

4.2 State of the Art for Prosthetic Socket, Manufacturing Techniques

The interface between the prosthesis and the stump is called the prosthesis socket (see Fig. 4.2) (Asif et al. 2021). This part is the most important part that determines the comfort, energy efficiency, and usefulness of the prosthesis.

However, amputees need more than artificial joints; they also need outlets connected to the remaining limbs. A knee prosthesis is connected to a socket, which is a bucket shell that encloses the limb. Prosthesis sockets can also be designed to be less comfortable and more functional, for example, due to rigid ischial restrictions that limit relative motion between the prosthesis and the stump. Prostheses are often prescribed during post-amputation rehabilitation to meet the patient's unique functional, occupational, and recreational needs. People who lose their lower limbs face lifelong functional limitations and ongoing health risks such as falls and falls, even with a prosthetic leg. They also require reduced activity levels, have difficulty climbing hills and stairs, and suffer from skin damage, joint

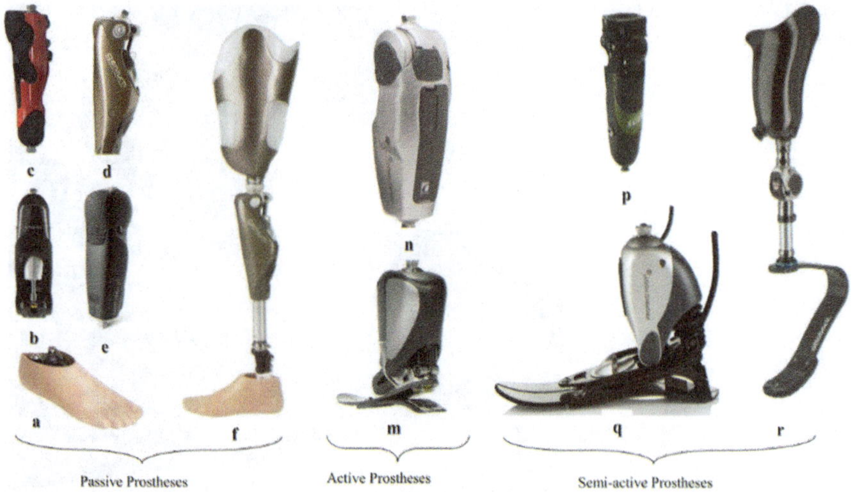

Fig. 4.2 Images of commercially available passive, active, and semi-active prostheses from left to right (Asif et al. 2021)

degeneration, and pain (Hafner and Sanders 2014). Despite improvements in wearable robotic platforms and prosthetic designs, the majority of amputees still express discomfort with sockets (Paternò et al. 2021).

Amputees can walk normally with a prosthesis that meets the requirements; their gait should correspond to that of a healthy person. Evaluation of socket fit currently focuses on verbal feedback on patient comfort and visual observation of walking performance and cutaneous irritation of the stump. A lower-leg prosthesis is manufactured to replace the function of an amputated leg and is important for facilitating daily activities such as standing and moving. Prosthesis sockets are made from a variety of materials. High chemical stability, heat resistance, abrasion resistance, and environmental resistance are just some of the unique properties of silicone rubber. Interest in the production and development of silicone rubber has increased in recent years, and the use of silicone rubber in many applications, including medical applications (Hassan and Abdul Ameer 2022; Anuar et al. 2022), and 3D printing techniques have helped find solutions.

The most important part of the prosthesis is the prosthesis socket. The effectiveness of a prosthesis depends on how well it is made. No matter how well the prosthetic module works, prosthetic results with well-designed sockets are good. This idea also applies to additive manufacturing technology. The following process is used when manufacturing sockets using additive technology, scanning of molds, computer processing of electronic geometric models (EGMs), and additive manufacturing of receiving sleeves. The widespread use of digitization in various aspects of human existence is reflected in medicine, especially in prosthetics for people who have lost their limbs. The advantage of this technique lies in the automated work of the prosthetist. This reduces the role of human factors in the manufacturing of prosthetic and orthopedic products (Ahsan 2016; Ahmad et al. 2019).

4.3 Sensor Technology

At the heart of socket sense technology is a series of sensors rigidly attached to the inner wall of the socket. Sensing and monitoring technologies have great potential to improve the standard of care for amputee patients. A key idea in the rehabilitation process is to understand how sensor technology can be integrated into prosthetics to transmit real-time biological and mechanical data to amputees. Today's sensors often have a single measurement parameter and are point sensors. Forthcoming socket prostheses may benefit from better sensor options, thanks to nanotechnology sensors. Karamousadakis et al. (2021) recorded the pressure distribution at the human socket interface and created a tissue-based sensor adapted inside the socket prosthesis (see Fig. 4.3). Shaft liners can be integrated with carbon nanotube-based thin-film sensors, but electrical impedance tomography can only map pressure distributions from a small number of remarks.

Prosthetic limbs are the perfect vehicle for sensing technology for amputees, especially for applications such as ambulatory monitoring. Attaching or integrating the sensor into the prosthesis seems like a logical way to circumvent the compliance issues with remote sensing noted by normal users. This is especially true when the slight weight gain required for such devices does not seem to affect exercise or energy expenditure.

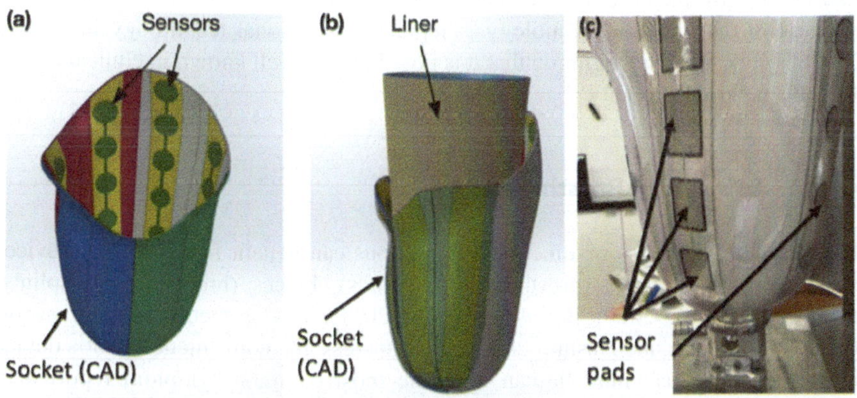

Fig. 4.3 Socket with sensors: (**a**) CAD of sensors on the inner wall; (**b**) CAD of liner with socket; (**c**) actual socket with socket sense sensors (Karamousadakis et al. 2021)

4.4 Smart Prosthetic Socket and Comfort

4.4.1 Smart Prosthetic

Much research has been done on the design of intelligent prostheses, with control systems still receiving the most attention and neglecting the prosthetic framework or foundation, which is the bone equivalent of biological inspiration (Manganyi and Mpofu 2011). Thanks to active stiffness modulation and sensor-controlled control circuitry, such intelligent sockets can handle pressure, temperature, and volume related issues simultaneously. The realization of smart socket prostheses allows the development of a 'digital twin' of the whole patient or stump and socket system. A digital twin is a representation of a physical system or object in the digital world (Gupta et al. 2020). As such, next-generation smart socket designs are enabled by the creation and integration of advanced materials, electronic systems, distributed sensors, and efficient actuators. These smart sockets can self-adjust in real-time to reduce interfacial stress, volume fluctuations, temperature fluctuations, and measure the level of amputees' discomfort.

The modernization of the manufacture of sockets for upper limb prostheses has not progressed much. Still highly dependent on manual labour, the casting methods used in clinics today are similar to those developed more than 50 years ago (Olsen et al. 2021). Public impressions are strongly influenced by superficial media representation and advertising. They often present modern manufacturing techniques such as 3D scanning and printing as off-the-shelf solutions for manufacturing inexpensive functional devices. Modern socket manufacturing technology has the potential to increase patient satisfaction, shorten manufacturing cycles, and reduce clinical burden. Misconceptions about the use of digital technologies such as additive manufacturing in the manufacture of upper extremity prostheses is exacerbated by media coverage (Paternò et al. 2021; Van Der Stelt et al. 2022), suggesting that modern technology is replacing traditional technology in clinics. There is widespread recognition that it is possible. It is well known in clinical circles that this is far from reality.

4.4.2 Comfort in Prosthetic

People with disabilities or functional limitations can benefit from medical devices such as prosthetic legs (prostheses and hands), braces (bracelets and splints) (Al-Zubaidi et al. 2020; Bertassoni et al. 2011), and/or metal frame transport (wheelchairs) (Ijaz and Hashmi 2022). Nevertheless, the convenience of this device is important in sustaining human life. The most common symptom reported in prosthetic clinics is socket discomfort. Despite various descriptive terms used by both patients and professionals, 'comfort' remains difficult to measure, describe and document. An important factor affecting prosthesis wearer comfort is the pressure at the socket interface. Several researchers have studied interfacial pressure using various modalities to assess socket structure and function (Meng et al. 2020).

Despite improvements in wearable robotic platforms and prosthetic designs, the majority of amputees still express discomfort with the physical human-machine interface of prosthetics (Walsh 2018). Conventional prosthesis users rely on painful tactile feedback when the residual limb makes contact with the ground. As a result, there is an increased risk of falls and limited range of motion. Prostheses are thought to increase the cognitive load on the brain from the presence of foreign bodies during exercise (Tan et al. 2022). As such, the main source of stress is now the abandonment problem of many psychological and mechanical limbs.

4.4.3 Sensor Design in Prosthetic Joints

Human movements are also coordinated and consistent in their diversity. These properties have been known for many years and are well described in Bernstein's pioneering work (Bernstein 1967). The human body is a collection of multimodal sensory systems that control bodily movements and functions. It is also important to remember that the mechanical performance of the muscle itself does not depend solely on motor neuron activation. Unlike torque motors in robots, the torque that a muscle produces at a joint at a given activation level is highly dependent on posture and movement. Multiplicative noise affects both human motor control and sensory feedback. This means that the variability of the control signal increases in proportion to the amplitude of the signal. The inability of traditional outlets to meet the daily needs of amputees has short and long-term consequences.

Sensing and monitoring technologies therefore offer great potential to improve the quality of care for individuals who have lost lower extremities. Sensor technology is evolving to satisfy the demanding needs of the burgeoning connected medical industry, with new breakthroughs in personal devices and medical equipment. By incorporating these technologies into the rehabilitation process, opportunities for the multifaceted interchange of timely, relevant, and useful health information between patients, prostheses, and physicians are created. Approximately 43% of amputees use myoelectric prostheses (Hafner and Sanders 2014), which utilize muscle contraction of the stump to control hand position. Myoelectric prostheses have improved functional grip patterns and overall appearance compared to body-powered prostheses, but lack tactile sensory feedback, leaving users with visual and auditory. A piezoresistive force sensing resistor (FSR) is a thin, flexible and malleable structure that makes it suitable for medical applications (Gupta et al. 2020). In addition to piezoresistive pressure sensors, capacitive sensors were also used to monitor the pressure distribution at the stump-prosthesis interface (Arjun Hari and Rajan 2021). Meier et al. presented the design and implementation of the first capacitive interface tension sensor for this application. A flexible capacitive sensor with a thickness of 2 mm showed an accuracy of 20%.

Subsequently, another prototype capacitive pressure sensor was developed by Polliack et al. (2002). In the prosthetic socket insert, 16 sensors are mounted in a 4×4 matrix on a $2.5 \times 2.5 \times 0.064$ cm^3 silicon substrate. There are few reports in the literature regarding the importance and evaluation of sensor efficacy and reliability for prosthetic use. The development of more powerful and real-time sensors that provide distributed measurements and more data will ultimately provide more detailed information about hip health. Failure of the socket to function as expected may be accentuated by changes in pressure distribution at the stump socket interface. This is caused by the normal diurnal variation in stump volume, soft tissue adaptation during postoperative recovery. To address this issue, field adjustable sockets with intelligent manual control systems have been developed (Ko et al. 2021). Robotic testing has emerged as a practical approach for performing repeatable dynamic tests for evaluating and comparing prototypes (Etoundi et al. 2022). Larsen et al. designed a new socket adjustment mechanism for limb volume management of external prostheses (Larsen et al. 2020).

A mechanism called Panel Pull helps stabilize stump volume in prosthesis wearers who experience volume loss throughout the day when applied while seated. Various coding strategies have been used to convert readings from sensors implanted or attached to the prosthesis into stimulation parameters (i.e., amplitude, pulse width, repetition rate, and duration of biphasic pulse trains). Recent studies have shown that direct nerve stimulation can be used to provide sensory feedback to hand amputees (Valle et al. 2018). The intensity of the evoked sensation can be modulated using the amplitude or frequency of the injected stimulus. These findings imply that selecting specific sensory feedback encodings can affect a user's grip performance. Furthermore, the results will prompt the development of new approaches to provide users with a more natural feel. This may be addressed by more biomimetic strategies in the future.

4.5 Challenges/Limitation of Prosthetic Socket

4.5.1 Production

Increased risk of long-term health problems, which may be directly related to amputation surgery and/or prosthetic rehabilitation, or indirectly related to a sedentary lifestyle due to the disability, increases the difficulty of living with lower limb loss. Prosthetic components such as physician-prescribed knees and foot/ankle units are designed to facilitate dynamic movement. However, the components in use have their limits. Shaft measurement and manufacturing is often done manually. First, a negative impression of the residual stump is made with a plaster model, and the positive impression of the residual limb is made by pouring it into this negative mold. The final socket will be made using this male mold. This male mold is contoured to correspond to the pressure points. Unfortunately, there are some limitations, such as the fact that this procedure is time- and labor-intensive and highly dependent on the knowledge and skills of those involved. Additive manufacturing is used to manufacture prosthetic sockets. Selective Laser Sintering (SLS) and Fused Filament Fabrication (FFF) are his two most commonly used printing processes for manufacturing medical devices (Van Der Stelt et al. 2022). Today, the SLS process is primarily used to manufacture additively manufactured prosthetic sockets. A fundamental problem with FFF printed shafts is that the bonding area between layers is small, which reduces the elasticity and toughness of the material in the vertical direction of the print. Most of the nanomaterials used in prosthesis fabrication have so far been discovered through limited trials (Ijaz and Hashmi 2022; Tan et al. 2022). Some components have not yet been used in actual prosthesis design due to extraction processes, manufacturing costs, stability, and other factors. Therefore, in order to conclusively confirm the efficacy and viability of these nanomaterials, the industry will focus on specific iterations of material renewal, fabrication of new functions (not only on a theoretical level), and impaired motor function. Additional relevant studies, including data on recovery, are needed.

Despite advances in technology, the delay between amputation and prosthesis fitting contributes to the high dropout rate of prosthesis fittings. Overall, the results of previous studies and the current case study demonstrate that 3D-printed prostheses outperform standard prostheses in functional activities involving compound grasps, individual finger movements, and differential grasps patterns, and that they are not functional in activities that require a strong grasp (Copeland et al. 2022). Additionally, the perceived low durability of 3D-printed prosthetics is an ongoing concern. Additionally, 3D-printed trans-radial prostheses require a stump that is at least 3–4 cm long for proper elbow flexion and finger articulation. People with short stumps can wear additional thermoplastic around their limbs that are inserted into 3D-printed sockets to allow longer lever arms. Nevertheless, the main advantages of 3D-printed prostheses are the devices' visual appeal, rapid and inexpensive manufacturing methods, and the ability to remotely customize these devices.

The development of flexible, sensitive, inexpensive and durable prosthetic tactile sensors is of great importance for prosthetic rehabilitation (Arjun Hari and Rajan 2021). Finally, the feasibility of designing the brace, performing structural simulations based on finite element analysis (FEA), and using biomimetics to ensure a structurally viable product was evaluated. In addition to comparing the methods of the current orthotic manufacturing process with conventional ones, we obtained prototype designs for lightweight, removable orthoses with the potential for upper extremity ventilation for factors such as time and manufacturing costs. The use of cellular structures has been suggested by additive manufacturing motivated by the desire to place material only where it is needed (Agudelo-Ardila et al. 2019). Voronoi diagrams are presented as an alternative to modeling cellular structures. These usually consist of shapes found in nature, sometimes ranging to light and strong structures. The main advantage of these structures is their high mechanical strength, even in relatively low-mass geometries.

4.5.2 Critical Needs

Due to the altered and excessive tissue stress during movement, people who have lost their lower limbs often suffer from osteoarthritis, back pain, and other chronic health problems. Through improvement of socket development, the prosthetists strive to maximize function while minimizing discomfort. However, finding the right balance between function and pain requires time and iteration and it is complicated by the lack of quantitative evidence. However, these are inherently manufacturing solutions. The final product, still common, is a hard device that provides a snapshot window of limb volume, size, and shape. However, prosthetic socket technology has not advanced much in the last 50 years (Gupta et al. 2020).

Variations in pressure distribution at the socket/stump interface, local body temperature (limb), and stump mass should all be considered to ensure proper fit of the socket. Hot spots that lead to pain and skin problems can be caused by irregular contact pressure. Sweating can be caused by increased temperature of the stump caused by excess blood and changes in metabolic rate. In these situations, excessive sweating can irritate the skin and cause maceration, exacerbating the situation and leading to serious infections and skin breakdowns, which may alter the gait pattern of amputees. Gait instability can be caused by abnormal gait patterns. Another researcher proposed a modified bushing with a heat pipe with working fluid and a wick structure. The heat pipe had a socket section and an extended heat sink that ran through the entire wall of the socket. The boiling point of the working medium was in the range of about 0–90 °C. The working fluid can be selected such that heat from the remaining rim in the pan vaporizes and converts to vapor, thereby drawing latent heat of vaporization from the remaining rim.

4.5.3 The Current Issues and Challenges of Prosthetic Joints

The use of implantable peripheral interfaces to activate remaining nerves and re-establish phantom hand sensation in amputees of the upper limb has received a lot of attention in the past (Valle et al. 2018). The feedback from users of orthoses and prostheses helps inspire new development concepts. The objective right now is to develop orthoses and prostheses that can be controlled by the brain while also improving how they appear and feel. The quality of prosthetic and orthotic sockets and designs has improved thanks to advancements in materials. To evenly transfer mechanical stresses over the afflicted limb and stump, total contact sockets are currently used. The weight of the prosthesis is also controlled through 3D manufacturing and the use of lightweight materials. It also costs nothing and provides an opportunity for resource-poor amputees to gain some functionality. Variation in stump shape and quantity is common and varies with changes in weather and activity levels.

Even during a physiotherapy session, the stump can change to the extent that the socket becomes uncomfortable or impossible to wear (Turner et al. 2022). Once properly seated, the socket can become loose, allowing the limb to move within the socket and damage the residual limb. The socket becomes very narrow, and it may not be possible to wear the prosthesis due to pain or skin conditions. Another problem is that the residual limb heats up inside the prosthesis because the socket is usually made of a non-breathable material and socks or liners are added to improve comfort and fit. Increased temperature in the socket is often accompanied by moisture build-up from perspiration, which can cause further problems with the health of the stump (skin damage, infection, etc.) as well as the use of the prosthesis. In addition to the physical influencing factors of the body, the psychology of prosthetic rehabilitation is a decisive success factor. People are looking to make big changes in their lives, but many don't want amputation to hold them back. It's not uncommon for people to become discouraged when they don't see the progress they hoped for.

4.6 Future Scope and Scope for Improvements

Many technical fields have seen improvements over the last few decades, including biotechnology, defense, and machine learning (Ngwangwa and Nemavhola 2021; Shayan et al. 2022; Kang et al. 2020). The prosthetic industry has made similar progress. Similar improvements are being made in the prosthetic industry. Our knowledge of human muscles has increased. In addition, improved electronic components and motors were created. But putting all these parts together to create a complete robotic prosthesis presents many challenges. There is much room for improvement in lower limb prostheses, motivating many researchers to use state-of-the-art technology for all prosthetic leg components. Research and development of lower limb prostheses require a multidisciplinary approach to collaboration between various departments, thus facilitating improved prosthesis manufacturing. In addition, better electronic components and motors have been developed. However, putting all these parts together to create a complete robotic prosthesis presents some challenges.

There is room for progress in lower extremity prostheses, and many researchers are encouraging the full adoption of state-of-the-art technology (Loucas et al. 2017). Improving prosthetic manufacturing is facilitated because lower limb prosthetic research and development require a multidisciplinary approach for cross-industry collaboration. Researchers are working on a transplantable stump that could eliminate the need for sockets. Thanks to these initiatives, parallel breakthroughs in robotics, bioprinting, prosthetics and superhuman body parts are no longer just science fiction. Future socket designs can be created based on knowledge of how prosthetic socket modifications affect the biomechanics of residual bone and skin, and that process can be used to study and improve existing designs. This not only saves time and money, but also improves the fit of prosthetic sockets for a large number of patients, improving patient mobility, participation and overall quality of life in terms of health (Anderst et al. 2022; van Houtum et al. 2012). The field of prosthetics is growing with new technologies, from exoskeletons to prosthetic limbs, designed to improve the quality of life of patients. The use of additive manufacturing in medical device manufacturing is increasing rapidly (Lebea et al. 2021, 2022a, b). Collaboration between volunteers and experts faces particular challenges due to the amateurish design of 3D-printed assistive technologies (Hofmann et al. 2016). The design of the liner and its printing should be considered when choosing a material for the 3D-printed socket, biocompatible, lightweight, and comfortable socket design. In addition, additive manufacturing techniques (Ahsan 2016; Edith et al. 2010;

Londono et al. 2018) and the biomaterial properties of PLA (polylactic acid) or acrylonitrile butadiene styrene for the manufacture of prostheses and braces are described (Durham et al. 2016). One of the major challenges in designing lower limb prostheses is to provide self-actuating capabilities similar to their biological counterparts, as it is currently difficult for prosthesis wearers to make their movements appear natural (Adamczyk 2020). Overcoming this obstacle may require formal studies and computer modeling of the biomechanical behavior of the limb. To solve these problems, the idea of soft robotics (soft sensors) has been proposed (Asif et al. 2021). Investigation of limb loss at birth and at a young age is also very important for the effective use of doctors and researchers. Due to frailty and other psychological problems, older people often have problems with their lower extremities. Counselling should emphasize the importance of special attention and awareness for life. An important part of client-centric support is continuous evaluation of customer satisfaction and incorporating the customer's perspective. The design and development of a compact, fully biocompatible mechanical frame that can be used to replace lost ligaments also enables full integration of smart prostheses (Asif et al. 2021; Manganyi and Mpofu 2011; Yankovskiy et al. 2022).

Polymethyl methacrylate (PMMA) bone cement is commonly used in orthopedics as the gold standard biomaterial for antibiotic treatment of surgical sites (Xie et al. 2022). Most rehab devices today are designed and handcrafted by orthopedic surgeons. Therefore, the quality of our products depends on the skill and experience of our experts. The manufacturing process is time consuming and relies on expert expertise to obtain a product with functional properties that correspond to each subject's unique gait dynamics. Paton et al. (2007) studied the physical properties of soft materials used to manufacture braces designed to prevent neuropathic diabetic foot ulcers. They concluded that the most clinically desirable cushioning materials tested were Poron® 96 and Poron® 4000 (6 mm thick), and the material with the best motion control properties was ethylene vinyl acetate (EVA). In addition, Walbran et al. (2016) compares the yield stress of custom braces made by SLS from FDM containing nylon with carbon fiber and PLA containing. While PLA was chosen for its mechanical properties and cost, AMT has the advantage of not only obtaining a consistent and reproducible model of the subject's affected limb, regardless of the subject's skill and constraints, but also of this AFO design. We concluded that there is a strong possibility to further automate the process. Previously, nano-silver-filled PMMA bone cement (BCAgNp) showed antibacterial activity but still lacked biodegradability and bioactivity. Hydroxyapatite, as a material with important biological activities and a molecular structure similar to bone mineral, has common clinical applications as a coating for prostheses. The combination of hydroxyapatite nanoparticle coating and baicalein was investigated to demonstrate its properties and attempts to improve antibacterial properties. Meanwhile, large companies are starting to use additive manufacturing by purchasing machines and hiring dedicated technicians to operate those machines. However, experts also point out that 3D-printed prosthetic parts have limited material options and limited structural strength of the printed parts. The materials used to laminate the final shaft, such as nyglas, carbon fiber, and fiberglass, are not commercially available for 3D printing. Furthermore, the structural strength and durability of 3D-printed load-bearing parts has not been systematically and rigorously validated by the literature or pertinent ISO standards.

4.7 Conclusion

Science and industry are working to improve systems and designs with technology solutions, but engineering and medicine have come a long way in recent decades and still have a long way to go. Promising recent discoveries have made professionals optimistic about the future of prosthetic legs. Lower limb prostheses require interdisciplinary research, which requires interdisciplinary collaboration between several disciplines. Lower extremity prostheses and orthoses are advanced, but they demand simplicity and elegance. The number of companies manufacturing these prostheses has increased significantly around the world. Products that increase the usefulness and credibility of amputees benefit society as a whole. Rapid prototyping has been viewed by many physicians as an advancement in prosthetic limb research. The ability of rapid prototyping technology to facilitate the integration of proprietary data acquisition sensors into prosthetics is one such example. The potential for prosthetic harness elimination is another important factor in developing comfortable and lightweight prosthetics. If harnesses were ruled out, intelligent prosthetics would have to connect directly to the biological host. Furthermore, considering that intelligence must be built into the machine frame to enable real movement and control, the frame will be equipped with motors, sensors, and similar devices later to induce vibrations. Because cancellous bone contains pores, the human body, especially the skeletal system, can withstand vibrations better than metallic structures.

References

Adamczyk PG (2020) Semi-active prostheses for low-power gait adaptation. Elsevier Inc.

Agudelo-Ardila CP, Prada-Botía GC, Rodrigues G PH (2019) Orthotic prototype for upper limb printed in 3D: a efficient solution orthotic prototype for upper limb printed in 3D: a efficient solution. In: 5th International week of science, technology and innovation, pp 1–7. https://doi.org/10.1088/1742-6596/1388/1/012016

Ahmad N et al (2019) 3D printing in medicine: current challenges and potential applications. 3D Print Technol Nanomed:1–22. https://doi.org/10.1016/B978-0-12-815890-6.00001-3

Ahsan M (2016) 3D printing and titanium alloys : a paper review. Eur Acad Res III(10): 11144–11154

Al-Zubaidi SM, Madfa AA, Mufadhal AA, Hameed OS, Yue X-G (2020) Improvements in clinical durability from functional biomimetic metallic dental implants. Front Mater 7. https://doi.org/10.3389/fmats.2020.00106

Anderst W, Fiedler G, Onishi K, Mckernan G, Gale T, Paulus P (2022) Within-subject effects of standardized prosthetic socket modifications on physical function and patient-reported outcomes. Trials 23:299

Anuar MAM, Sabi AR, Shuib S, Abdullah AH, Miswan MFM (2022) Effect of geometrical designs on mechanics of unicompartmental knee arthroplasty (UKA): a finite element study. Int J Emerg Technol Adv Eng 12(6):84–91. https://doi.org/10.46338/ijetae0622_12

Arjun Hari M, Rajan L (2021) Advanced materials and technologies for touch sensing in prosthetic limbs. IEEE Trans Nanobioscience 20(3):256–270. https://doi.org/10.1109/TNB.2021.3072954
Asif M et al (2021) Advancements, trends and future prospects of lower limb prosthesis. IEEE Access 9:85956–85977. https://doi.org/10.1109/ACCESS.2021.3086807
Bernstein N (1967) The Co-ordination and Regulation of Movements. New York, NY: Pergamon Press
Bertassoni LE, Habelitz S, Marshall SJ, Marshall GW (2011) Mechanical recovery of dentin following remineralization in vitro—an indentation study. J Biomech 44(1):176–181. https://doi.org/10.1016/j.jbiomech.2010.09.005
Copeland C, Reyes CC, Peck JL, Srivastava R, Zuniga JM (2022) Functional performance and patient satisfaction comparison between a 3D printed and a standard transradial prosthesis: a case report. Biomed Eng Online 21(1):1–12. https://doi.org/10.1186/s12938-022-00977-w
Durham J, Sychareun V, Santisouk P, Chaleunvong K (2016) Users' satisfaction with prosthetic and orthotic assistive devices in the Lao People's Democratic Republic: a cross-sectional study. Disabil CBR Incl Dev 27(3):24–44. https://doi.org/10.5463/DCID.v27i3.553
Edith F, Yong J, Shyan M, Nian P, Goh F, Wen C (2010) Printing of titanium implant prototype. Mater Des 31:S101–S105
Etoundi AC, Dobner A, Agrawal S, Semasinghe CL, Georgilas I, Jafari A (2022) A robotic test rig for performance assessment of prosthetic joints. Front Robot AI 8:1–10. https://doi.org/10.3389/frobt.2021.613579
Gupta S, Loh KJ, Pedtke A (2020) Sensing and actuation technologies for smart socket prostheses. Biomed Eng Lett 10(1):103–118. https://doi.org/10.1007/s13534-019-00137-5
Hafner BJ, Sanders JE (2014) Considerations for development of sensing and monitoring tools to facilitate treatment and care of persons with lower-limb loss: a review. J Rehabil Res Dev 51(1): 1–14. https://doi.org/10.1682/JRRD.2013.01.0024
Hassan AK, Abdul Ameer ZJ (2022) Effect of the cure time on the mechanical properties of silicone rubber used as socket liners. IOP Conf Ser Earth Environ Sci 961(1). https://doi.org/10.1088/1755-1315/961/1/012100
Hofmann M et al (2016) Clinical and maker perspectives on the design of assistive technology with rapid prototyping technologies. In: ASSETS 2016—Proceedings of the 18th international ACM SIGACCESS conference on computers and accessibility, Nov 2016, pp 251–256. https://doi.org/10.1145/2982142.2982181
Ijaz MF, Hashmi F (2022) Revisiting alloy design of al-base alloys for potential orthotics and prosthetics applications. Crystals 12:1699. https://doi.org/10.3390/cryst12121699
Kang D-Y, Duong HP, Park J-C (2020) Application of deep learning in dentistry and Implantology. Korean Acad Oral Maxillofac Implantol 24(3):148–181. https://doi.org/10.32542/implantology.202015
Karamousadakis M, Porichis A, Ottikkutti S, Panagiotis DC, Vartholomeos P (2021) A sensor-based decision support system for transfemoral socket rectification. Sensors 21:1–18
Ko ST, Asplund F, Zeybek B (2021) A scoping review of pressure measurements in prosthetic sockets of transfemoral amputees during ambulation: key considerations for sensor design. Sensors 21(15). https://doi.org/10.3390/s21155016
Larsen BG et al (2020) Does actively enlarging socket volume during resting facilitate residual limb fluid volume recovery in trans-tibial prosthesis users? Clin Biomech 78:105001. https://doi.org/10.1016/j.clinbiomech.2020.105001
Lebea L, Ngwangwa HM, Desai D, Nemavhola F (2021) Experimental investigation into the effect of surface roughness and mechanical properties of 3D-printed titanium Ti-64 ELI after heat treatment. Int J Mech Mater Eng 16:16
Lebea L, Ngwangwa HM, Desai DA, Nemavhola F (2022a) Corrosion resistance of 3D-printed titanium alloy Ti64-ELI parts for dental application. Appl Bionics Biomech 2022:1–8
Lebea L, Ngwangwa H, Desai D, Nemavhola F (2022b) Investigation on 3D printed dental titanium Ti64ELI and lifetime prediction. In: Eighth international conference on structural engineering, mechanics and computation (SEMC 2022, Cape Town, South Africa, 5–7 Sept 2022), pp 613–617

Londono J, Tadros M, Salgueiro M, Baker PS (2018) Digital design and 3D printing of an implant-supported prosthetic stent for protecting complete arch soft tissue grafts around dental implants : a dental technique. J Prosthet Dent 120(6):801–804. https://doi.org/10.1016/j.prosdent.2018.01.009

Loucas CA, Brand SR, Bedoya SZ, Muriel AC, Wiener L (2017) Preparing youth with cancer for amputation: a systematic review. J Psychosoc Oncol 35(4):483–493. https://doi.org/10.1080/07347332.2017.1307894

Manganyi UN, Mpofu K (2011) Biological considerations in the structural design of smart prosthetics. In: 4th Robotics and mechatronics conference of South Africa (ROBMECH), Nov 2011, pp 23–25. https://doi.org/10.13140/2.1.1523.9683

Meng Z, Wong DWC, Zhang M, Leung AKL (2020) Analysis of compression/release stabilized transfemoral prosthetic socket by finite element modelling method. Med Eng Phys 83:123–129. https://doi.org/10.1016/j.medengphy.2020.05.007

Nemavhola F (2017) Fibrotic infarction on the LV free wall may alter the mechanics of healthy septal wall during passive filling. Biomed Mater Eng 28(6):579–599. https://doi.org/10.3233/BME-171698

Nemavhola F (2021) Study of biaxial mechanical properties of the passive pig heart: material characterisation and categorisation of regional differences. Int J Mech Mater Eng 16:1

Ngwangwa HM, Nemavhola F (2021) Evaluating computational performances of hyperelastic models on supraspinatus tendon uniaxial tensile test data. J Comput Appl Mech 52(1):27–43. https://doi.org/10.22059/jcamech.2020.310491.559

Olsen J, Day S, Dupan S, Nazarpour K, Dyson M (2021) 3D-printing and upper-limb prosthetic sockets: promises and pitfalls. IEEE Trans Neural Syst Rehabil Eng 29:527–535. https://doi.org/10.1109/TNSRE.2021.3057984

Paternò L et al (2021) Residual limb volume fluctuations in transfemoral amputees. Sci Rep 11(1): 1–12. https://doi.org/10.1038/s41598-021-91647-9

Paton J, Jones RB, Stenhouse E, Bruce G (2007) The physical characteristics of materials used in the manufacture of orthoses for patients with diabetes. Foot Ankle Int 28(10):1057–1063. https://doi.org/10.3113/FAI.2007.1057

Polliack AA, Craig DD, Sieh RC, Landsberger S, McNeal DR (2002) Laboratory and clinical tests of a prototype pressure sensor for clinical assessment of prosthetic socket fit. Prosthetics Orthot Int 26(1):23–34. https://doi.org/10.1080/03093640208726618

Shayan S, Carpentieri B, Shriram D, Holzapfel GA (2022) Multi-fidelity surrogate modeling through hybrid machine learning for biomechanical and finite element analysis of soft tissues. Comput Biol Med 148:105699. https://doi.org/10.1016/j.compbiomed.2022.105699

Tan Q, Wu C, Li L, Shao W, Luo M (2022) Nanomaterial-based prosthetic limbs for disability mobility assistance: a review of recent advances. J Nanomater 2022. https://doi.org/10.1155/2022/3425297

Turner S, Belsi A, McGregor AH (2022) Issues faced by prosthetists and physiotherapists during lower-limb prosthetic rehabilitation: a thematic analysis. Front Rehabil Sci 2. https://doi.org/10.3389/fresc.2021.795021

Valle G, Petrini FM, Strauss I, Iberite F, Anna ED, Granata G (2018) Comparison of linear frequency and amplitude modulation for intraneural sensory feedback in bidirectional hand prostheses. Sci Rep 8:1–13. https://doi.org/10.1038/s41598-018-34910-w

Van Der Stelt M, Verhamme L, Slump CH (2022) Strength testing of low-cost 3D-printed transtibial prosthetic socket. Proc Inst Mech Eng H 236:367. https://doi.org/10.1177/09544119211060092

van Houtum WH, Lavery LA, Harkless LB (2012) The costs of diabetes-related lower extremity amputations in the Netherlands. Diabet Med 12(9):777–781. https://doi.org/10.1111/j.1464-5491.1995.tb02079.x

Walbran M, Turner K, McDaid AJ (2016) Customized 3D printed ankle-foot orthosis with adaptable carbon fibre composite spring joint. Cogent Eng 3(1). https://doi.org/10.1080/23311916.2016.1227022

Walsh C (2018) Human-in-the-loop development of soft wearable robots. Nat Rev Mater 3(6): 78–80. https://doi.org/10.1038/s41578-018-0011-1

Xie H et al (2022) Recent advances in prevention, detection and treatment in prosthetic joint infections of bioactive materials. Front Bioeng Biotechnol 10:1–16. https://doi.org/10.3389/fbioe.2022.1053399

Yankovskiy VM, Chernikova MV, Kuzicheva AD, Fogt EV (2022) Medical aspects of prosthetics in lower limb amputees with use of digital technologies. Genij Ortop 28(4):495–502. https://doi.org/10.18019/1028-4427-2022-28-4-495-502

Zapen B (2021) An examination of current prosthetic technologies and areas for innovation. Bashar Zapen Muthesius Kunsthochschule, SS 21 Design Science Hausarbeit Paula Ellert

Integrating Advanced Technologies in Post-operative Rehabilitation: 3D-Knitting, 3D-Printed Electronics, and Sensor-Embedded Textiles

5

Rahul Gorka, Anand Kumar Subramaniyan, and Rajkumar Velu

Contents

Abstract

Introduction: The recovery phase following surgery, termed "rehabilitation," plays a vital role in aiding patients to regain their preoperative state. Monitoring and understanding the post-operative recovery phase is crucial for healthcare professionals to identify deviations from the typical recovery curve and for caregivers to integrate long-term functional outcomes. Digital post-operative care leverages mobile devices to share rehabilitation advice and collect patient data, enhancing post-operative recovery by remotely educating, monitoring, and data collection.

R. Gorka (✉)
All India Institute of Medical Sciences Vijaypur, Jammu, Jammu and Kashmir, India
e-mail: rahul.gorka@aiimsjammu.edu.in

A. K. Subramaniyan · R. Velu
Additive Manufacturing Research Laboratory, Mechanical Engineering, Indian Institute of Technology Jammu, Jammu, Jammu and Kashmir, India

R. Velu et al. (eds.), *Digital Design and Manufacturing of Medical Devices and Systems*, https://doi.org/10.1007/978-981-99-7100-8_5

Benefits of Digital Post-operative Care: Automated rehabilitation education, real-time patient data collection, and early detection of complications are advantages of digital post-operative care. It reduces unnecessary visits, paper communication, and phone calls while enhancing patient confidence.

Modern Rehabilitation Systems Based on Textiles: Textile-based solutions are prevalent in the realm of medical rehabilitation, particularly within compression therapy and orthopedics. Knitting technology contributes to the manufacturing of compression products, offering tailored pressure to body parts for diverse health functions. Compression orthoses aid children's health and provide venous blood flow control. Pantyhoses with anti-varicose properties and stabilizing bands for joints are other applications. Textiles are vital in orthoses composition, enhancing comfort and moisture removal. Anti-bedsore protection textiles create a breathable layer to prevent pressure ulcers. The integration of sensor technology in textiles enhances pressure ulcer prevention. Customized 3D-knitted garments improve hand therapy, with gloves aiding rehabilitation exercises and sensory-motor movement. Muscle electro-stimulation using conductive textiles activates muscles, promoting rehabilitation.

Challenges and Prospects: Challenges include cost-effectiveness, air breathability, eco-friendliness, and sensor integration. Overcoming these challenges could lead to more affordable, multi-functional, and sustainable healthcare solutions.

Summary and Conclusions: Textiles significantly impact post-operative rehabilitation, particularly in compression therapy and orthopedics. Advances in textiles, such as 3D knitting and sensor integration, offer innovative solutions for patient comfort and effective rehabilitation. Overcoming challenges and enhancing textile-based rehabilitation systems will improve patient outcomes and quality of life.

Keywords

3D-knitting · 3D-printed electronics · Sensor-embedded textiles · Post-operative rehabilitation · Compression therapy · Muscle electro-stimulation

5.1 Introduction

The pivotal time period following surgery, during which patients return to or exceed their preoperative state, is called the "Recovery phase" (Bergman and Drudi 2019). The training and therapy aimed at helping a patient during the "recovery phase" are called "rehabilitation." Follow-up and staying connected with patients after discharge are vital for the surgical care pathway. At the same time, there is a definite need to monitor, analyze, and understand the "post-operative recovery phase." This might be useful for the surgeon or primary care physician to understand any deviation from the typical recovery curve and any need for further investigations. Additionally, the caregivers would like to recognize and integrate the long-term functional outcomes in the setting of personal practice audits, measuring the effectiveness of the intervention, or even when comparing new procedures/techniques. Patients receive care-related medical advice on their mobile devices. Simultaneously, the caregivers' dashboard collects medical data and provides a detailed clinical overview of patients' recovery. They can collect digital pain scales or other VAS measurements from patients and, at the same time, share rehabilitation advice and counseling (Delgado et al. 2018; Mura et al. 2022). Hence, it is possible to enhance the post-operative recovery of patients by digitally educating, collecting medical data, and monitoring remotely.

5.1.1 Benefits of Digital Post-operative Care

- Supports automated rehabilitation education sharing and monitors patients after discharge.
- Automatically collects real-time patient data.
- Helps in identifying post-operative complications.
- Reduces unnecessary post-surgical visits and hospital readmissions through early tracking of complications or the length of hospital stay.
- Reduces or even eliminates telephone calls and paper letters.
- Patients feel relaxed, knowing they are monitored remotely after discharge (Digital Postoperative Care 2023)

5.2 Modern Rehabilitation Systems Based on Textiles

5.2.1 Medical Compression

Knitting technology plays a crucial role in the production of compression products, utilizing the row-knitted fabrics technique on double-bearing cylindrical machines with elastomeric yarn (Digital Postoperative Care 2023). These products, crafted either as whole garments or tailored for specific body parts, undergo rigorous scrutiny to ensure precise design and compression features that serve defined health functions in terms of pressure on the body (Lim and Davies 2014; Zmyt 2018; Xiong and Tao 2018; Carneiro 2004; Sigrist et al. 2013; Delph et al. 2013; Vromansa and Faghria 2018; Curteza et al. 2016; Zieba et al. 2011; Kutlu et al. 2016; Yang et al. 2014). A notable application involves enhancing children's well-being through sensory-focused solutions, such as flexible orthoses designed to conform to the child's body (Fig. 5.1). These orthoses provide support, improve muscle tone control, and enhance respiratory mechanics by applying deep pressure. Their efficacy extends to reducing reaction time, involuntary movements, and autostimulation behaviors. Compression orthoses prove highly advantageous for children dealing with conditions such as cerebral palsy, Down syndrome, muscular atrophy, or sensory integration disorders. Additionally, these orthoses are vital in enhancing physical stability and posture control in children with motor function

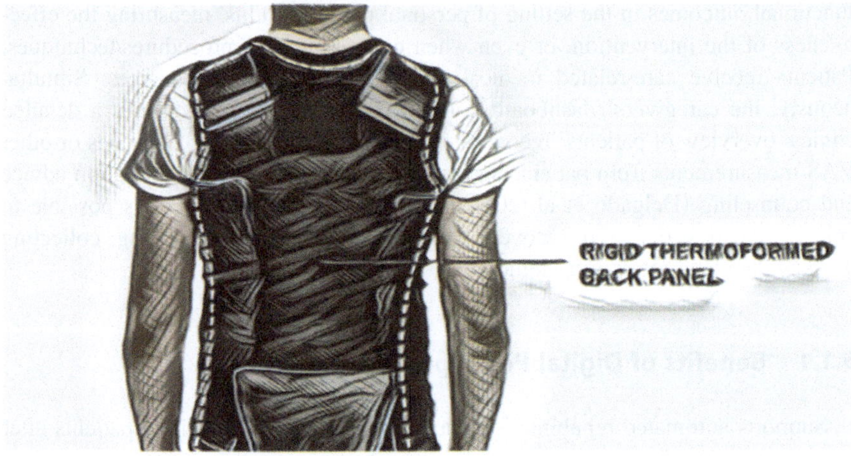

Fig. 5.1 Compression orthosis of the torso

disorders. They achieve this by promoting increased coordination, heightened body awareness, and improved speed and responsiveness in the movements.

One of the groups among products with compressible properties is pantyhoses which have anti-varicose and anti-edema properties. Crafted with the intent to apply customizable and targeted compression pressure on the patient's legs, these products aim to facilitate the movement of venous blood from the lower extremities towards the heart (Mura et al. 2022; Digital Postoperative Care 2023; Lim and Davies 2014; Delph et al. 2013). They are engineered to deliver optimal pressure ranging from 10 to 32 mmHg, ensuring proper circulation in the lower body (Fig. 5.2). These items come in seamless designs as well as those incorporating flat seams (Fig. 5.3). Whether, in the form of pantyhoses, stockings, or knee-length socks, they offer a preventive effect, particularly beneficial for individuals engaged in prolonged standing or sitting positions. This is especially relevant for those with specific medical indications for treating lower limb varicose veins.

The products fitted to the user's body include knitted bands in seamless form. They are used for stabilizing parts of the body such as wrists or other joints (knee, ankle) (Fig. 5.4). They provide adequate stiffening and compression at the early stages of degenerative disease as well as during chronic, post-traumatic or post-operative irritations in the joint area (Zmyt 2018). They also prevent injuries, for example, while practicing competitive sports. These products ensure the comfort of use while performing the assumed function. This is attributable to the use of a variety of raw materials. There are additional features such as moisture dissipation, which ensures antibacterial properties, as well as the introduction of the anti-rheumatic function through the addition of a natural ingredient such as amber (enrichment or fiber) or minerals providing a thermal effect by increasing the body temperature, which can further contribute to the process of improving health.

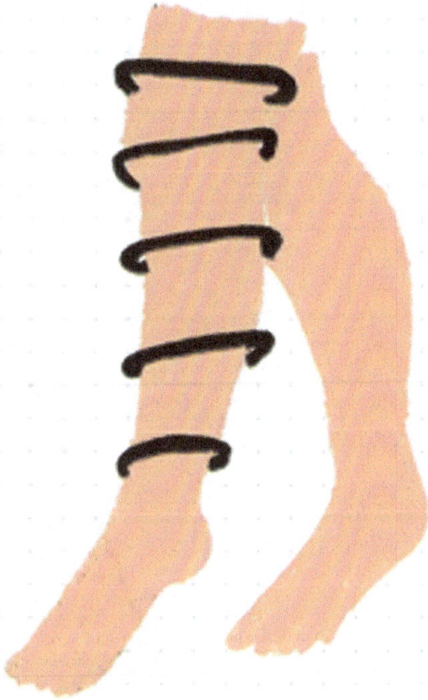

Fig. 5.2 Stockings for varicose veins

When exploring the functions of textile products in rehabilitation with a focus on immobilizing specific body parts, it is crucial to underscore the role of textiles in producing a diverse array of stabilizing orthoses. These orthoses serve as rehabilitation devices functioning as orthopedic aids to immobilize joints, body segments, or muscle groups, often replacing traditional plaster casts (Fig. 5.5). Their primary objective is to maintain a stable position for the joints in the injured limb, particularly in cases of sprains, dislocations, or torn ligaments (Xiong and Tao 2018; Carneiro 2004). Irrespective of their structural classification into rigid, semi-rigid (semi-flexible), or soft (elastic) categories, textile materials in the form of woven fabrics, knitted fabrics, and tapes are integral components of these orthotic devices.

In conjunction with the rigid composite components of orthoses, the inclusion of elastic and soft textile materials in close proximity to the skin enhances wearing comfort and establishes an air layer that facilitates moisture removal from the immobilized body part. To achieve this, spacer fabrics with a three-dimensional (3D) structure are employed, typically crafted from polyamide and produced using both warp and weft knitting technologies. The spatial structure and elasticity of (3D) spacer-knitted fabrics make them particularly suitable for this purpose. Entire textile orthoses are connected using flat seams along with lacing elements or Velcro fasteners, ensuring convenient injury stabilization. Furthermore, the compression effect of textiles not only aids in temperature regulation around the affected joint but also helps maintain a consistent level of warmth. Compression therapy plays a vital

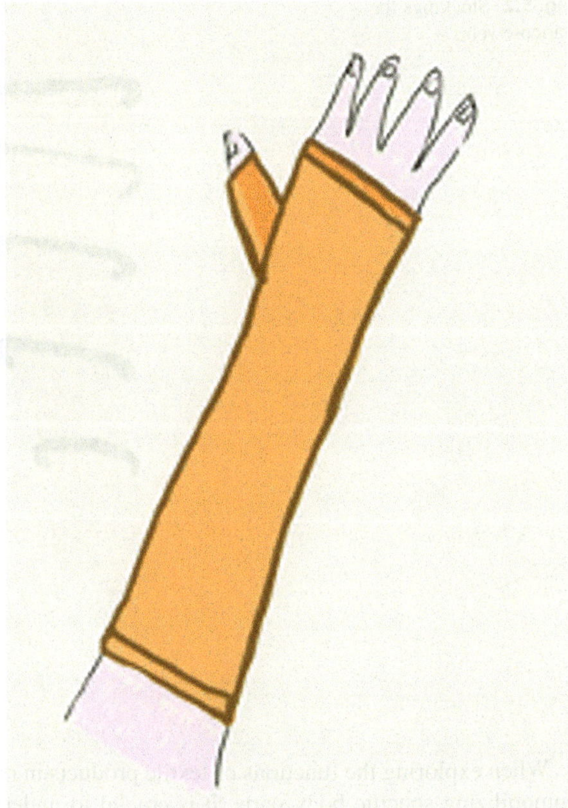

Fig. 5.3 Compression product with visible seams

role in scar treatment, representing a significant application of textiles, including knitted fabrics, in the field of rehabilitation. Particularly crucial in addressing burn wounds and post-operative scars post wound healing, specialized devices tailored to the patient's structure and needs are employed (Sigrist et al. 2013; Delph et al. 2013). Research papers (Vromansa and Faghria 2018; Curteza et al. 2016; Zieba et al. 2011) delve into the challenges of compression products, emphasizing the importance of the individual pressure exerted by the product on various body parts to ensure its therapeutic efficacy.

The analysis extends to the impact of seams and the tolerance performance of compression products, considering the stiffness of the stretching (compression) fabric in relation to the complexity of the female and male figures. Achieving optimal results in patient treatment requires selecting the appropriate pressure level on the scar, a determination made by the medical professional. Excessive pressure may lead to tissue necrosis due to circulatory issues, while insufficient pressure fails to yield the desired therapeutic effect.

Garments tailored to individual wearers with flat seams, minimizing the risk of irritation, possess an appropriate compression value (Fig. 5.6) to enhance treatment

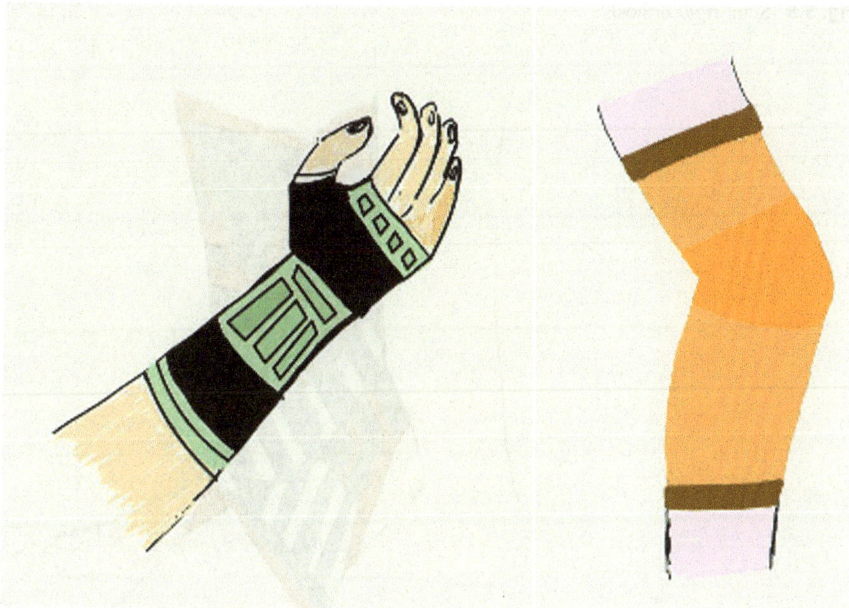

Fig. 5.4 (**a** and **b**) Stabilizer of the wrist and knee

effectiveness. These devices find application on healed burns or scars and should be worn consistently throughout the day for a recommended period of 6–24 months, ensuring sustained positive outcomes such as scar flattening, fading, and softening.

5.2.1.1 Anti-bedsore Protection

An important aspect of rehabilitation is safeguarding patients' health and supporting treatment, particularly in terms of preventing pressure ulcers when patients are immobilized in prolonged sitting or lying positions, leading to skin pressure (Smart Textiles Recognize Body Movements 2023, Guttmann 1955). Under these circumstances, patients may experience pressure loads that result in impressions on the skin, potentially leading to the formation of pressure ulcers.

A practical solution to mitigate the formation of pressure ulcers involves the use of a textile product crafted from technical knitted fabric. This product takes the form of a "full body" 3D spacer-knitted fabric with dimensions of 90 cm × 200 cm. Its spatial shape and structure, composed of closely arranged monofilaments connecting the upper and lower layers of the flat-knitted fabric, impart elasticity to the product, serving as an effective alternative to foam. The product's openwork and highly deformable structure create an air and moisture-permeable layer between the patient's body and the bed. These characteristics contribute to protecting the patient from pressure sores and, if such discomforts exist, can improve the overall state of health (Tong et al. 2016).

Fig. 5.5 Semi-rigid orthosis

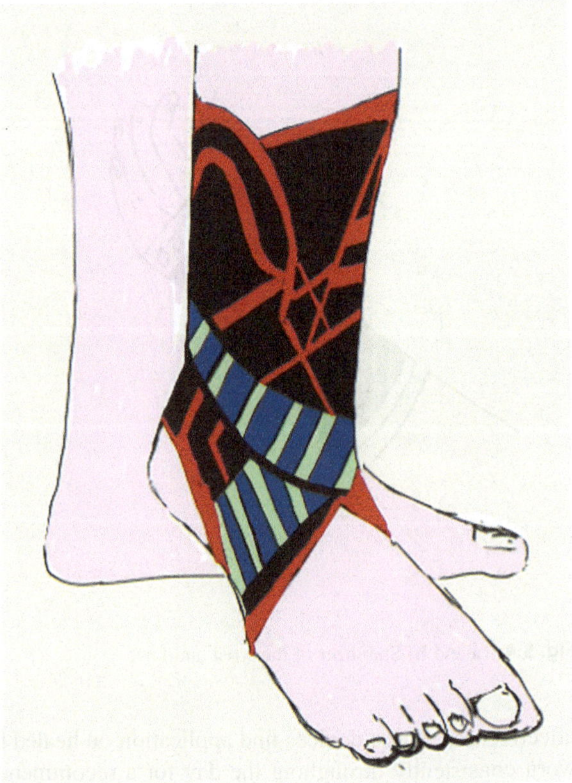

The mat ensures a uniform distribution of pressure across the patient's body, mitigating the risk of concentrated point loads. Following successful testing in hospital conditions at the Rehabilitation and Physical Medicine clinic in Łódź, the product has garnered favorable feedback from both patients and doctors. Consequently, it has earned registration as a medical device. There are the following technical challenges that need to be addressed:

(a) Pressure Distribution: Bedsore prevention involves distributing pressure evenly across the body to avoid excessive pressure on specific areas. Designing 3D-knitted garments that can effectively distribute pressure requires careful consideration of the garment's structure, stitch patterns, and material properties. Achieving optimal pressure distribution while maintaining comfort and mobility is a technical challenge.
(b) Moisture Management: Moisture management is critical for preventing bedsores as excessive moisture can increase the risk of skin breakdown. 3D-knitted fabrics should have good breathability and moisture-wicking properties to keep the skin dry and comfortable. Ensuring effective moisture management

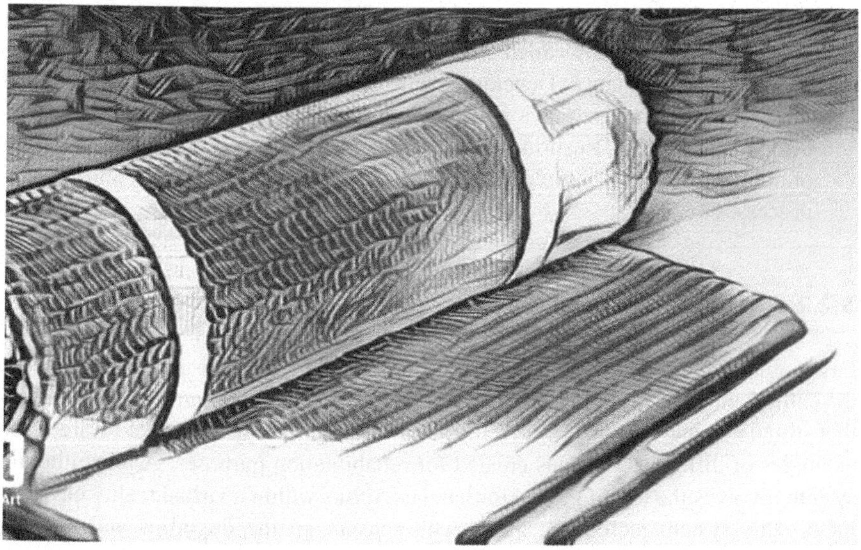

Fig. 5.6 The anti-bedsore overlay

in the knitted garments through appropriate material selection and construction techniques can be challenging.

(c) Friction and Shear Reduction: Friction and shear forces can contribute to the development of bedsores. 3D-knitted garments for anti-bedsore protection should incorporate features that minimize friction and shear, such as incorporating smooth and low-friction surfaces or utilizing padding in high-risk areas. Designing these features within the 3D knitting process requires careful consideration of the garment's construction and material properties.

(d) Customization and Personalization: Each patient's needs for anti-bedsore protection may vary based on their specific condition and body shape. 3D knitting technology has the potential to create customized garments that fit individual patients, but it presents challenges in terms of design complexity and manufacturing scalability. Developing techniques to efficiently customize and personalize 3D-knitted anti-bedsore garments for each patient is a technical challenge.

(e) Durability and Longevity: Anti-bedsore protection garments need to withstand repeated use, washing, and wear without compromising their effectiveness. Ensuring the durability and longevity of 3D-knitted fabrics while maintaining their desired properties, such as pressure distribution and moisture management, is a technical challenge. Selecting appropriate materials and optimizing the knitting parameters can contribute to achieving the desired durability.

(f) Integration of Sensor Technology: Integrating sensor technology into 3D-knitted anti-bedsore protection garments can provide real-time monitoring of pressure, temperature, and other relevant parameters. However, embedding sensors or electrodes without compromising the garment's comfort, flexibility, and functionality is a technical challenge. Ensuring reliable and accurate data collection from the embedded sensors adds another layer of complexity.

(g) Regulatory Compliance: Developing anti-bedsore protection garments using 3D knitting technology requires adherence to regulatory standards and guidelines for medical devices. Ensuring compliance with safety, performance, and quality requirements adds complexity to the design, manufacturing, and testing processes.

5.2.2 Rehabilitation Gloves

Fascinating solutions to enhance patient health include knitted garments covering the entire hand, such as gloves. These garments are designed to carry motor elements that stimulate hand and finger movements towards specific actions. Below are some examples of different solutions created for rehabilitation purposes. A rehabilitation system involves the use of gloves for hand exercises within a virtual reality environment. This system includes a glove with sensors on the fingertips and a tether running along each finger, connecting to the control system. It addresses hand injuries by monitoring and guiding hand movements through a predefined set of exercises. For instance, an orientation sensor in the glove tracks the hand's position in the room, while the tether's position enables accurate detection of each finger's bending and movement, as illustrated in Figs. 5.7 and 5.8a, b. This setup allows patients to engage in exercises aligned with the rehabilitation program displayed on the virtual reality environment screen [19].

They are paired with virtual reality headsets to enhance patient motivation and promote the consistent use of gloves for hand exercises. In this simulated environment, hand movements are replicated to provide visual and physical feedback, making the activities more enjoyable and compelling.

In the realm of using textiles to incorporate stimulation elements, a notable application for the hand and forearm involves a tool designed to assist visually impaired individuals in hand operations. This device serves as a valuable aid for coaches of visually impaired athletes participating in the Paralympic Games,

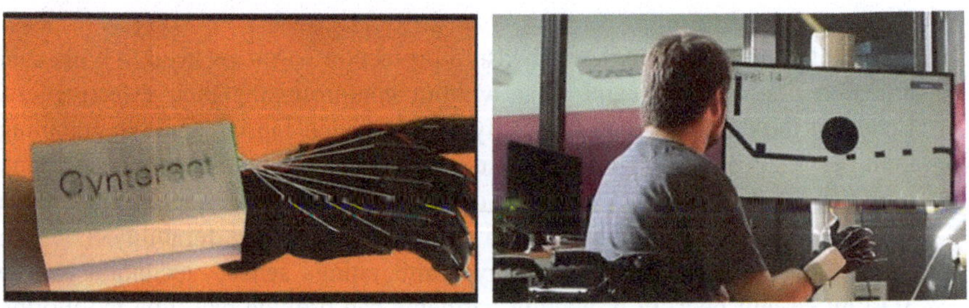

Fig. 5.7 Cynteract glove for rehabilitation exercises aimed at improving the motor performance of the hand. (Source: https://cynteract.com/en/)

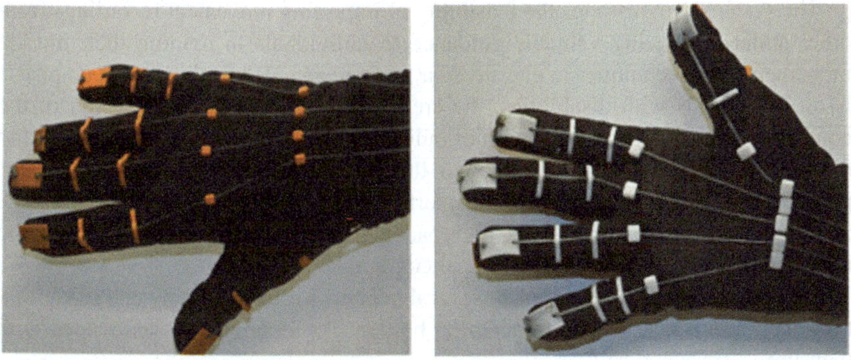

Fig. 5.8 (**a**, **b**) Prototype of the hand rehabilitation device

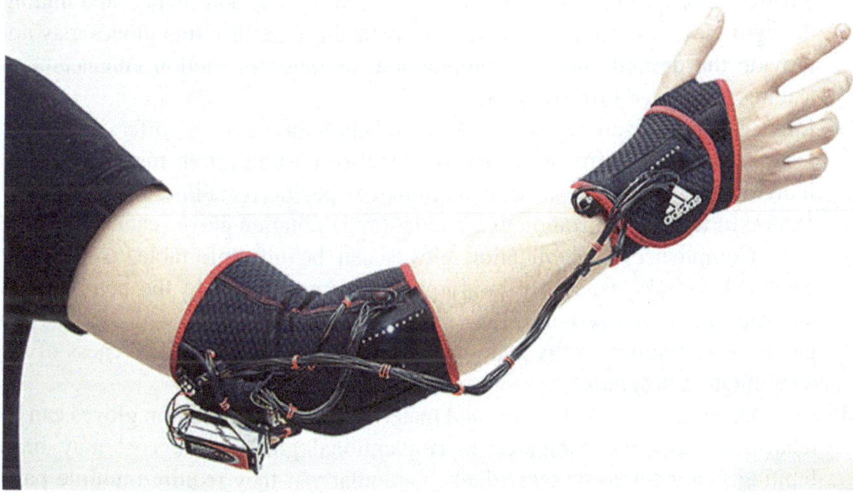

Fig. 5.9 The "Ghost" system for stimulation of blind people's hand movements. (Source: www.medgadget.com)

facilitating the learning of precise muscle movements. Traditionally, training for visually impaired individuals involved physical manipulation of their hands and legs, allowing them to memorize specific movements and muscle activities with the guidance of a trainer.

Addressing this, researchers at Imperial College London have developed a vibratory feedback device known as the "Ghost" system. This innovation enables visually impaired individuals to learn and execute movements precisely and consistently without the need for a trainer. The "Ghost" system has the capability to store specific activities demonstrated by a trainer, allowing athletes to practice these movements while receiving continuous monitoring for accuracy through vibration and sound signals (Fig. 5.9).

The system demonstrates the feasibility of importing movement recordings from other athletes, offering valuable guidance to individuals in refining their muscle movements and techniques to elevate their performance. While the current emphasis is on individuals with disabilities, the creators envision a future extension of the concept to assist in the rehabilitation of individuals who have undergone strokes and other neurological disorders. Although the system has been custom-tailored for people with disabilities at present (Smart Textiles Recognize Body Movements 2023), the future direction aims to broaden its application to contribute to the rehabilitation of those with neurological conditions.

While rehabilitation gloves offer several benefits for hand therapy and rehabilitation, there are a few following potential bottlenecks or limitations associated with their use.

(a) Individual Fit and Sizing: Ensuring the proper fit and sizing of rehabilitation gloves can be a challenge. Hands come in various sizes and shapes, and finding the right glove size for each individual can be difficult. Ill-fitting gloves may not provide the desired support, compression, or range of motion enhancement, leading to reduced effectiveness.
(b) Limited Customization: While some rehabilitation gloves offer adjustable features, such as straps or inserts, the level of customization may be limited. Individuals with unique hand conditions or specific rehabilitation needs may require further customization that standard rehabilitation gloves cannot provide.
(c) User Compliance: Rehabilitation gloves can be uncomfortable to wear for extended periods, especially in warm environments, due to the compression and snug fit. This discomfort may reduce patient compliance with wearing the gloves as recommended by therapists, affecting the overall effectiveness of the rehabilitation program.
(d) Cost: Depending on the features and materials used, rehabilitation gloves can be relatively expensive compared to conventional gloves. The cost may be a limiting factor for some individuals, particularly if they require multiple pairs or long-term use.
(e) Limited Evidence and Research: While rehabilitation gloves are commonly used in hand therapy, the scientific evidence supporting their efficacy is still evolving. More research is needed to validate their effectiveness, determine optimal design features, and establish specific guidelines for their use in various rehabilitation contexts.
(f) Functional Limitations: Rehabilitation gloves may have limitations in addressing certain hand conditions or functional goals. Some conditions may require more targeted therapy interventions or specialized devices beyond what rehabilitation gloves can provide.

Despite these bottlenecks, rehabilitation gloves continue to be valuable tools in hand therapy and rehabilitation. Ongoing advancements in materials, design, and customization options, as well as further research and evidence may help address these limitations and enhance the effectiveness of rehabilitation gloves in the future.

5.3 Muscle Electro-stimulation

Using textiles in rehabilitation finds a prominent application in the electro-stimulation of nerves and muscles. This technique is designed to activate specific muscles with the overarching goal of enhancing their condition and functionality. It encompasses activities such as re-educating lost muscle function, preserving or augmenting joint mobility, improving local blood circulation, and contributing to sports training during post-injury rehabilitation. The desired effects are achieved by using electrodes that rapidly alternate AC with varying frequency and pulse width. Research has played a crucial role in experimentally determining optimal conditions for stimulating muscles of different sizes by manipulating specific parameters of Functional Electrical Stimulation (FES), including stimulation intensity and frequency (Delgado et al. 2018).

Various innovative solutions, currently at the research level, offer alternatives to traditional electrodes by incorporating conductive textiles composed of conductive yarns in fabric and knit applications (Curteza et al. 2016). An intriguing approach to muscle electro-stimulation involves using silkscreen printing technology to create a system of electrodes (Zieba et al. 2011; Kutlu et al. 2016).

The flexible stimulative device for muscle electro-stimulation is crafted from woven fabric, boasting a notable advantage in that it eliminates the need for a hydrogel layer. This characteristic makes it a convenient therapeutic element, enabling direct contact with dry skin (Fig. 5.10). Programmable patterns were employed for muscle stimulation, allowing the recreation of three distinct hand gestures. Notably, the device demonstrated more effective recreation of hand gestures compared to the widely used printed circuit board containing a hydrogel layer. Consequently, it was deduced that this new textile electrode could facilitate therapeutic interventions at a level comparable to that of a typical stimulation electrode. These findings have set the stage for further exploration into integrating such electrodes into clothing, commonly referred to as e-textiles.

To improve the effectiveness and usability of a muscle electro-stimulation system, the following improvisations could be adopted:

(a) Targeted Stimulation: Enhance the system's capability to provide targeted stimulation to specific muscle groups or areas. This can be achieved through the use of electrode placement guides or specialized electrode arrays that allow for precise positioning on the target muscles.
(b) Programmability and Customization: Develop a system that offers programmability and customization options. Users should be able to adjust stimulation parameters such as frequency, pulse duration, and intensity to suit their specific needs and comfort levels. Pre-set programs tailored to different rehabilitation or training goals can also be included.
(c) Wireless and Wearable Design: Create a wireless and wearable design for the MES system, allowing for increased freedom of movement during therapy or training sessions. This eliminates the restrictions posed by wired connections

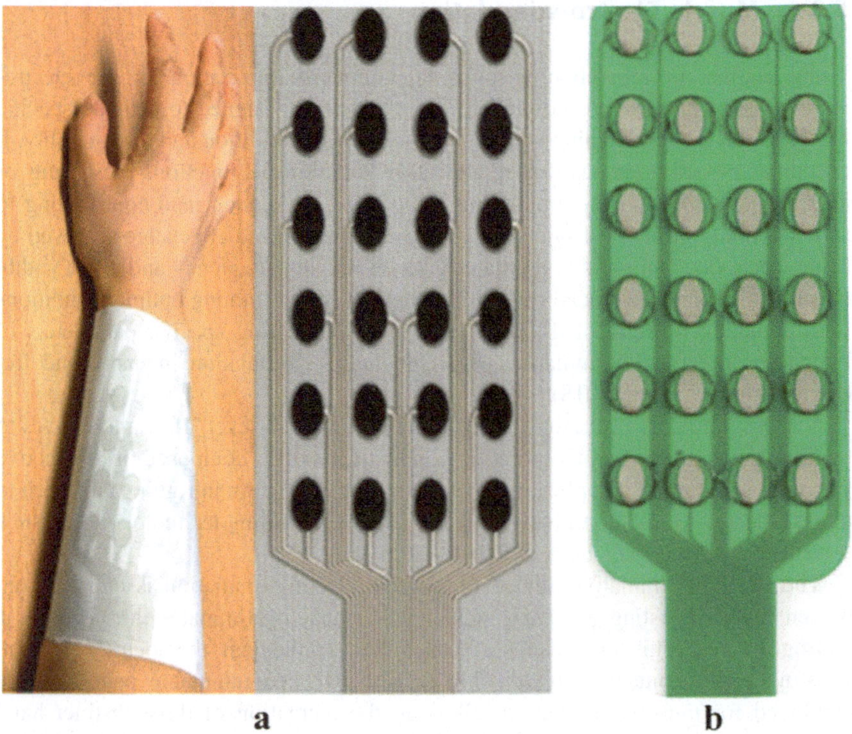

Fig. 5.10 Flexible printed matrix of electrodes. Source: (Yang et al. 2014)

and enables users to engage in functional activities while receiving muscle stimulation.

(d) Feedback and Monitoring: Incorporate sensors or feedback mechanisms into the system to provide real-time data on muscle activation, fatigue levels, or performance metrics. This information can help users and healthcare professionals monitor progress, optimize training parameters, and prevent overexertion or muscle imbalances.

(e) User-Integrated Therapy Programs: Develop MES systems with integrated therapy programs that combine muscle stimulation with other rehabilitation techniques. For example, integrating functional exercises, range of motion exercises, or biofeedback mechanisms can enhance the effectiveness of rehabilitation protocols.

(f) User-Friendly Interfaces: Design user-friendly interfaces for easy operation and control of the system. Intuitive displays, touchscreens, or mobile applications can simplify the user experience and provide clear instructions and feedback during therapy or training sessions.

(g) Safety Features: Ensure the system incorporates safety features to prevent misuse or excessive stimulation. This can include built-in timers, automatic shut-off mechanisms, and intensity limits to prevent muscle fatigue or injury.
(h) Portable and Compact Design: Make the MES system portable and compact, allowing users to use it conveniently at home or during travel. Consider the use of lightweight materials and a compact form factor without compromising functionality or durability.
(i) Longevity and Battery Life: Optimize the system's power management and battery life to ensure extended use between recharges or battery replacements. This is particularly important for wireless systems, where longer battery life allows for uninterrupted therapy or training sessions.
(j) Evidence-Based Approach: Base the design and functionality of the MES system on scientific evidence and research findings. Collaborate with healthcare professionals, therapists, and researchers to ensure that the system aligns with established rehabilitation or training protocols. It is crucial to involve healthcare professionals, engineers, and end-users in the development and testing of any improvisations to ensure safety, effectiveness, and usability of the improved muscle electro-stimulation system.

5.4 Challenges and Prospects

The requirement for patient-comfort knitting for post-operative rehabilitation and monitoring is increasing due to its demand. However, it offers multifold associated challenges that need to be dealt with from the viewpoint of affordability, multi-functional characteristics, biodegradable and smartness, etc. Therefore, the features mentioned above give engineers and medical professionals opportunities to work coherently to achieve tangible outcomes. The following are most relevant but not limited to salient points worth mentioning as a prospect to be resolved.

- Cost-effectiveness is significant for any innovative medical product, especially in developing countries with limited resources and funds.
- Air breathability is a desirable property of 3D-knitted material to be used as an anti-bedsore mattress, pad for surgery, and mattress on a wheelchair.
- Eco-friendly material paves the way for developing a sustainable healthcare system that is lean and green, with minimal waste production, preferably biodegradable or recyclable.
- Sensor integration and IoT-enabled textiles are the advanced versions of these revolutionary 3D-knitted textiles with multi-functional capabilities.

5.5 Summary and Conclusions

Textiles play a pivotal role in medical rehabilitation, particularly in areas such as compression therapy and orthopedics. The use of shaped and designed products with customized pressure, delivering specific and consistent unit pressure to targeted body parts, contributes significantly to enhancing motor and sensory functions in children with congenital malformations. Additionally, this approach aids in promoting health by treating conditions like varicose veins, addressing the effects of accidents such as burn wounds, and managing injuries like wrist joint injuries.

In orthopedics, integrating knitted fabrics into elements provides improved patient comfort, particularly in cases of minor joint injuries. These fabrics contribute to enhancing skin condition by offering protection against abrasions, ensuring proper ventilation, and facilitating moisture wicking. Spatial tight-knit forms are also employed to prevent and treat pressure ulcers, thereby enhancing the well-being and health of immobilized patients.

Beyond traditional applications, textiles are integral to advanced textronic solutions for monitoring vital signs. Moreover, textile-based devices are crucial in improving hand and arm movements and functions. This is achieved through various glove structures and muscle stimulation therapies, showcasing the versatility and significance of textiles in diverse rehabilitation contexts.

The 3D-knitted healthcare fabrics are a prevalent phenomenon in technical textiles, possessing considerable added value and technological complexity. A plethora of structures and materials are incessantly being innovated to satisfy medical use needs. Nonetheless, there are still formidable complications for implanted devices in the human body, as certain fabrics have exhibited inclinations towards eliciting adverse reactions and device malfunction after prolonged usage. As the elderly population grows, injuries escalate, and an enhanced quality of life is demanded, diverse woven healthcare fabrics and materials must be furnished to meet crucial requirements in medical sectors.

References

Ališauskienė D, Mikučionienė D (2012) Influence of the rigid element area on the compression properties of knitted orthopaedic supports. Fibres Text East Eur 20(6A(95)):103–107

Allman RM, Laprade CA, Noel LL, others (1986) Pressure sores among hospitalized patients. Ann Intern Med. 105(3):37–42

Belbasisa A, Fussa FK, Sidhua J (2015) Muscle activity analysis with a smart compression garment, 7th Asia-Pacific Congress on Sports Technology. Procedia Eng 112:163–168

Bergman S, Drudi LM (2019) Postoperative recovery and rehabilitation. In: Rosenthal RA, Zenilman MF, Katlic MR (eds) Principles and practice of geriatric surgery. Springer International Publishing, Cham, pp 1–17. https://doi.org/10.1007/978-3-319-20317-1_30-1

Carneiro MM (2004) Assistive interfaces for the visually impaired using force feedback devices and distance transforms. ITD J. http://easi.cc/itd/volume10/number2/carneiro.html

Curteza A, Cretu V, Macovei L, Poboroniuc M (2016) The manufacturing of textile products with incorporated electrodes. AUTEX Res J 16(1):13–18

Delgado DA, Lambert BS, Boutris N, McCulloch PC, Robbins AB, Moreno MR et al (2018) Validation of digital visual Analog scale pain scoring with a traditional paper-based visual Analog scale in adults. J Am Acad Orthop Surg Glob Res Rev 2(3):e088

Delph MA, Fischer SA, Gauthier PW, Martinez Luna CH, Clancy EA, Fischer GS (2013) A soft robotic exomusculature glove with integrated SEMG sensing for hand rehabilitation. In: 13th International Conference on Rehabilitation Robotics (ICORR), Seattle, WA

Digital Postoperative Care (2023). Cited 2023 Feb 16. Available from: https://www.buddyhealthcare.com/en/digital-post-operative-care

Guttmann L (1955) The problem of treatment of pressure sores in spinal paraplegics. Br J Plast Surg 8:196–213

Ilska A, Kowalski K, Kłonowska M, Kowalski TM (2014) Influence of stress and relaxation characteristics of knitted fabrics on the unit pressure of compression garments supporting external treatment. Fibres Text East Eur 22(4(106)):87–92

Ilska A, Kowalski K, Kłonowska M, Kowalski TM, Sujka W (2016) Issues regarding the design of textile compression products for small body circumferences. Fibres Text East Eur 24(6 (120)):116–120

Kowalski K, Karbowski K, Kłonowska M, Ilska A, Sujka W, Tyczyńska M, Włodarczyk B, Kowalski TM (2017) Influence of a compression garment on average and local changes in unit pressure. Fibres Text East Eur 25(6(126)):68–74

Kutlu M, Freeman CT, Hallewell E, Hughes A-M, Laila DS (2016) Upper-limb stroke rehabilitation using electrode-array based functional electrical stimulation with sensing and control innovations. Med Eng Phys 38:336–379

Lim CS, Davies AH (2014) Graduated compression stockings. CMAJ Can Med Assoc J 186(10): E391–E398

Liu R, Kwok Y-L, Li Y, Lao T-T (2010) Fabric mechanical-surface properties of compression hosiery and their effects on skin pressure magnitudes when worn. Fibres Text East Eur 18(2 (79)):91–97

Macintyre L, Baird M (2006) Pressure garments for use in the treatment of hypertrophic scars—a review of the problems associated with their use. Burns 32:10–15

Maklewska E, Nawrocki A, Ledwoń J, Kowalski K (2006) Modelling and designing of knitted products used in compressive therapy. Fibres Textiles East Eur 14(5 (59))

Mura A, Maier M, Ballester BR, De la Torre CJ, López-Luque J, Gelineau A et al (2022) Bringing rehabilitation home with an e-health platform to treat stroke patients: study protocol of a randomized clinical trial (RGS@home). Trials 23:518

Senthilkumar M, Kumar LA, Anbuman N (2012) Design and development of a pressure sensing device for analysing the pressure comfort of elastic garments. Fibres Textiles East Eur 20(1 (90)):64–69

Sigrist R, Rauter G, Riener R, Wolf P (2013) Augmented visual, auditory, haptic, and multimodal feedback in motor learning: a review. Psychon Bull Rev 20(1):21–53

Smart Textiles Recognize Body Movements (2023) Medgadget. https://www.medgadget.com/2022/07/smart-textiles-recognize-body-movements.html

Szmyt J (2018) Modern rehabilitation systems based on textiles. Acta Innov 27:5–13

Tong SF, Yip J, Yick KL (2016) The possibility of using weft knitted spacer fabric as the wound dressing for pressure ulcer. Int J Adv Sci Eng Technol 4(4) Spl. Issue-1:13–19

Trümper W, Sachse C, Diestel O, Cherif C (2011) Innovative flat-knitted spacer fabrics for orthoses. Tech Text 54(4):171

Vromansa M, Faghria PD (2018) Functional electrical stimulation-induced muscular fatigue: effect of fiber composition and stimulation frequency on rate of fatigue development. J Electromyogr Kinesiol 38:67–72

Wang L, Felder M, Cai JY (2011) Study of properties of medical compression fabrics. J Fiber Bioeng Inform 4(1):15–22. Acta Innovations • ISSN 2300-5599 • 2018 • no. 27: 5-13 • 12 https://doi.org/10.32933/ActaInnovations.27.1 • ISSN 2300-5599 • Ó 2018 RIC Pro-Akademia – CC BY

Xiong Y, Tao X (2018) Compression garments for medical therapy and sports. Polymers 10(6):663
Yang K, Freeman C, Torah R, Beeby S, Tudor J (2014) Screen printed fabric electrode array for wearable functional electrical stimulation. Sensors Actuators A Phys 213:108–115
Zieba J, Frydrysiak M, Tokarska M (2011) Research of textile electrodes for electrotherapy. Fibres Text East Eur 19(5):70–74

Augmented Reality Interface for Additive Manufacturing of Biomedical Applications

6

S. Rimer, T. Berman, M. Gololo, T. Pandelani, and K. Ouahada

Contents

Abstract

The digital divide has deepened in the last few years. The rapid pace of technological progress combined with the focus on biotechnology and vaccines due to the Covid-19 pandemic has resulted in less time and resources being given to supplying more fair access to technological innovation's benefits. The developing world, especially Sub-Saharan Africa, (where most people have limited access to technology that could improve their lives), is affected by multiple issues that limit their ability to provide their populations with access to adequate healthcare services and biomedical equipment compared to developed countries.

S. Rimer (✉) · T. Berman · M. Gololo · T. Pandelani · K. Ouahada
Department of Electrical and Electronic Engineering Science, University of Johannesburg, Johannesburg, South Africa
e-mail: suvendir@uj.ac.za

R. Velu et al. (eds.), *Digital Design and Manufacturing of Medical Devices and Systems*, https://doi.org/10.1007/978-981-99-7100-8_6

The advent of emerging technologies such as augmented reality and 3D printing supplies a unique opportunity to address healthcare inequities using innovative solutions to rapidly transfer knowledge and improve health outcomes. In the developing world, 3D printing technology can lead to the fabrication of cost-effective patient-specific models and the development of innovative implants. 3D printing technology has various uses in different fields of application in biomedical engineering. In pre-operation planning for complex surgeries, the technology has enhanced success by enabling surgery visualization and understanding of complex patient-specific anatomy prior to the surgical operation. The technology has also helped educate trainee surgeons understand the complex 3D anatomy of different organs. It also aids better communication across different departments within a hospital working on the same patient. Patients are also able to understand the risks involved in their surgical procedure.

This chapter supplies a brief overview of additive manufacturing (AM) and augmented reality (AR) and the application of these technologies in biomedical engineering. Possible techniques and applications using either AM or AR or both to develop biomedical applications in developing countries are described. The challenges in implementing practical solutions in developing countries are considered, and possible strategies to overcome them are discussed.

Keywords

Biomedical engineering · Augmented reality · Additive manufacturing · 3-D printing

6.1 Introduction

Healthcare systems and services available in developing countries are under enormous strain due to limited medical and technical skills and resources, inadequate or non-existent transport and communication infrastructure to support the development and transfer of knowledge, and scarce manufacturing capability to rapidly produce biomedical equipment. These factors combined with the fact that most developing countries historically imported all biomedical equipment and did not enter into any form of knowledge transfer agreements with suppliers to ensure that the equipment is correctly maintained result in biomedical equipment often not reaching its intended lifespan capability and underperforming or being relegated to scrapheaps because the parts and/or technical knowledge to fix the equipment are non-existent. This means that poorer countries are continuously spending more money to achieve diminishing health outcomes for their populations.

The term "factory of the future" is widely used to allude to additive manufacturing (AM), also known as 3D printing (Eiríksson et al. 2017). AM is a promising, highly automated, and digital manufacturing technique (Eiríksson et al. 2017). The versatility of AM techniques means it can be used to rapidly manufacture and print-on-demand parts required for maintenance as well as the ability to supply access to prosthetics that are designed and built from real-time feedback of a patient's biological and health details. The combination of augmented reality (AR) applications and artificial intelligence (AI) to aid technicians in the design and manufacturing of biomedical equipment parts removes the restrictive requirement that the operators of AM technology are required to be highly trained and skilled individuals, which is often not achievable in developing countries. AI expert systems that are trained in specific AM techniques can direct an AR application to help a technician in accurately building parts and prosthetics.

In this chapter, we will supply a review of the present-day state-of-the-art in using AR and AM in biomedical engineering. An analysis of the technology, its applications, appropriateness, and usability in developing countries is discussed. Various innovative possibilities and solutions using 3D manufacturing and AR in biomedical engineering in developing countries are explored. Finally, the challenges in implementing practical solutions in developing countries are considered, and possible strategies to overcome them are discussed.

6.2 Review of AR

The current interaction between technology and digital information is two-dimensional. Products are designed in the virtual space using software and then manufactured in the physical space. In AR, real-world elements in the user's physical surroundings are combined with digital information (including text, graphics, photos, audio, and videos) to create three-dimensional computer-generated things that are only visible to the user (Gartner Glossary 2022; Wikipedia 2022; Gillis 2022).

AR connects the digital and physical worlds together, making it easier and faster for humans to interact with both simultaneously and to process, understand, and interpret digital information and designs (nothing gets lost in translation). The information may be gathered and shown on the physical aspects of the object or machine using AR. This information can be found in a range of applications, including maintenance records, inspection and repair instructions, and technical specifications. AR can include views of various pieces of equipment, allowing people to physically compare products and understand dimensions. Different perspectives and up-to-date information about the object's attributes will be revealed as the AR-enabled device moves around the object. Applications for AR might be as straightforward as a text message or as complex as a guide on how to do a life-threatening surgical procedure. They can provide clear and timely information while highlighting certain characteristics and improving comprehension. Through the supply of more contextual and operationally relevant data layered over a live image of a machine or item, AR applications will power the next generation of workplace productivity (Hunter 2017; Papagiannis 2022). AR can be used as a tool that benefits society, as well as individual companies. In order to increase the maintainability and dependability of machinery and equipment, AM and AR

Table 6.1 Categories of AR technology

Category	Technology
Marker AR	Uses a camera and visual markers, such a QR/2D code, to only deliver a result when the marker is detected by a reader
Markerless AR	Obtains location data from the device using either a GPS, digital compass, velocity meter, or accelerometer
Projection-based AR	Human engagement is achieved by projecting light onto a real-world surface and then detecting the human interaction, touch, of that light. By distinguishing between an expected (or known) projection and the changed projection (produced by the user's interaction), the user's interaction may be detected
Superimposition based AR	Uses object recognition algorithms to either completely or partially swap out the original view of an object for a more enhanced version of the same thing

technologies and services will be merged. Table 6.1 outlines the current categories of AR technology:

In order to render AR content, a variety of technologies are utilized, such as optical projection systems, monitors, portable devices, and headgear or display systems that project data into the user's field of vision in order to correlate with a real item or location the user is witnessing (Hunter 2017). The three main characteristics of an AR system are (Taqvi 2013) as follows:

- Combines physical and digital items in a genuine setting
- Aligns real and virtual objects to one another
- Operates in real-time and three dimensions interactively

The technology components needed for AR applications are hardware, software that is embedded into the hardware, and communications to convey to that machine what is happening digitally. The information about what is occurring within the machine may be found in databases, analytics, platforms, and applications on the cloud or in the real world. The user is given the opportunity to interact with that hardware data in a distinctive way, since AR also supports video communication and video augmentation.

The AR application employs artificial and natural light to project or overlay pictures on a screen or a set of transparent goggles or glasses, allowing the visuals and interactive virtual objects to layer on top of the user's perception of the outside environment. The primary hardware elements are built into a device that wirelessly transmits data to a display, including the tracking system, mobile processing power, and visual display system (such as glasses, lenses, or a head-mounted display). It overlays the user's field of view with pictures of both the real environment and registered virtual graphical items. AR hardware includes smartphones, tablets, sensors, head-up visual displays, eyewear, optical headsets, and perceptual systems that are evolving and getting smaller and cheaper.

A developer can link animation or contextual digital data in a computer program to an AR "marker" in the actual environment using AR software applications. When an AR application or browser plug-in on a computer device gets digital data from a recognized marker, it starts to run the marker's code and overlay the appropriate picture or images.

6.3 Review of AM of Biomedical Applications

AM is the technique of assembling materials in a layer-by-layer configuration based on a 3D computer-aided design model to make an item. Powder bed fusion (PBF), material extrusion, directed energy deposition (DED), vat photopolymerization, binder jetting, material jetting, and sheet lamination are the seven subcategories of the current AM technique. New processes are being invented due to ongoing research efforts (Lhachemi et al. 2019; Sreeraj et al. 2022).

AM has applications in different biomedical engineering fields. In pre-operation planning for complex surgeries, the technology has enhanced success by enabling surgery visualization and understanding of complex patient-specific anatomy prior to the surgical operation. The technology has also helped educate trainee surgeons understand the complex 3D anatomy of different organs. It also aids better communication across different departments within a hospital working on the same patient. Patients are also able to understand the risks involved in their surgical procedure.

Due to their excellent mechanical qualities, biocompatibility, and hemocompatibility, AM employs polymers and metals to create implanted medical devices. 3D printing, a technique within AM, is employed to fabricate medical implants such as catheters and cardiovascular devices, etc. that are specifically tailored to meet specific anatomical, mechanical, and biological criteria. To induce the desired response in the host tissue, pores' size, shape, and overall dimensions can be modified. By carefully adjusting the scaffold, it is possible to optimize vascularization, oxygenation, and food delivery to guarantee a positive outcome once the device is implanted in a clinical context. In the biomedical industry, being able to manage the architecture is significant since it enables the production of bespoke, patient-specific implants as well as the repeatability and reproducibility of a variety of implants.

The biomaterials market has four categories: metallic biomaterials, polymeric biomaterials, ceramic biomaterials, and natural biomaterials. In 2021, the metallic biomaterials category held the greatest proportion of the global market in the healthcare industry (Thompson et al. 2015). AM technology has led to the fabrication of cost-effective patient-specific models and the development of innovative implants. AM technology helps to avoid material wastage, and manufacturing errors are less costly to fix.

In order to achieve positive clinical outcomes, reconstructive surgery seeks to correct tissue abnormalities by replacing them with equivalent autologous tissue. To restore the anatomical shape and partial function, however, synthetic materials are frequently needed because the lesion is too wide or the available tissue is insufficient. Traditional manufacturing of bone implants faced challenges, notably in-terface failure as per Hoffman's criterion. This included concerns about wear particles infiltrating confined spaces and the lack of implant fixation, which mechanically hindered bone growth (Surjadi et al. 2019; Hench and Jones 2005; Thompson et al. 2015).

AM proposes addressing the above issues and improving the manufacturing of complex structures, resulting in saving manufacturing time and labour costs. AM has the capacity to enable design for specialized applications or take into account unique features to meet the necessary patient demands. In addition to resolving the issue of various anatomical shapes, AM technology offers the ability to alleviate the lack of organ donors available for transplantations.

6.3.1 AM for Prosthesis and Orthosis

Prosthesis (artificial legs and hands) and orthosis (braces and splints) are fundamental devices to aid physical impairments people or people with functional limitations to live a better social life. WHO estimates that only 10% of people in need have access to assistive devices, including prosthesis and orthoses, because of their excessive cost (WHO 2022).

Tissue engineering, organ bioprinting, and assistive devices like prostheses or orthoses to fulfill the biomechanical demands of persons with physical limitations are all significantly impacted by AM technology. Traditional production methods for orthoses and prostheses waste materials take a long time and involve a lot of labor.

Prosthesis or orthosis can receive help from the AM technology by customizing the assistive device for patients. Using current traditional manufacturing processes, patients have a limited choice of off-the-shelf replacement components. These solutions can be uncomfortable for the patient, especially as they are often quite heavy and need to fit perfectly. The AM components are often customizable, lightweight, and more comfortable for the patient.

6.3.2 AM for Medical Device Maintenance

Medical devices that are physically similar to the natural bone are beneficial. The use of AM technologies to fabricate patient-specific devices will reduce the need for replacement and maintenance. Furthermore, certain customized product designs are more cost-effective when produced by AM technologies and reduce lead time to manufacture. Through an optimal design, AM lowers material usage and material waste and builds weight. Due to this, AM has a lower environmental effect than conventional production techniques.

6.3.2.1 Application AM Biomedical Devices in Developing Countries

The concept of AM is indeed making a substantial contribution to the medical practices of developing countries. AM is widely employed in the production of customizable prosthetics and implants from a wide range of materials, including biomedical materials, and is enhancing orthopedic technology and treatment benefits using polymers, ceramics, and metals. Both patients and manufacturers are beginning to experience significant enhancements in product quality and profitability.

It is also important to note that timescales for bespoke AM products are often lower than for conventional manufacturing, which benefits patients even more. A cost-benefit analysis of implementing AM technology in medical facilities revealed that such advances improve complex procedures and would be a vital tool in alleviating time and budgetary strains for healthcare.

It is clear that the possibilities for AM application in the healthcare business are limitless, with the potential to improve society's quality of life, minimize healthcare expenditures, and also saving lives in developing countries.

6.4 Use of AR Interface for AM of Biomedical Applications

6.4.1 AR as an Assistive Technology in Design and Manufacturing

The use of engineered materials with new properties and performance created and prepared by microstructure and composition design can be used in the AM process, which offers significant opportunities for designing and fabricating complex structures with various functionalities, such as complex curved surfaces, hierarchical lattice, and thin wall/hollow structures. Another beneficial design technique is part consolidation, which involves turning several printed pieces from an assembly into a single part (Tian et al. 2022).

For designers and operators, augmented reality (AR) offers an immersive modeling environment or an interactive virtual assembly environment that enables intuitive interaction with the information of the creation/production process in their actual surroundings (Lhachemi et al. 2019). The conventional unidirectional AM technique is one through which a digital 3D model of the component is created. The technique does not permit design changes during the printing process, and the item is then fabricated. AR allows an iterative approach to the design and AM of components.

6.4.2 AR as an Assistive Technology in Training in the Use of AM of Biomedical Applications

A broader control framework is necessary for large-scale manufacturing that employs multiple AM systems and highly automated machine tools. Managing multiple types of machinery and checking their performance using their traditional physical user interfaces is often challenging. However, with an AR control interface, these interfaces can be dynamically scaled. Such an interface allows for constant modification and iterative adaptation to the various use cases. Controlling several devices through a single AR user interface is one example (Eiríksson et al. 2017).

The capacity of AM to create parts with complicated geometry makes it unique and suited for producing specialized, one-of-a-kind products for biomedical applications (Obeidi et al. 2022). In the biomedical industry, AR is a crucial training tool for biomedical applications and usage in AM. These two technologies working together is a step toward the Industrial 4.0 workplace. For machines equipped with sensors and connected to other machines and the cloud, this next-generation industrial area will be the ideal setting. It will be a perfect space for machines enabled with data analytics. The desire for access to such capabilities and data will redefine the role of people. New methods for engagement, feedback, and monitoring will also be created as a result of this transformation (Borish and Westfall 2020).

The potential for AR in AM training is significant, as it can supply a more realistic and interactive experience for users. The use of AR in AM training can help improve efficiency and accuracy while reducing costs. AR can also be used to train multiple users simultaneously, which is not possible with traditional methods such as manual or computer-based training. AR has the potential to revolutionize the way that AM training is conducted, making it more efficient and effective. AR can be used in the medical manufacturing industry and various other industries.

AR has been identified as a potentially transformative technology for training in the use of AM for biomedical applications. It has been shown to improve learning outcomes and the transfer of knowledge in various domains, and it has the potential to supply similar benefits for trainees in AM biomedical applications. AR can be used to supply contextualized information and feedback to trainees, which can help them understand and visualize complex processes. It can also be used to create virtual environments in which trainees can practice using AM equipment and techniques. Furthermore, AR can be used to create customized training programs tailored to each trainee's individual needs. Overall, AR has immense potential to improve training in the use of AM for biomedical applications, and it is a promising new area of research.

In a variety of applications, including biomedical ones, AR can be used as a feedback tool to enhance the production process. Through the use of immersive computer-generated information like sights, audio, touch interactions, and more, users' real-world surroundings can be enhanced. The ability to naturally engage with information about the creation/production process in their immediate physical surroundings is provided by AR for designers and operators (Lhachemi et al. 2019).

Additionally, AR can ease maintenance. For instance, technicians can display the information they need at once onto the part they are working on when inspecting or repairing a machine. By doing away with the need to go through charts and instruction manuals, time is saved. Additionally, the projected information supports the operator, enabling even a worker with basic ability to complete the required repair. Additionally, AR can be used to deliver expert advice without the requirement for professionals to fly halfway around the world. Anyone wearing AR glasses can receive remote guidance from a qualified individual, who helps by simulating the actions that the employee should perform. Additionally, new hires can be trained using this manner. Additionally, AR can be quite beneficial in preparing staff for emergency operations (Nikolaidou 2022).

Technologies like AR and three-dimensional printing have a variety of uses in the medical industry. In the case of AR, its interaction with virtual 3D models and real-world surroundings supports doctors' education and training, communication with other medical experts, and direction during clinical procedures. The development of patient-specific, adaptable tools and the production of 3D models of a patient's anatomy have both received help from 3D printing, which can enhance preoperative planning and therapeutic treatments.

The next obvious step is to combine AR with 3D printing technology, as both aid in enhancing orientation, guidance, and spatial abilities during medical procedures. According to earlier study, their combined usage can improve patient education, make it easier to explain medical issues and recommended therapies optimize surgical workflow, and improve patient-to-model registration. Despite the exponential growth of these technologies in recent years, physicians have not yet adopted them in large numbers since doing so requires substantial technical and software development ability (Moreta-Martinez et al. 2020).

6.4.3 Types of AR Interfaces for AM of Biomedical Applications

A variety of AR interfaces are used in AM for different biomedical applications. A 3D-printed construct is developed from Microtomographic Images for bone tissue engineering with an excellent biological response (Pérez-Sánchez et al. 2021). The scaffold design involves the generation of digital imaging and communication in medicine (DICOM) images. These images are generated using Albira Reconstructor software, which generates a 558 × 558 × 516 image matrix with a voxel size of 125 μm^3. Layer-by-layer extrusion melt deposition was used to print the scaffold using polylactic acid (PLA) (FDA approved) filament with a 1.75 mm thickness that was acquired from 3D Printers Puebla. The scaffold has a 3D, uniform, close-pore, shape and a 130 μm square pore size and the size of the calvaria defect. The scaffold has a thickness of 1.90 mm and an overall diameter of 9 mm.

A 3D-printed, customized brachytherapy applicator for vaginal topography and guided needle source channels can be used for gynecological cancer patients. Customized applicators (Laan et al. 2019) were created using the MRI data of two women with gynecological cancer. For intracavitary and guided interstitial needle implantation, the applicators have curved needle canals. Increased normal forces and friction are the results of driving needle deflections within applicators. This friction may start to dominate the insertion force for designs with large or multiple curves.

Porous metal structures with lower strength and ingrowth tendency, akin to bones, are now being used for biomedical implants in the field of orthopedic regenerative medical investigations. Such replicable topology or designable microarchitecture porous metal structures can be created via AM. The biomedical sector uses these synthetic pore geometries primarily to increase the product's biocompatibility by simulating bone (Balcı et al. 2021).

In a computer environment, the 3D models of the trabecular bone and samples were aligned to look for changes in the size and angle of the arms in the trabecular structure. It was shown that the deviations decreased when the angle was over 60°; nevertheless, when the size was below 150 μm, they sharply increased. The size distribution and interconnectivity ratio of the pores created during manufacture were determined using PNMs. Given that the mean equivalent diameters of the vertebral and femoral pores, as determined by the pore network models, are 767 ± 265 m and 623 ± 245 m, respectively, it was demonstrated that the samples made in the scales of 1:1 and 1:1.25 may represent the pore size distribution in the bone.

Fixation plates are created using easily accessible, biocompatible metals including stainless steel, titanium, and its alloys. The stiffness mismatch between these plates and bone, however, causes stress shielding and bone loss. It is necessary to look into using topology optimization and AM together to produce fixation plates that are less stiff and have better biological performance (Al-Tamimi et al. 2020). Fixation plates were developed using the solid isotropic microstructure with penalization (SIMP) approach under various loading situations (compression, bending, torsion, and combinations of all these loads) (Al-Tamimi et al. 2017).

Utilizing computed tomography (CT) scan data and DICOM files, implants can be created that are unique to a patient (Modi and Sanadhya 2018). To create the tailored implants, these models were imported into the Geomagic Freeform program from 3D Systems. The strength of the cranium implant was determined by finite element analysis. It was found that the maximum von Mises stress and deformation were far below the material's permissible limit. Physical models of the skull, pelvic bone, and implant prototypes, including the cranial, ilium, pubic symphysis, and ischium, were made using a selective laser-sintering machine. One of the main clinical difficulties in orthopedics is the correction of osteochondral abnormalities. Large abnormalities, however, have had less success, mostly due to the joint's mechanical environment and the tissue's heterogeneity. A multi-layered osteochondral scaffold is produced utilizing AM technology, which combines the heterogeneous character of osteochondral tissue with cutting-edge laser sintering and material extrusion methods (Tamaddon et al. 2021). The created scaffold is built on a composite system that consists of a titanium and polylactic acid matrix-reinforced collagen "sandwich." An ovine condyle model was used to investigate the scaffold's safety and effectiveness in repairing significant osteochondral lesions, as well as its microstructure and mechanical characteristics.

6.5 Trends and Future Possibilities

Cai et al. employed AR to create a cyber-physical link between a reconfigurable AM system and its matching digital twin for toolpath planning and simulation to exchange layout data. The spatial relationships between various physical objects (camera, robotic arms, component substrate, etc.) are discovered using the AR marker tracing approach, which also directs the user to place the robotic arms in the simulation's predetermined places. This system allowed for fast retrieval of position information from the physical system layout into the digital twin optimization simulation; this facilitated the deployment of an optimized layout determined in the digital twin into the physical system (Caia et al. 2020). The increasing use of AR as a visual tool bridge between data acquired from IoT sensors in the physical environment and digital twin simulation models, can lead to personalized and rapid manufacturing of medical prosthesis artifacts.

Furthermore, bioengineering and the medical sciences have experienced major advancements because of nanomaterials (Velu 2020). Although nanomaterials have been used in medical implants for a few decades already, it is still challenging to make them compatible with new AM technologies, especially for specialized medical applications. Researchers from a range of disciplines, including bioengineering and mechanical engineering, now have the chance to gain insight into the selection of the best materials for 3D printing based on the type of application. The quick commercialization of AM technology for medical implant applications will be made possible by a thorough analysis of the physics of material selection, process optimization, and design/geometry requirements (Velu 2020).

6.6 Conclusion

In this chapter, we provided an overview of AR and AM and discussed the uses of AM for biomedical applications and how AR can be used as an assistive tool to assist in the design and manufacturing of biomedical artifacts. The examples provided are incomplete as this research field is developing rapidly, and innovative techniques to combine the two fields will be developed in the future.

References

Al-Tamimi AA, Fernandes PR, Peach C, Cooper G, Diver C, Bartolo PJ (2017) Metallic bone fixation implants: a novel design approach for reducing the stress shielding phenomenon. Virtual Phys Prototyping 12:141–151. https://doi.org/10.1080/17452759.2017.1307769

Al-Tamimi AA, Hernandez MA, Omar A, Morales-Aldana DF, Peach C, Bartolo P (2020) Mechanical, biological and tribological behaviour of fixation plates 3D printed by electron beam and selective laser melting. Int J Adv Manuf Technol 109:673–688. https://doi.org/10.1007/s00170-020-05676-1

Balcı A, Küçükaltun F, Aycan MF, Usta Y, Demir T (2021) Reproducibility of replicated trabecular bone structures from Ti6Al4V. Arab J Sci Eng 46:2527–2541. https://doi.org/10.1007/s13369-020-05145-7

Borish M, Westfall J (2020) Additive and subtractive manufacturing augmented reality interface (ASMARI). In: 2020 SoutheastCon, pp 1–6

Caia Y, Wangb Y, Burnetta M (2020) Using augmented reality to build digital twin for reconfigurable additive manufacturing system. J Manuf Syst 56:598–604

Eiríksson ER, Pedersen DB, Frisvad JR, Skovmand L, Heun V, Maes P, Aanæs H (2017) Augmented reality interfaces for additive manufacturing. In: Scandinavian conference on image analysis, Lecture notes in computer science, vol 10269. Springer, pp 515–525

Gartner Glossary (2022) Augmented reality (AR), 2022-10-5. Retrieved from Gartner Glossary: https://www.gartner.com/en/information-technology/glossary/augmented-reality-ar

Gillis AS (2022) What is augmented reality (AR)? 2022-10-5. Retrieved from TechTarget: https://www.techtarget.com/whatis/definition/augmented-reality-AR

Hench LL, Jones JR (2005) Biomaterials, artificial organs and tissue engineering. Woodhead Publishing

Hunter L (2017) Augmented reality for the industrial enterprise. O'Reilly Media

Laan RC, Nout RA, Dankelman J, van de Berg NJ (2019) MRI-driven design of customised 3D printed gynaecological brachytherapy applicators with curved needle channels. 3D Print Med 5. https://doi.org/10.1186/s41205-019-0047-x

Lhachemi H, Malik A, Shorten R (2019) Augmented reality, cyber-physical systems, and feedback control for additive manufacturing: a review. IEEE Access 7:50119–50135

Modi YK, Sanadhya S (2018) Design and additive manufacturing of patient-specific cranial and pelvic bone implants from computed tomography data. J Braz Soc Mech Sci Eng 40. https://doi.org/10.1007/s40430-018-1425-9

Moreta-Martinez R, García-Mato D, García-Sevilla M, Pérez-Mañanes R, Calvo-Haro JA, Pascau J (2020) Combining augmented reality and 3D printing to display patient models on a smartphone. J Vis Med. https://doi.org/10.3791/60618

Nikolaidou N (2022) Augmented and virtual reality in advanced manufacturing. Digital transformation in advanced manufacturing, 8 Apr 2022. Retrieved from https://dtamproject.eu/augmented-and-virtual-reality-in-advanced-manufacturing/

Obeidi MA, Karazi S, Kinahan D, Culliton D, Brabazon D (September 2022) Additive manufacturing virtual reality lab for training industry employees and engineering students. In: Eighth international symposium for engineering education. The University of Strathclyde

Papagiannis H (2022) Designing beyond screens to augment the full human sensorium, 2022-10-5. Retrieved from O'Reilly: https://www.oreilly.com/ideas/designing-beyond-screens-to-augment-the-full-human-sensorium

Pérez-Sánchez L, Ortiz de la O MA, González-Alva P, Medina LA, Masuoka-Ito D, Alvarez-Perez MA, Serrano-Bello J (2021) In vivo study on bone response to 3D-printed constructs designed from microtomographic images. J Mater Eng Perform 30:5005–5012. https://doi.org/10.1007/s11665-021-05585-8

Sreeraj PR, Mishra SK, Singh PK (2022) A review on non-destructive evaluation and characterization of additively manufactured components. Progress Addit Manuf 7:225

Surjadi JU, Gao L, Du H, Li X, Xiong X, Fang NX, Lu Y (2019) Mechanical metamaterials and their engineering applications. Adv Eng Mater 21:1800864

Tamaddon M, Blunn G, Tan R, Yang P, Sun X, Chen SM (2021) In vivo evaluation of additively manufactured multi-layered scaffold. Biodesign Manuf 5:481. https://doi.org/10.1007/s42242-021-00177-w

Taqvi Z (2013) Reality and perception: utilization of many facets of augmented reality. In: 23rd International conference on artificial reality and telexistence (ICAT). IEEE, pp 11–12

Thompson SM, Bian L, Shamsaei N, Yadollahi A (2015) An overview of direct laser deposition for additive manufacturing; part I: transport phenomena, modeling and diagnostics. Addit Manuf 8: 36–62

Tian X, Wu L, Gu D, Yuan S, Zhao Y, Li X et al (2022) Roadmap for additive manufacturing: toward intellectualization and industrialization. Chin J Mech Eng Addit Manuf Front 1:100014

Velu RC (2020) A comprehensive review on bio-nanomaterials for medical implants and feasibility studies on fabrication of such implants by additive manufacturing technique. Materials 13:92

WHO (2022) Retrieved from WHO standards for prosthetics and orthotics, 14 Oct 2022. https://www.who.int/publications/i/item/9789241512480

Wikipedia (2022) Augmented reality, 2022-10-5. Retrieved from Wikipedia: https://en.wikipedia.org/wiki/Augmented_reality

Design Tools and Methods for Design for Additive Manufacturing (AM) of Medical Devices

7

Yojana Sharma, Parnika Shrivastava, and Mohit Pant

Contents

Abstract

With today's rapid market growth, new opportunities and challenges are emerging in the medical sector. Additive manufacturing (AM) has been used to create geometrically complicated shapes as a flexible and economic method that allows for personalised and adaptable design solutions. It's a digital manufacturing process that's reshaping the healthcare industry by printing customised medical devices and unique body parts with inherent structures. It also represents a huge step forward in the development of patient-specific

Y. Sharma · M. Pant
Department of Mechanical Engineering, National Institute of Technology Hamirpur, Hamirpur, Himachal Pradesh, India

P. Shrivastava (✉)
Department of Mechanical Engineering, Dr. B.R. Ambedkar National Institute of Technology, Jalandhar, Punjab, India
e-mail: shrivastavap@nitj.ac.in

R. Velu et al. (eds.), *Digital Design and Manufacturing of Medical Devices and Systems*, https://doi.org/10.1007/978-981-99-7100-8_7

medications. The chapter lays out the understanding of AM technologies and is classified as per the American Society for Testing and Materials (ASTM) standards. The chapter, in particular, focuses on the capabilities of AM in the creation of medical devices and technology. The medical devices are classified as medical equipment, bio-fabricated implants and drug delivery systems, which are further elaborated in this chapter. Different types of design tools and methods for designing medical devices by AM are explained. AM technology is ushering in a new age, particularly in the production of medical devices, enabling designers to push the limits of design complexity. Still, there are significant technological limitations with AM that must be worked around throughout the design and manufacturing stages. The purpose here is to highlight the benefits of AM applications in the medical field while also elucidating their current limitations. Future research prospects regarding the use of AM in the medical field are discussed in the chapter's conclusion.

Keywords

Medical device · Additive manufacturing · Design tools and methods · CAD/CAM/CAE · FEA · Structure optimisation · 3D printers · 3D scanners

7.1 Introduction to AM Processes

Additive manufacturing (AM) is a production process. Through layer-by-layer deposition of materials, AM converts a computer-aided design (CAD) model into a 3D object. AM revolutionised manufacturing in the 1980s. It has advantages over traditional approaches. AM is rapid and cost-effective, and its design ability enables complex geometries. AM was quickly built to meet the needs of patients and doctors, and it was used in medical engineering soon after its conception. ASTM and ISO standards recognise seven additive manufacturing methods that have been modified for healthcare: sheet lamination, material extrusion, material and binder jetting, powder bed fusion, vat photopolymerisation and direct energy deposition are examples (Culmone et al. 2019).

7.2 Medical Device

Any item created with the intent of aiding in medical treatment is considered a medical device. Devices used in medicine encompass anything from needles and syringes to X-ray machines and surgical instruments to pacemakers and artificial limbs. AM has developed in recent years to become a versatile and cost-effective method for creating medical equipment with complex geometrical shapes (Thanigaiarasu 2020).

Definition and Concepts
Any hardware, software or substance designed to aid in the medical analysis, prognosis, monitoring or treatment of an illness is considered a 'medical device', where 'illness' includes any adverse health changes, including injuries and mental health (Santos 2013).

Medical devices can be classified as follows:

7.2.1 Medical Equipment

Essentially, medical equipment is a tool used to examine and treat patients. Such a tool comes into direct contact with the patients. AM has created various types of medical equipment that can be used for both diagnosing and treating patients. Various types of medical equipment are discussed in the following subsections.

7.2.1.1 Diagnostic Tools

Diagnostic tools are used for the detection of various diseases. The application of AM has made it possible for better evaluation and assessment as well as more precise diagnosis. CT scans and other medical imaging techniques are non-invasive diagnostic tools. The visualisation of organ anatomy specific to a patient is also made easier by AM. Liver models, tumours, kidneys and a 3D-printed brain system are some examples of anatomical models made with AM techniques. Such anatomical models are very helpful for surgical planning and teaching (Li et al. 2020).

7.2.1.2 Therapeutic Tools

Therapeutic tools are mainly of three types: prostheses, orthoses and surgical tools. Prostheses are an alternative to missing body parts. Various prosthetics are known as above elbow (AE), below elbow (BE), above knee (AK) and below knee (BK) prosthetics (Li et al. 2020). Patients with bone injuries often benefit from orthoses, which provide support based on biomechanical requirements to alleviate pain and improve mobility. Plaster, splints and braces are examples of orthopaedic devices. Surgical instruments are used for surgical treatment. Surgical tools can be general-purpose or specific-purpose. General-purpose tools are intended for use with small incisions. Surgical kits are examples of general-purpose surgical instruments (Fig. 7.1). A thermo-coagulator, which is used in the treatment of gynaecological cancer, and an MRI-compatible device, which is used to alleviate the pain of bone cancer, are examples of specific-purpose surgical tools.

7.2.2 Medical Implants

Medical implants are artificial devices that partially or completely reside in the human body for monitoring, diagnosis or therapeutic purposes. Implants can be either hard or soft in structure. Dental implants, orthopaedic implants and cardiovascular stents are hard-structure implants. Tissue implants are soft-structure implants.

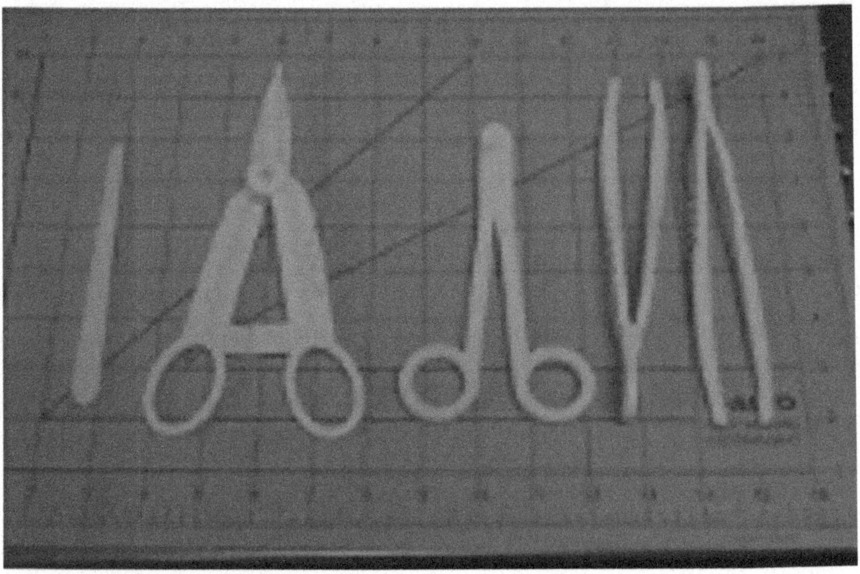

Fig. 7.1 Surgical kit (scalpel handle, haemostats, needle drivers, forceps) (George et al. 2017. Copyright 2016. Reproduced with permission of Springer Nature)

Hard structures often support mechanical loads, whereas soft constructs or structures primarily support biological and chemical functions, such as neural processing and skeletal muscle contraction. Different types of medical implants are discussed below.

7.2.2.1 Dental Implants

Dental decay is a very common issue in humans. Dental implants are inserted to replace missing or decayed teeth. Dental implants can be produced using a lot of AM, a relatively new and developing technique. There are four main types of dental implants used today (Selvaraj et al. 2022). Kshirsagar and Dhatrak presented CAD model of dental implant and its parts (Fig. 7.2):

(a) Sub-periosteal shape
(b) Blade design
(c) Ramus structure
(d) Endo-osseous form

7.2.2.2 Orthopaedics

Orthopaedic implants are substitutes for defective bones and joints. There are two categories of orthopaedic implants: one is permanent joint replacement, and the other is temporary fracture fixation devices. Knee, elbow, hip, wrist and shoulder are examples of permanent joint replacement, and plates, wires, screws and pins are

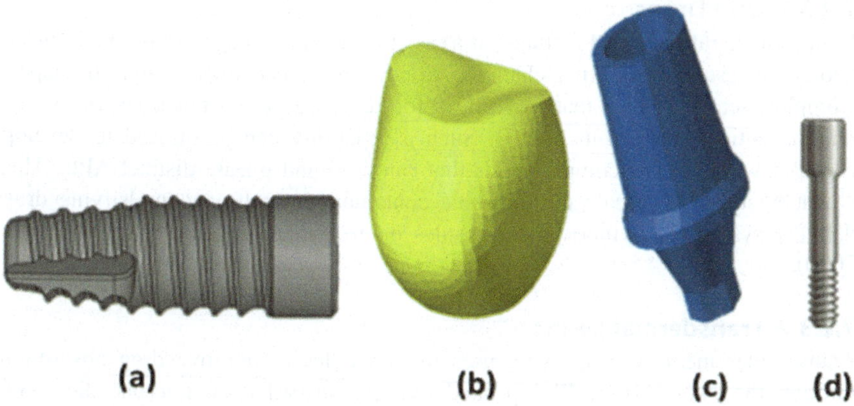

Fig. 7.2 CAD model of (**a**) dental implant, (**b**) crown, (**c**) abutment, (**d**) screw (Kshirsagar and Dhatrak 2023. Copyright 2023. Reproduced with permission of Elsevier)

examples of temporary fracture fixation devices. AM allows for the simple fabrication of complex orthopaedic implant shapes (Jin and Chu 2019).

7.2.2.3 Cardiovascular Stents

Coronary heart disease is dangerous, and it is a leading cause of mortality in our growing world. It occurs when arteries become narrowed due to plaque buildup. Stents are used for treating such diseases. Cardiovascular stents are expandable tubular mesh constructions that may be inserted into constricted arteries to widen and open the lumen without requiring open-heart surgery. Cardiovascular stents come in bare metal (BMS), drug-eluting (DES) and bio-resorbable (BRS) varieties (Scafa Udrişte et al. 2021).

7.2.2.4 Tissue Implants

Tissue implants are soft, structured medical implants used for the reconstruction of tissue voids. Due to an accident or any harmful disease, tissues get damaged. Different types of biomaterials are used to make tissue scaffolds. The reconstruction of the intricate structure of tissue is easy with the help of AM technologies.

7.2.3 Drug Delivery System

A growing number of papers discuss the development of pharmacological formulations using AM methods, including transdermal and oral medications. AM is especially helpful for promoting the release of insoluble molecules that can't be released. Using AM technology, oral and transdermal medication delivery techniques to the body are capable of development (Li et al. 2020).

7.2.3.1 Oral Drugs

Using a wide range of AM methods, it's easy to construct dosage forms with intricate geometries, such as internal channels, honeycombs, networks or gyroid shapes. Complex scaffolds and matrices allow for drug-loaded formulations or Active pharmaceutical Ingredients (APIs). Such a capability can be utilised to develop capsules with specific compartments that can hold and release distinct APIs. This characteristic helps create customisable containers for self-nanoemulsifying drug delivery systems, polymeric nanocapsules or drug-filled alginate beads (Li et al. 2020).

7.2.3.2 Transdermal Drugs

Transdermal medication delivery uses microneedles to improve drug absorption through the skin barrier. SLA-printed pyramid-shaped resin microneedles with insulin-xylitol coatings demonstrated fast insulin release and protein integrity. Post-fabrication chemical etching was used to optimise the microneedles' geometrical properties. A microneedle-customised splint was used to treat trigger finger by adjusting medication administration for skin curvature. A bioinspired needle was manufactured using AM to resemble honeybee stinger barbs to lessen percutaneous extraction and insertion forces (Li et al. 2020).

7.3 Design Tools and Methods for Designing Medical Devices by AM Technique

Design for additive manufacturing (DfAM) is a collection of principles, guidelines, tools and expertise that encourages designers to incorporate additive manufacturing during the product design phase. DfAM requires design considerations. These included manufacturing process, material, layer thickness, support structure placement (if needed) and component production orientation. Recent advancements in the accuracy, dependability, range of processable materials and commercial availability of AM processes make them ideal candidates for the creation of parts that are used in the medical industry. The complexity-for-free property of AM makes it possible to create extremely complicated designs, and batch-size independence facilitates the creation of customised medical equipment (Zadpoor 2017). DfAM strategies aim to maximise the use of these aspects in the development of medical devices with significantly improved performance. Moreover, the form freedom and simplicity characteristics of AM make it possible to use design optimisation strategies that aim to minimise weight, maximise stiffness, improve fatigue life and extend the lifespan of medical devices.

For the effective and efficient design of medical devices using AM, the following DfAM tools and techniques are utilised:

7.3.1 Designing for Structure Optimisation

With the help of AM techniques, very complex structures can be made, and the complexity of the part has no effect on the cost of production. Bulky products are usually not desired, so to mitigate the weight of the product, the structure of the product can be optimised. Some tools for structure optimisation are given below.

7.3.1.1 Topology Optimisation

To alleviate the waste and weight of the product, topology optimisation is an effective technique. Topology optimisation is an objective function-driven technique in which constraints are defined to maximise or minimise the objective function. AM techniques are the best for the fabrication of optimised designs due to their ability to manufacture complex structures. But manufacturing constraints also should be considered in topology optimisation; otherwise, it may result in a significant increment in cost and geometry, which will be difficult to manufacture. Topology optimisation is an iteration-based technique in which optimum material use is achieved without compromising strength (Jankovics et al. 2018). There are various methods of topology optimisation, like solid isotropic material with penalisation (SIMP), bi-directional evolutionary structural optimisation (BESO), the level set method and the geometry projection method. Different software is used for topology optimisation. ANSYS, ABAQOUS and MATLAB are some of them. Wu et al. described the orthopaedic use of topology optimisation (Wu et al. 2021). Iqbal et al. formulated a method of topology optimisation for designing a pelvic prosthesis with low weight and high strength (Iqbal et al. 2019). Silva et al. optimzed the topology of the core geometry of the dental bridge (Fig. 7.3).

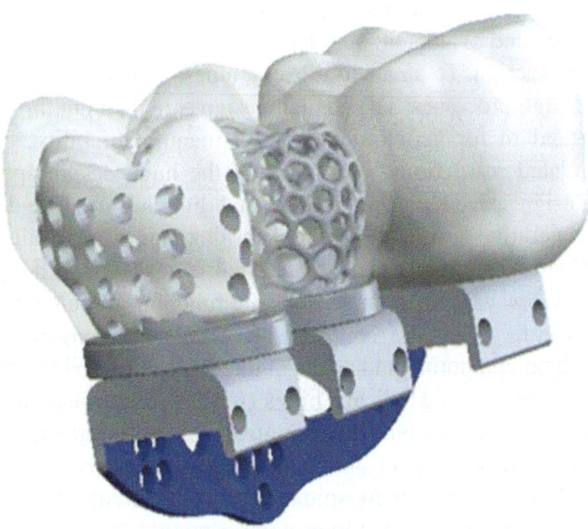

Fig. 7.3 Topology optimisation of the core geometry of the dental bridge (Silva et al. 2017. Copyright 2017. Reproduced with permission of Elsevier)

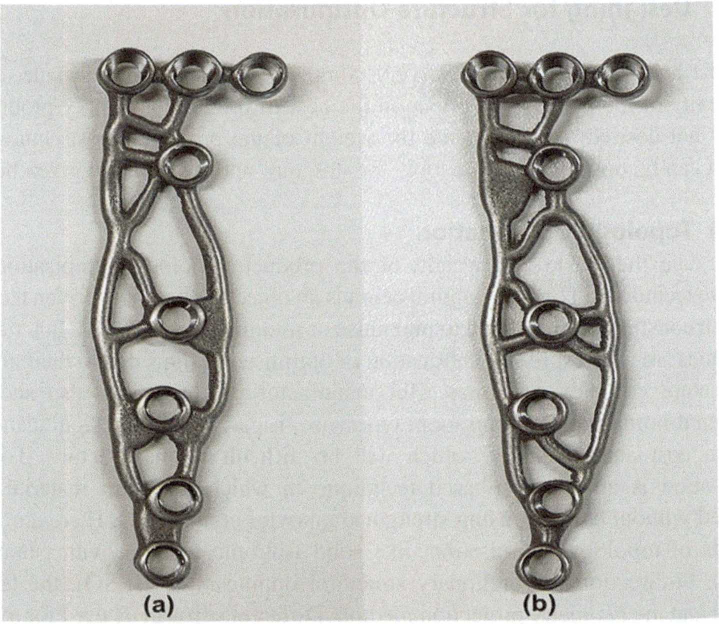

Fig. 7.4 Generatively designed high tibial osteotomy fixation plates (a) plate a and (b) plate b (Kanagalingam et al. 2022. Copyright 2022. Reproduced with permission of Springer Nature)

7.3.1.2 Generative Design

Generic design is 'the rules for making form, not the shapes' (Leary 2020). This method comprises three phases: problem description, where the issue's limitations and goals are outlined; embodiment design, where high-level solutions are developed and evaluated; and detail design, in which the chosen solution is specified for production. To create usable outcomes, generative design must supplant one or more design processes. The created designs are then put through constraint envelopes that stand in for geometric viability, manufacturability, cost and other performance-related restrictions, which shrink the huge design space into a more manageable design space represented by outstanding designs. The designer can improve them. In generative design, a machine-learning algorithm produces outputs that comply with limits. This method generates biomedical device design possibilities. Biomedical devices vary in complexity and function. When generative design and additive manufacturing are coupled, biomedical equipment is more useful and cheaper. Cloud computing and artificial intelligence (AI) algorithms enable generative design for Internet of Medical Things (IoMT)-based medical devices (Dilibal et al. 2021). Zhang et al. employed generative design to reduce a dental component's support structure (Zhang et al. 2020). Using generative design, Murzac et al. created a patient-specific smart spinal orthosis (Murzac et al. 2021). Kanagalingam et al. generatively designed high tibial osteotomy fixation plates (Fig. 7.4).

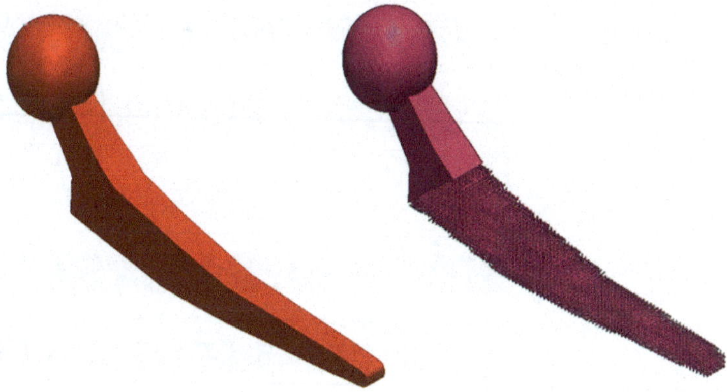

Fig. 7.5 CAD of a hip implant (**a**) conventional implant and (**b**) integrated lattice designed implant (Burton et al. 2019. Copyright 2019. Reproduced with permission of Elsevier)

7.3.1.3 Lattice Structure Filling

Material may be added to or subtracted from the design space directly using topology optimisation or generative design approaches, but there are problems. Human knowledge can be used in generative design to connectively select alternative solutions in order to establish a compromise and minimise the complexity of the problem. Filling pre-determined unit structures or lattices in place of solid volumes in a way that is equivalent to the optimal design solution is another technique to find a middle ground.

One of two strategies can be used to build lattice structures: (1) homogenisation or (2) density-based mapping. The lattice structure in the first is homogenised into volume elements that resemble solid substances. The lattice structures resemble a typical solid structure's microporosity in homogenised volumes. The special volumes can then be operated using traditional topology optimisation or alternative optimisation techniques after the representative volumes have been given specific features.

The second technique, which improves mechanical response approximation, transfers density values from non-penalised topology optimisation onto explicit, preset lattice structures with optional adaptability. This method can be used to produce uniform or graded lattice structures (Vaneker et al. 2020). Burton et al. designed the conventional and integrated lattice designed implant (Fig. 7.5).

7.3.1.4 Methods for Optimising Surface Structure

Finding the universal ideal for structural design is often difficult. In similar circumstances, one might look to nature for a solution. Natural porous structures, like artificial lattice structures, serve as a collection of distinct features to address particular design requirements. Lightweight infill, porous scaffolds, energy

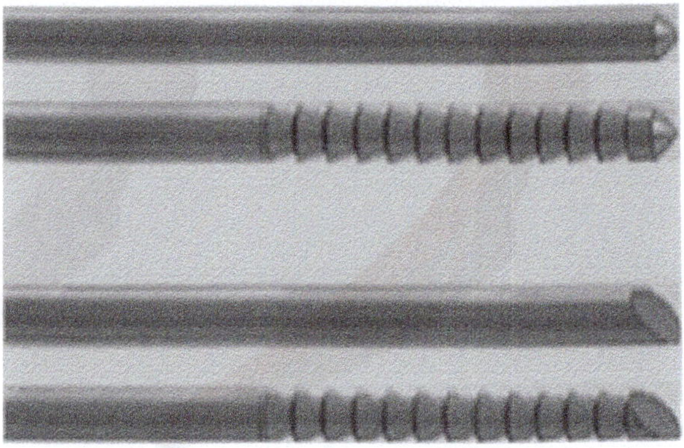

Fig. 7.6 Honeybee-inspired needle (Ma et al. 2022. Copyright 2022. Reproduced with permission of Elsevier)

absorbers and self-adapting constructions are a few examples. These structures and how they work have been understood for some time, but because of AM's capacity to create such sophisticated structures, they are now incorporated into the design principles that product developers can use. As a result, a new design technique known as 'bio-inspired' or 'biomimetic design' is created by the imitation and post-processing of complex topologies that are inspired by nature or are produced randomly. Its objective is to produce either multifunctional surface structures or lightweight structures with surprising mechanical properties. In this field, two design methodologies are typically used: general bio-inspiration using design principles or guidelines and direct or indirect replication of natural topologies using reverse engineering.

The main methods for fabricating irregular porous structures from an initial design with complex interior surface topologies include either filling or hollowing materials using specific algorithms. Triply periodic minimal surface (TPMS), an implicit surface with complex structures, is an example of a filling technique (Vaneker et al. 2020). Ma et al. designed honeybee-inspired needle (Fig. 7.6).

7.3.2 Product Design Tools

The following sections will discuss the various types of design tools used in the additive manufacturing of medical devices:

7.3.2.1 Integrated CAD-CAM Tools

CAD is the use of computer technology to facilitate the conception, modification, analysis and optimisation of a design. The orthotic and prosthetic industry has benefited from the use of CAD/CAM technology by raising the calibre of medical equipment. Maxillofacial traumatology and reconstructive surgery have lately benefited from the effective use of CAD and CAM to enhance the accuracy and predictability of surgical methods in difficult clinical circumstances. CAD/CAM technology allows surgeons to model the process on a computer, conduct virtual

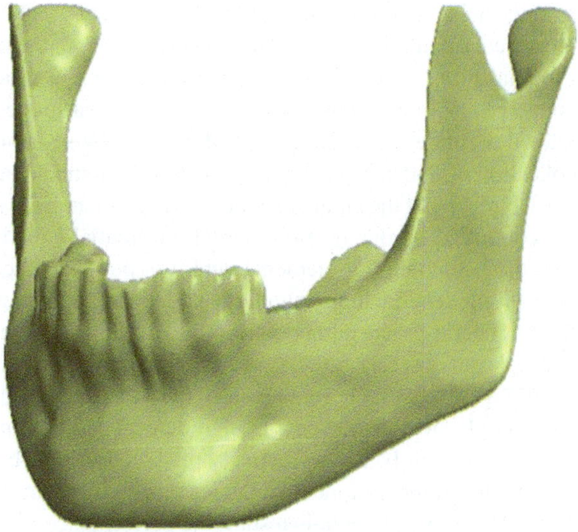

Fig. 7.7 3D CAD model of maxilla (Silva et al. 2017. Copyright 2017. Reproduced with the permission of Elsevier)

fragment repositioning, choose the optimum fixation technique and improve surgical precision by producing and immediately applying navigation guides or patient-specific implants.

Microvascular-free flap restoration has remained the gold standard for repairing major tissue defects after ablative head and neck oncologic surgery, especially for bony structures. Three-dimensionally printed models and tools, as well as CAD/CAM, provide inventive solutions for the reconstruction of bony anomalies (Nyirjesy et al. 2022). The 3D model can be created and modified using CAD software such as 3D Systems, Geomagic, Freeform, Materialise 3-Matic and others. Materialise mimics, 3D Systems D2P, Simpleware scanIP, Vitrea and 3D slicers are used to convert DICOM images to 3D models. Nyirjesy et al. explained the role of these systems in head and neck oncologic surgery. Abbas used UG-NX-5 software for designing (Abbas 2012). Ardila et al. used the softwares Invesalius, 3D Slicer, Solid Works and Rhinoceros for developing customised craniofacial devices (Ardila et al. 2018). Moiduddin et al. also used mimics and 3-Matics for designing customised porous plates for mandibular reconstruction (Moiduddin et al. 2017). Mortadi et al. employed Free Form software for the manufacturing of dental appliances (al Mortadi et al. 2012). Sickel et al. used a CAD system that is similar to Magics and Shell Designer for designing a hearing aid device (Sickel et al. 2011). Silva et al. produced 3D CAD model of maxilla (Fig. 7.7).

7.3.2.2 CAE Tools

Design analysis and synthesis methods utilising computers and information technology are referred to as Computer Aided Engineering (CAE) (Bi 2018). The purpose of CAE tools is to aid designers in addressing increasingly complex, open-ended and/or interconnected design issues in the actual world. One of the most crucial methods among the several CAE tools is Finite Element Analysis (FEA). FEA is a sort of numerical calculation used to roughly estimate a mathematical model's solution. It is essential to accurately model design challenges in order for the approximation to converge. A continuous area of interest is partitioned into discrete sub-regions known as finite elements as part of the piecewise approximation used in FEA. A collection of nodes is used to represent each element, and the nodes' behaviours are used to represent the elements' behaviours, which in the relevant physical disciplines are controlled by one or more partial differential equations. Element models represent the behaviours of elements, and it is possible to create a system model using element models. Include boundary and load conditions in the system model to solve the engineering issue numerically. An FEA tool can numerically simulate any design concept and forecast how a system will behave and react under any conceivable operating condition. It enables designers to make final design adjustments before creating physical prototypes. Design defects can be found, and the performance of new designs can be cost-effectively predicted using FEA on computer models.

FAE has improved medical device design for years throughout product development. This typically entails testing the performance of a medical design in a virtual environment that simulates its intended use in the real world. A user may make informed recommendations for improving and optimising device performance using the findings of such a study (Driscoll 2019). ANSYS, ABAQOUS, HyperMesh and MATLAB are some CAE software frequently used in medical applications (Liu and Tovar 2014; Wu et al. 2021).

7.3.2.3 Reverse Engineering by 3D Scanners (Imaging Techniques)

Using a 3D scanner or image technology for medical purposes, reverse engineering is a method for creating a 3D virtual model of an object. 3D scanners are categorised based on attributes like resolution, accuracy, portability and price. In terms of technology adoption, 3D scanners and magnetic resonance imaging (MRIs) both have advantages and disadvantages. The undeformed geometry of a body component can be accurately captured with a 3D scanner, but the interior structure of the body part cannot be shown. MRI pictures make it possible to gather insightful information about a bodily part's internal tissues (Colombo et al. 2018). Rodin, Willowood and Vorum Spectra scanners are popular because they accurately recognise features in 3D models. On the other hand, affordable options are available to achieve the same result. A computed tomography (CT) scan is a type of diagnostic imaging exam that uses X-ray technology to create images of the body's internal structures. MRI is used for 3D reconstruction in many medical fields to help medical personnel diagnose patients more accurately. There are currently software solutions designed to create 3D models of specific objects. These applications rely on the application of sophisticated image processing techniques that enable the extraction of profiles related to a specific object from each 2D image of the MRI volume. Some open-source applications for 3D reconstruction have been created, including 3D Slicer, MITK, DeVide and Invesalius. Osirix and 3D Slicer, which may be used for diagnostics, surgery and 3D organ reconstruction for 3D printing and medical evaluation, are two of the most crucial tools among them (Fig. 7.8).

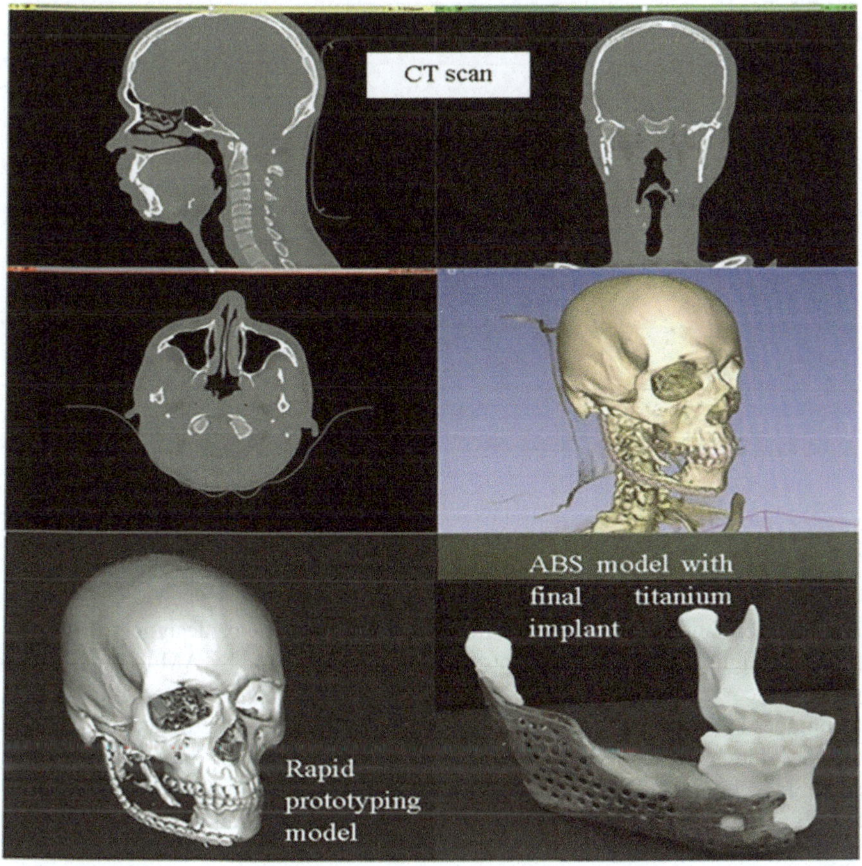

Fig. 7.8 CT scanned data to mandibular implant conversion (Popov et al. 2018. Copyright 2018. Reproduced with permission of Springer Nature)

7.3.2.4 Rapid Prototyping by 3D Printers

Clinicians can now investigate the use of 3D printing for pre-procedural planning, biomedical tissue modelling and direct fabrication of implantable devices thanks to recent advancements in the 3D printing sector. Although rapid prototyping and additive manufacturing methods are increasingly being used in the medical industry, many doctors lack the skills necessary to utilise this exciting and useful technology. A growing number of 3D printers and printable materials are also a result of the 3D printing industry's expansion. Therefore, in order to profit, it is crucial for clinicians to stay current with this fast-evolving profession. Digital surface models may easily be converted into physical models using 3D printers to enable quick prototyping. Medical fields that significantly rely on understanding complicated anatomical structural links for therapeutic interventions are increasingly using 3D printing (Fig. 7.9).

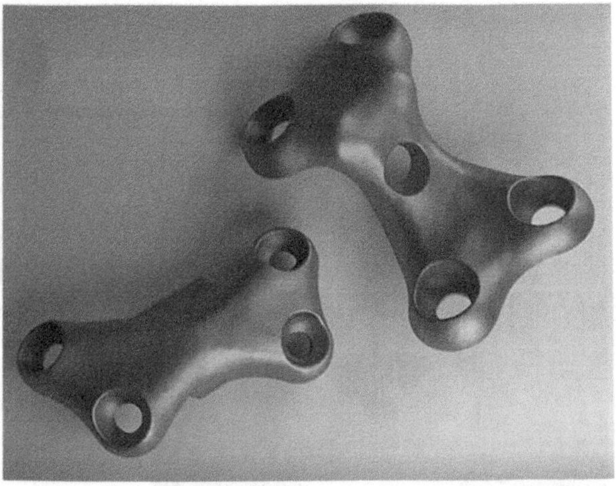

Fig. 7.9 Bone implants made by 3D printer (Popov et al. 2018. Copyright 2018. Reproduced with permission of Springer Nature)

7.4 Future Challenges and Opportunities

AM provides unrivalled degrees of freedom to medical device designers. The main goal of design for AM is to maximise the potential afforded by AM to improve the performance of medical devices. A variety of medical devices and imaging techniques have constraints. AM's main drawbacks are its limited material selection and accuracy. Additive bio-manufacturing materials must be biocompatible and sometimes biodegradable. Future AM techniques and biomaterials must solve those constraints. High-resolution medical images demand longer scanning periods, which increase ionising radiation and cost. Future imaging modalities and protocol design could alleviate some of these restrictions, giving higher-resolution pictures and increasing patient-specific design accuracy. Topology optimisation allows solutions beyond lightweight design to minimise support utilisation, thermal deformation, local heat input, material characteristics, porosity and strength. Most research in these domains is still immature and unavailable to product designers. TO approaches need improvement to address optimisation as a 3D challenge in all product development stages. Like TO, generative design methodologies create many design possibilities, but few manufacturing and inspection limitations are included. Methods and tactics should be developed to enable designers to select among the numerous, frequently comparable design possibilities. Absorption of energy and conduction of heat are aided by lattice structures. However, lattice structures are computationally demanding, limiting large lattice optimisation parameters.

7.5 Conclusion

An outline of the AM of medical devices is given in this chapter. We divided the medical devices into categories based on their clinical applications, innovation, justifications for adopting additive manufacturing and the specifics of the AM technology employed. The AM technology is paving the way for a customised treatment that will benefit people with unique anatomy or rare diseases. The design of medical devices makes extensive use of integrated CAD/CAM software, CAE tools, 3D printers and 3D scanners. To create a lightweight medical device, a variety of structural optimisation techniques are beneficial. The potential for generating patient-specific medical equipment is increased by AM, computer-aided simulations and FEA. A new generation of medical devices can be created by designers using AM in conjunction with the tools and processes previously stated.

References

Abbas AT (2012) Reconstruction skeleton for the lower human jaw using CAD/CAM/CAE. J King Saud Univ Eng Sci 24(2):159–164. https://doi.org/10.1016/j.jksues.2011.10.003

al Mortadi N, Eggbeer D, Lewis J, Williams RJ (2012) CAD/CAM/AM applications in the manufacture of dental appliances. Am J Orthod Dentofac Orthop 142(5):727–733. https://doi.org/10.1016/j.ajodo.2012.04.023

Ardila CC, López CI, Martínez JM, Meléndez GL, Navarro DC, Galeano CF (2018) Study for development of a patient-specific 3D printed craniofacial medical device: design based on 3D virtual biomodels/CAD/RP. Proc CIRP 70:235–240. https://doi.org/10.1016/j.procir.2018.03.335

Bi Z (2018) Overview of finite element analysis. In: Finite element analysis applications. Elsevier, pp 1–29. https://doi.org/10.1016/b978-0-12-809952-0.00001-7

Burton HE, Eisenstein NM, Lawless BM, Jamshidi P, Segarra MA, Addison O, Shepherd DET, Attallah MM, Grover LM, Cox SC (2019) The design of additively manufactured lattices to increase the functionality of medical implants. Mater Sci Eng C 94:901–908. https://doi.org/10.1016/j.msec.2018.10.052

Colombo G, Rizzi C, Regazzoni D, Vitali A (2018) 3D interactive environment for the design of medical devices. Int J Interact Des Manuf 12(2):699–715. https://doi.org/10.1007/s12008-018-0458-8

Culmone C, Smit G, Breedveld P (2019) Additive manufacturing of medical instruments: a state-of-the-art review. Addit Manuf 27:461–473. https://doi.org/10.1016/j.addma.2019.03.015

Dilibal C, Davis BL, Chakraborty C (2021) Generative design methodology for internet of medical things (IoMT)-based wearable biomedical devices. In: HORA 2021—3rd international congress on human-computer interaction, optimization and robotic applications, proceedings, 11 Jun 2021. https://doi.org/10.1109/HORA52670.2021.9461370

Driscoll M (2019) The impact of the finite element method on medical device design. J Med Biol Eng 39(2):171–172. https://doi.org/10.1007/s40846-018-0428-4

George M, Aroom KR, Hawes HG, Gill BS, Love J (2017) 3D printed surgical instruments: the design and fabrication process. World J Surg 41(1):314–319. https://doi.org/10.1007/s00268-016-3814-5

Iqbal T, Wang L, Li D, Dong E, Fan H, Fu J, Hu C (2019) A general multi-objective topology optimization methodology developed for customized design of pelvic prostheses. Med Eng Phys 69:8–16. https://doi.org/10.1016/j.medengphy.2019.06.008

Jankovics D, Gohari H, Tayefeh M, Barari A (2018) Developing topology optimization with additive manufacturing constraints in ANSYS®. IFAC-PapersOnLine 51(11):1359–1364. https://doi.org/10.1016/j.ifacol.2018.08.340
Jin W, Chu PK (2019) Orthopaedic implant. In: Narayan R (ed) Encyclopedia of biomedical engineering, vol 2. Elsevier, pp 425–439
Kanagalingam S, Dalton C, Champneys P, Boutefnouchet T, Fernandez-Vicente M, Shepherd DET, Wimpenny D, Thomas-Seale LEJ (2022) Detailed design for additive manufacturing and post processing of generatively designed high tibial osteotomy fixation plates. Progress Addit Manuf 8:409. https://doi.org/10.1007/s40964-022-00342-2
Kshirsagar M, Dhatrak P (2023) Strain based in vitro analysis of dental implant using artificial bone model and validation by numerical technique. Med Eng Phys 111:103931. https://doi.org/10.1016/j.medengphy.2022.103931
Leary M (2020) Generative design. In: Design for additive manufacturing. Elsevier, pp 203–222. https://doi.org/10.1016/b978-0-12-816721-2.00007-5
Li C, Pisignano D, Zhao Y, Xue J (2020) Advances in medical applications of additive manufacturing. Engineering 6(11):1222–1231. https://doi.org/10.1016/j.eng.2020.02.018
Liu K, Tovar A (2014) An efficient 3D topology optimization code written in Matlab. Struct Multidiscip Optim 50(6):1175–1196. https://doi.org/10.1007/s00158-014-1107-x
Ma Y, Xiao X, Ren H, Meng MQ-H (2022) A review of bio-inspired needle for percutaneous interventions. Biomimetic Intell Robot 2(4):100064. https://doi.org/10.1016/j.birob.2022.100064
Moiduddin K, Anwar S, Ahmed N, Ashfaq M, Al-Ahmari A (2017) Computer assisted design and analysis of customized porous plate for mandibular reconstruction. IRBM 38(2):78–89. https://doi.org/10.1016/j.irbm.2017.01.003
Murzac R, Doicin CV, Ulmeanu ME (2021) Data acquisition and generative design for a smart spinal orthosis. Macromol Symp 396(1). https://doi.org/10.1002/masy.202000297
Nyirjesy SC, Heller M, von Windheim N, Gingras A, Kang SY, Ozer E, Agrawal A, Old MO, Seim NB, Carrau RL, Rocco JW, VanKoevering KK (2022) The role of computer aided design/computer assisted manufacturing (CAD/CAM) and 3-dimensional printing in head and neck oncologic surgery: a review and future directions. Oral Oncol 132:105976. https://doi.org/10.1016/j.oraloncology.2022.105976
Popov V, Muller-Kamskii G, Kovalevsky A, Dzhenzhera G, Strokin E, Kolomiets A, Ramon J (2018) Design and 3D-printing of titanium bone implants: brief review of approach and clinical cases. Biomed Eng Lett 8(4):337–344. https://doi.org/10.1007/s13534-018-0080-5
Santos, I. C. T. (2013). Product development methodologies: the case of medical devices
Scafa Udrişte A, Niculescu AG, Grumezescu AM, Bădilă E (2021) Cardiovascular stents: a review of past, current, and emerging devices. Materials 14(10):2498. https://doi.org/10.3390/ma14102498
Selvaraj SK, Prasad SK, Yasin SY, Subhash US, Verma PS, Manikandan M, Dev SJ (2022) Additive manufacturing of dental material parts via laser melting deposition: a review, technical issues, and future research directions. J Manuf Process 76:67–78. https://doi.org/10.1016/j.jmapro.2022.02.012
Sickel K, Baloch S, Melkisetoglu R, Bubnik V, Azernikov S, Fang T (2011) Toward automation in hearing aid design. Comput Aided Des 43(12):1793–1802. https://doi.org/10.1016/j.cad.2011.06.005
Silva M, Felismina R, Mateus A, Parreira P, Malça C (2017) Application of a hybrid additive manufacturing methodology to produce a metal/polymer customized dental implant. Proc Manuf 12:150–155. https://doi.org/10.1016/j.promfg.2017.08.019
Thanigaiarasu P (2020) Biomimetics in the design of medical devices. In: Trends in development of medical devices. Elsevier Inc., pp 35–41. https://doi.org/10.1016/B978-0-12-820960-8.00003-4
Vaneker T, Bernard A, Moroni G, Gibson I, Zhang Y (2020) Design for additive manufacturing: framework and methodology. CIRP Ann 69(2):578–599. https://doi.org/10.1016/j.cirp.2020.05.006

Wu N, Li S, Zhang B, Wang C, Chen B, Han Q, Wang J (2021) The advances of topology optimization techniques in orthopedic implants: a review. Med Biol Eng Comput 59:1673. https://doi.org/10.1007/s11517-021-02361-7

Zadpoor AA (2017) Design for additive bio-manufacturing: from patient-specific medical devices to rationally designed meta-biomaterials. Int J Mol Sci 18(8):1607. https://doi.org/10.3390/ijms18081607

Zhang Y, Wang Z, Zhang Y, Gomes S, Bernard A (2020) Bio-inspired generative design for support structure generation and optimization in additive manufacturing (AM). CIRP Ann 69(1):117–120. https://doi.org/10.1016/j.cirp.2020.04.091

Modular Product Architecture to Design and Fabricate Prosthetic and Orthotic Products by 3D Printing

8

Mohit Teacher, Rajkumar Velu, and Surinder Kumar

Contents

Abstract

Modular design in prostheses and orthoses (P&O) fabrications is the overall cost-effective method from the product architecture standpoint. The design concept for additive manufacturing is aligned with the integral approach, whereby a singular product is produced to achieve all required functionalities. Simultaneously,

M. Teacher (✉) · R. Velu
Additive Manufacturing Research Laboratory, Mechanical Engineering, Indian Institute of Technology Jammu, Jammu, Jammu and Kashmir, India

S. Kumar
Acharya Shri Chander College of Medical Sciences (ASCOMS) and Hospital, Jammu, Jammu and Kashmir, India

R. Velu et al. (eds.), *Digital Design and Manufacturing of Medical Devices and Systems*, https://doi.org/10.1007/978-981-99-7100-8_8

modular product design entails portioning a particular product into distinct components based on its functionality. This approach effectively diminishes the overall cost of the product and enables the fabrication of damaged parts separately, thereby increasing the product's lifespan. Additionally, to reduce the product's weight, the topology optimization approach is employed, which permits the use of lattice structures without compromising the strength of the components. P&Os are the standard assistive devices that facilitate partial and complete movement of the body, and these devices need full customization. Consequently, additive manufacturing (AM) represents the most appropriate methodology for the fabrication of P&O. The present chapter briefs the process of fabricating P&O using a modular framework.

Keywords

Additive manufacturing (3D printing) · Prostheses and orthoses (P&O) · Product architecture · Modular architecture designs · Lattice structures

8.1 Introduction

8.1.1 Product Architecture

The concept of product architecture pertains to a systematic approach to arranging product features, converting them into component designs, and elucidating the interconnections among them. Based on the product fabrication approach, the product development architecture field encompasses two primary categories: integrated and modular, as depicted in Fig. 8.1.

8.1.1.1 Integral Architecture Design

Integral design refers to a configuration where multiple components perform their functions without necessarily being grouped or arranged into assemblies. The reduced interchangeability of components and component groups has financial ramifications for maintenance and service. The fabrication of distinctive configurations and components may require a longer duration and entail higher acquisition expenses.

8.1.1.2 Modular Architecture Design

The concept of modular design entails creating discrete subassemblies designed to perform specific functions, which are then integrated into a complete product. The standard interfaces between the assemblies are treated as discrete components. During the intensive design phase, comprehensive details regarding assemblies, such as physical dimensions, specifications, dependability, expenses, and support, are gathered and documented. This allows consumers to choose and acquire assemblies that are comparable to individual components (Ulrich 1995).

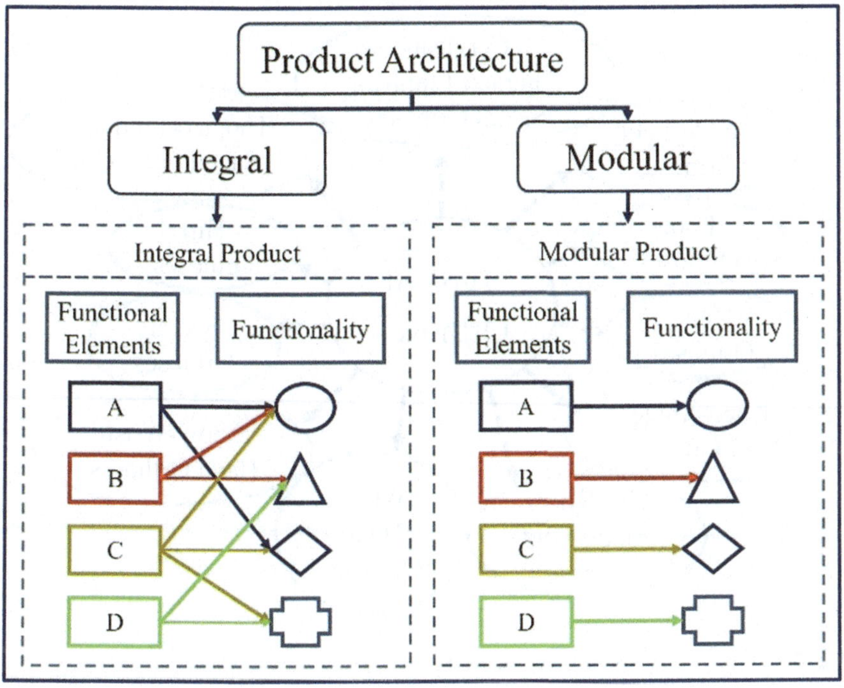

Fig. 8.1 Product architecture design. (Source: Authors)

8.1.2 Prostheses and Orthoses

Prostheses and orthoses (P&O) are the standard assistive devices that serve the biomechanical functions of the person (amputee) with impairment or disabilities. The prostheses are also known as "artificial legs," which include the prosthetic socket, pylon, and foot. The prosthetic socket is a cup-shaped component into which the amputees insert their residual limb, and the entire compression and shear loads are transferred to the prostheses. Orthoses are the devices used to support and adjust structural and functional features of the human musculoskeletal system; a few types are illustrated in Fig. 8.2. Extremities and amputations can be classified based on where they happen. Based on the back joint (as a reference point), extremities below this are defined as lower and above as upper extremities; a few examples are illustrated in Table 8.1. Due to the aging population, veterans injured in recent conflicts, and auto accidents, the demand for P&O is increasing. In 2013, Medicare approved payment for nearly 2.4 million orthotic codes, 2.07 million prosthetic services, and 5.9 million Ped orthic codes, resulting in expenditures of over $734 million, $664 million, and $255 million, respectively (Chen et al. 2016).

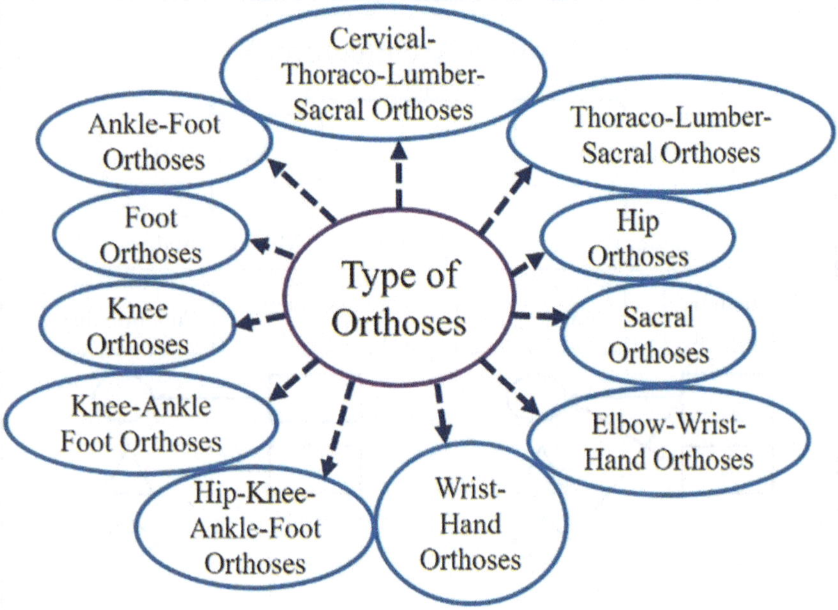

Fig. 8.2 Type of orthoses. (Source: Authors)

Table 8.1 Prostheses for the upper and lower extremities (Coombes et al. 1996)

Types of extremities	Types of amputees	Types of prostheses
Lower extremity	Trans-pelvic	Hip disarticulation
	Trans-femoral (above knee)	Knee disarticulation
	Trans-tibial (below knee)	–
	Ankle (Syme's)	Partial foot
Upper extremity	Forequarter	Shoulder
	Trans-humeral (above elbow)	–
	Elbow disarticulation	Trans radial (below elbow)
	Wrist disarticulation	Partial hand

8.1.3 Additive Manufacturing (3D Printing)

Additive manufacturing (AM), commonly called 3D printing, encompasses a range of techniques whereby a computer-aided design (CAD) model is transformed into a physical 3D object through a layer-by-layer fabrication process. AM techniques have the ability to produce intricate and complex geometries in a cost-effective and timely manner. This is because AM does not require a shaping mold and generates minimal waste (Herbert et al. 2005). These unique characteristics have led to the emergence of innovative applications of AM in the healthcare industry. AM has been employed in the medical and biomedical domain to fabricate personalized scaffolds or synthetic tissues and organs for transplantation, drug administration

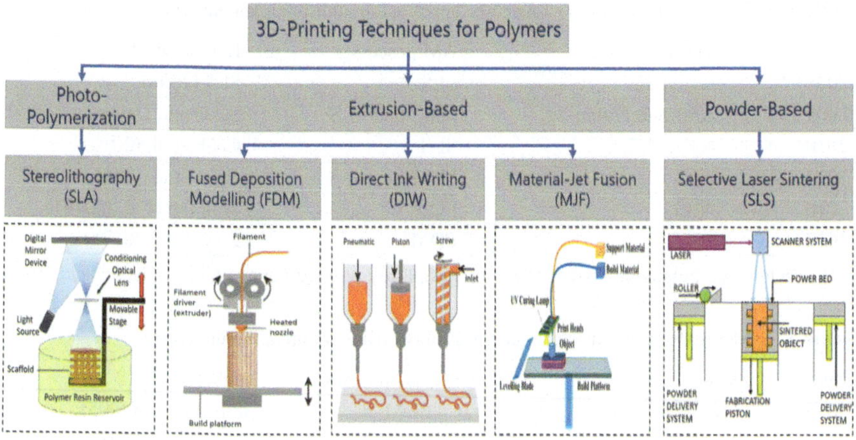

Fig. 8.3 Additive manufacturing techniques used for polymers (Silva et al. 2021; Saleh et al. 2020). (Re-use permission licensed under CC-BY/4.0 from both references)

Fig. 8.4 The various fabrication methods used to print the prostheses (Kate et al. 2017). (Re-use permission licensed under CC-BY-NC-ND/4.0)

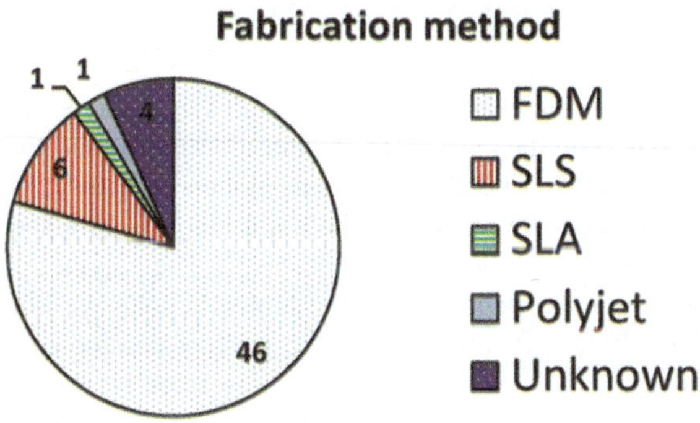

mechanisms, sensors, and devices to identify specific medical parameters, orthotic and prosthetic devices, implants, anatomical models, and medical tools for surgical and diagnostics purposes. According to estimates, the market share of AM technology attributed to biomedical applications is approximately 11%, and this percentage is steadily increasing. AM is a suitable method for fabricating customized prototypes or products in small quantities. This is especially beneficial as patient-specific products are frequently required. There is a variety of AM techniques based on photo-polymerization, extrusion-based, and powder deposition based. However, a few of those are related to the fabrication through polymers, illustrated in Fig. 8.3 (Silva et al. 2021).

According to the literature, it has been determined that among all additive manufacturing techniques, fused deposition modeling (FDM) is the most prevalent process for producing prostheses and orthoses, as depicted in Fig. 8.4. The procedure involves the extrusion of materials through filaments and their deposition onto the bed-plate in a sequential layer-by-layer process. Positioned atop the fabrication

Table 8.2 Materials required to produce orthoses using additive manufacturing

Year	Material	AM process	Reference
2008	Nylon-12	SLS	SLS (2008)
2009	ABS and Nylon-12	FDM and SLS	Saleh and Dalgarno (2009)
2010	Nylons-12	SLS	Cook et al. (2010)
2014	ABS	FDM	Chen et al. (2016)
2016	ABS	FDM	Walbran et al. (2016)
2017	TPU	FDM	Cha et al. (2017)

ABS acrylonitrile-butadiene-styrene, *TPU* thermoplastic polyurethane, *PLA* poly-lactic acid

Table 8.3 Materials required to produce prostheses using additive manufacturing

Year	Material	AM process	Reference
2005	Polyurethane (PU)	FDM	Herbert et al. (2005)
2007	Nylon-11	SLS	Rogers et al. (2007)
2017	PLA and TPU	FDM	Comotti et al. (2017)
2019	PLA	FDM	Pourfarzaneh et al. (2019)
2020	PLA	FDM	Owen and DesJardins (2020)
2021	Rigid PLA and elastic TPE	FDM	Górski et al. (2021)

platform within an extrusion apparatus with the ability to traverse along the *X* and *Y* axis. Polymer materials are introduced into the extruder, subjected to heat and subsequently extruded in a semi-molten state through a nozzle. The deposition of polymer by the head onto the build platform in a specific pattern to form a cross-sectional component layer is observed. The polymer materials undergo rapid solidification upon deposition and establish a cohesive bond with the underlying layer. The slicer software governs the process parameters, including temperature, infill density, support structures, deposition velocity, and wall thickness. Currently, there are 3D printers equipped with multiple nozzles that are capable of depositing multi-materials. This technology enables the fabrication of P&O by utilizing two distinct materials; a rigid material for the exterior and a flexible material for the interior (Jin et al. 2016). The material used to print orthoses and prostheses using AM is presented in Tables 8.2 and 8.3, respectively.

8.2 Fabrication of Prostheses and Orthoses via Conventional and 3D-Printing Techniques

8.2.1 Conventional Approach

In the context of conventional fabrication, individuals who have undergone amputation are required to seek medical attention at rehabilitation centers or hospitals. At these facilities and as discussed in Fig. 8.5, prosthetists apply a polyethylene (PE) sheet to cover the amputated limb, which is subsequently layered with cotton and POP (plaster of Paris) dressings. Upon completion of the curing process, the

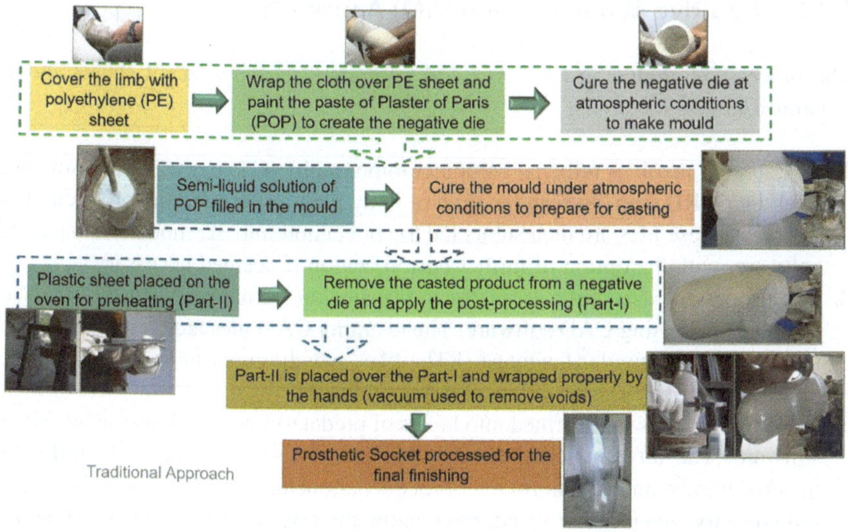

Fig. 8.5 Steps involved in prostheses fabrication through the conventional approach. (Source: Authors)

negative die is fabricated. Subsequently, the aforementioned adverse die or cavity is employed to fabricate a POP mold and a holder featuring a rapid detachment mechanism. After the process of curing is completed. Furthermore, the machining and finishing procedures are employed to achieve a POP limb mold. Concurrently, polycarbonate (PC) or polypropylene (PP) sheets are subjected to thermal treatment in an oven until they reach the glass transition temperature (T_g). Applying heat to the polymer sheet at its T_g includes transitioning to a rubbery state, facilitating its facile placement over the intricately shaped limb mold. Prosthetists manually apply polymers onto limbs, often leading to imperfections such as voids or irregularities. As a result, the utilization of a vacuum pump was deemed imperative to facilitate a seamless transition from the mold to the pliable plastic material. Upon completion of the procedure, employ machining techniques to eliminate surplus substances, such as POP mold and plastic debris. At times, supplementary finishing procedures may be necessary to finalize the socket.

To obtain prostheses, patients must make multiple visits to rehabilitation centers. The first visit is for the measurements, the second for the trial, and the third for the final prostheses, as revealed by an analysis of the patient's visits. This visit and socket add to the total cost of the prosthetic, which amputees pay for out of their own savings. Also, the comprehensive approach is patient-centered; consequently, the inability to process the customized design results in a prosthetic socket that is rigid in nature, creating a vacuum and leading to wounds and ulcers. Therefore, additive manufacturing addresses these issues, particularly in the medical field for P&O.

8.2.2 Additive Manufacturing (AM) Approach

The process of producing P&O via AM comprises the subsequent stages and is illustrated in Fig. 8.6:

1. The process involves utilizing computer tomography (CT) or magnetic resonance imaging (MRI) scans to scan the limb or body part, resulting in the production of 2D files. These files are then subjected to conversion into 3D models using CAD software, with the option of further customization if deemed necessary.
2. The process of assigning geometric properties and dimensions to an object is accomplished using CAD software. The resulting CAD files are then transformed into standard triangular language (STL) files, which represent the object's complete geometry as a series of small triangular facets.
3. The STL model is transformed into layers of predetermined thickness using Slicer software. The aforementioned software allows users to exercise flexibility in material allocation and control over process parameters, including wall thickness, infill density, and printing speed. Eventually, the resultant file is saved in the form of a G-code file, which serves as the machine-run file.
4. The G-code file is transferred to the AM setup, initiating the material deposition process in a layer-by-layer fashion. Additionally, a post-processing step is necessary to eliminate the support structure and achieve a polished finish.

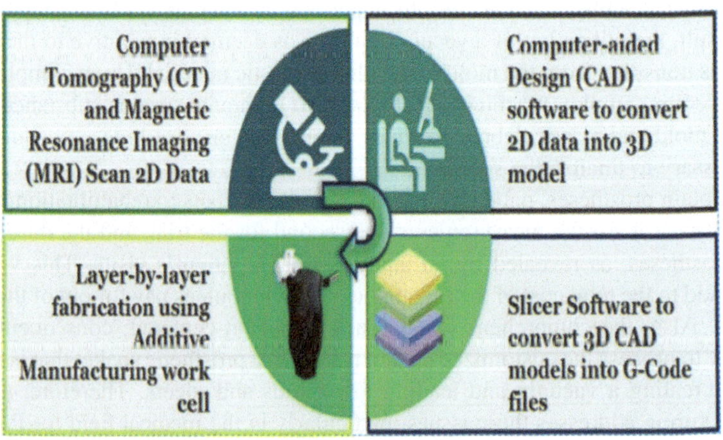

Fig. 8.6 Basic steps to fabricate models from AM (Rai et al. 2022; Górski et al. 2021). (Source: Modified from the authors' previous published work)

8.3 Topology Optimization

Topology optimization (TO) refers to the utilization of mathematical models to devise optimized configurations of microstructures within porous structures, intending to achieve desired and optimal properties. The utilization of algorithms in conjunction with computational models facilitates the identification of topologically optimized systems and local microstructural compatibility for designers. One of the potential objective functions involves maximizing the specific stiffness, which refers to the stiffness-to-mass ratio. This approach incorporates the design elements of topology optimization with AM characteristics, including the technique that focuses on enhancing the arrangement of support materials throughout the AM procedure. Incorporating this integration serves to mitigate the occurrence of stress concentrations at the struts and their junctions within lattice structures, as depicted in Fig. 8.7, both during and post-3D printing, when the support materials are being extracted. This results in a reduction of material usage and a decrease in the amount of time required to fabricate the P&O (Mirzaali et al. 2022).

8.4 Modular Designs of 3D-Printed Prostheses and Orthoses

Based on the challenges experienced by amputees in relation to dermatological concerns such as wounds and ulcers, it is imperative to explore the implementation of a multi-material in the production of P&O, focusing on customization. The current conventional approach is inadequate for these two solutions as it only

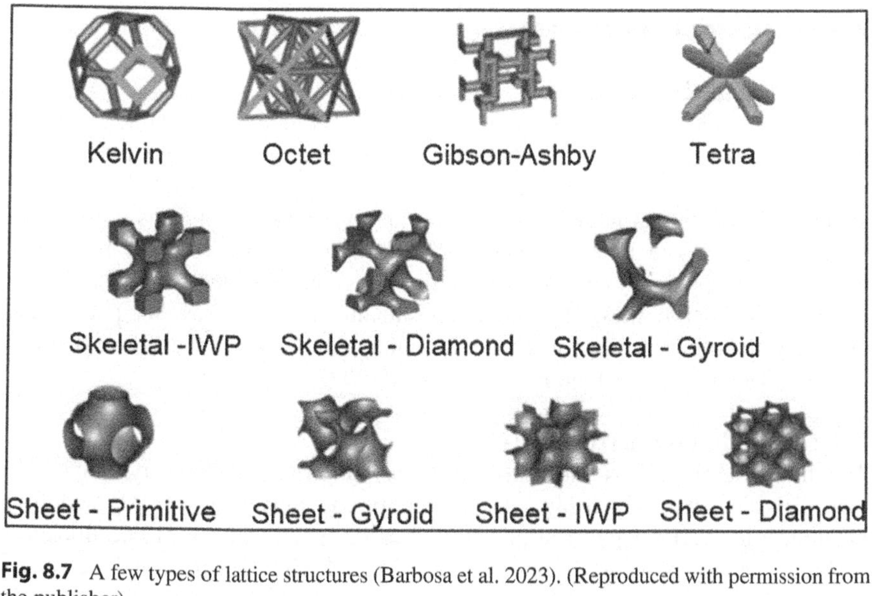

Fig. 8.7 A few types of lattice structures (Barbosa et al. 2023). (Reproduced with permission from the publisher)

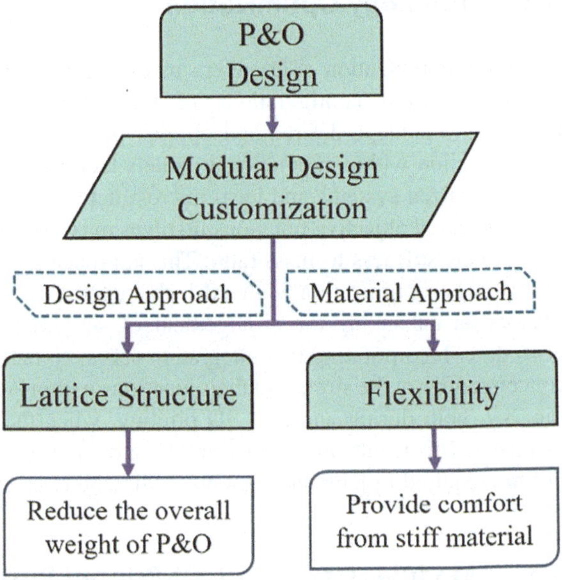

Fig. 8.8 Flowchart to fabricate modular designs in 3D printing. (Source: Authors)

permits the production of a single material that is rigid and patient-centered in design. Consequently, there is a necessity to implement additive manufacturing to produce a modular design of P&O, resulting in a significant reduction in weight, design complexity, and aesthetic consideration, as depicted in Fig. 8.8.

8.4.1 3D-Printed Orthoses

8.4.1.1 Spinal Orthoses

The technological advancements in the field of spinal deformity treatment, specifically highlighting the utilization of 3D printing for the creation of the spinal elements, are illustrated in Fig. 8.9. The treatment of spinal deformities is a highly subjective process that heavily depends on the expertise of orthotists, physicians, physiotherapists, and the willingness of patients to comply with the prescribed treatment. The proposed advancements aim to promote evidence-based practices in treating spinal deformities. The technologies mentioned above have the potential to ascertain the optimal timing for the implementation of bracing, enhance the standard of living, and augment patient results (Ali et al. 2021).

8.4.1.2 Ankle-Foot Orthoses (AFO)

The final prototype was fabricated using acrylonitrile-butadiene-styrene (ABS) thermoplastic material using fused deposition modeling (FDM) additive manufacturing technology. The prototype was designed using a plastic thickness of 4 mm from the previous design iterations. The selection of 4 mm thickness and a reduced toe section in comparison to earlier designs enabled the AFO to nestle

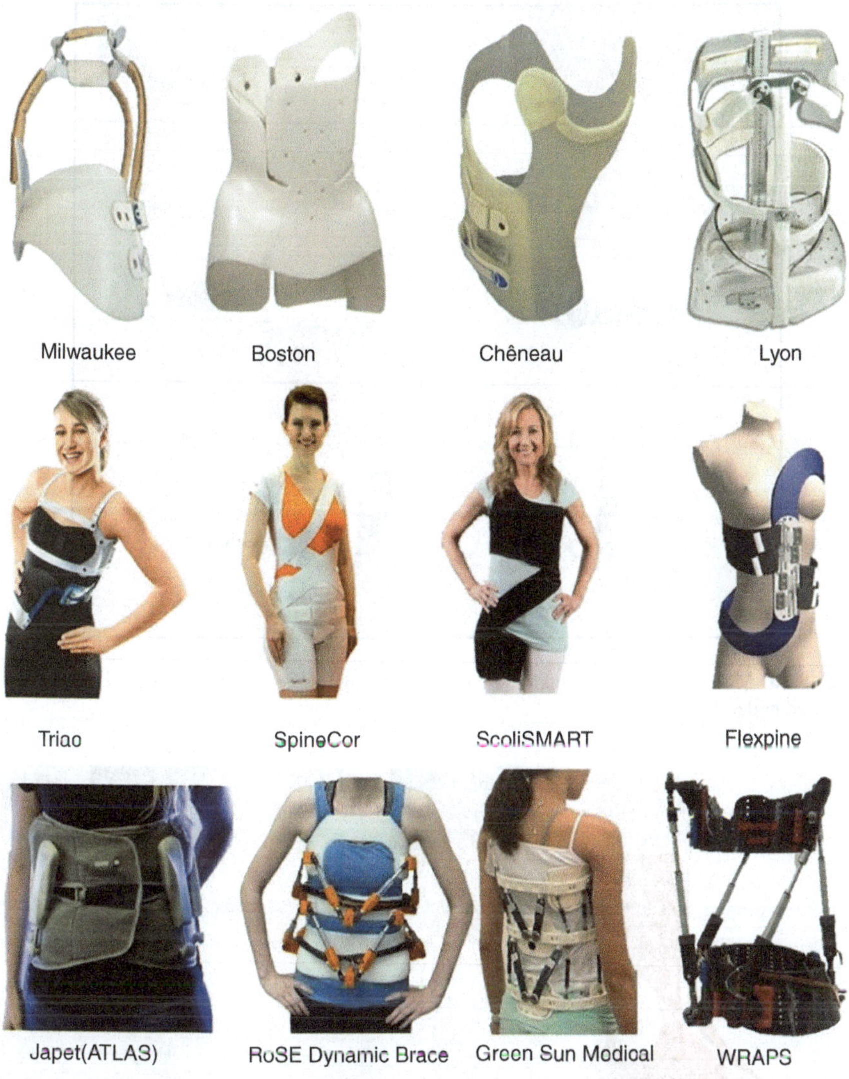

Fig. 8.9 Spinal orthoses (Ali et al. 2021). (Re-use permission licensed under the CC-BY)

comfortably inside a shoe for increased comfort. The posterior and side views of the AFO prototype are illustrated in Fig. 8.10 (Walbran et al. 2016). Yong Ho Cha et al. proposed an alternative design, as shown in Fig. 8.11, for AFO that prioritized weight, customization, and comfort over functionality. The AFO was designed for fabrication through the utilization of a fused filament fabrication (FFF) 3D printer by using thermoplastic polyurethane (TPU) (Cha et al. 2017).

Powered orthoses that are currently in development have the potential to restore normal leg biomechanics. However, these devices have yet to be widely adopted due

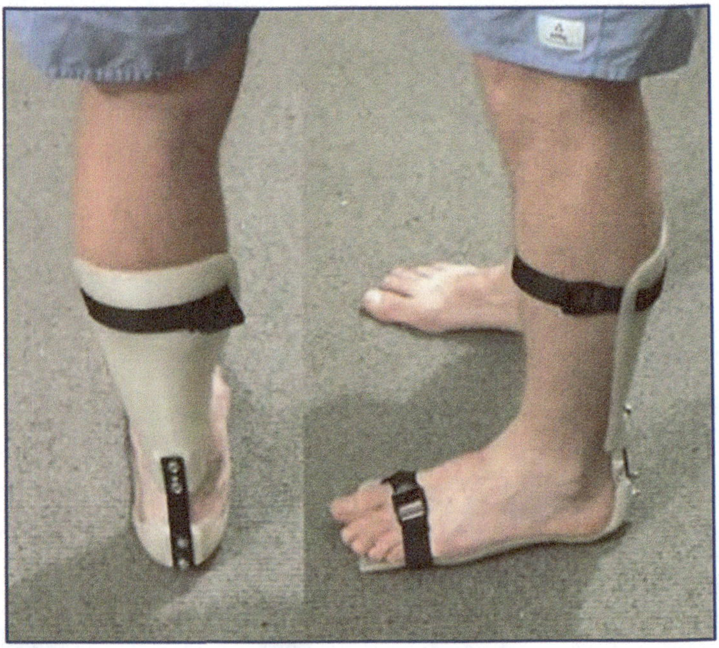

Fig. 8.10 Modular design of ankle-foot orthoses (Walbran et al. 2016). (Re-use permission licensed under the CC-BY)

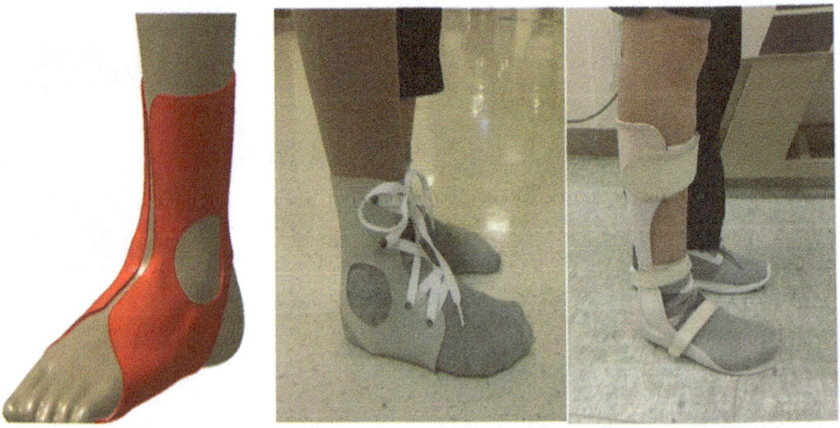

Fig. 8.11 Integrated design of ankle-foot orthoses (Cha et al. 2017). (Re-use permission licensed under the CC BY)

to their rigid joints, bulkiness, and designs that are specific to certain populations. Typically, these devices are equipped with actuators that inhibit the retrograde movement of the joint caused by the user's weight and facilitate the generation of significant output torques to fully restore the limb functionalities of individuals afflicted with spinal cord injury or severe stroke. To reduce both size and mass, the actuators have been designed with small, high-speed motors of low torque, necessitating a substantial gear ratio to attain torques-velocity regimes comparable to those of humans. The phenomenon whereby the motor's inertia is reflected through the gearbox is proportional to the square of the gear ratio, while the friction resulting from the meshing of parts is similarly magnified. The outcome of this phenomenon is the manifestation of elevated mechanical impedance at the joint, thereby impeding the user's ability to effortlessly back-drive the actuator for joint movement. Within this paradigm of actuation, users are often constrained to adhere to predetermined joint patterns of the robot rather than having agency over their own movements. However, certain drives, such as the Indego, may offer more outstanding back drivability compared to other options (Hip et al. 2022).

8.4.1.3 Hand, Forearm, and Wrist Orthoses

The two orthoses *depicted in* Fig. 8.12 have successfully achieved the goal of modularization. The integration of rigid (fabricated through PLA) and flexible (fabricated through TPU) components results in the formation of a distinctive product. The amalgamation of distinct material characteristics within a singular apparatus may be advantageous in the context of rehabilitating individuals who suffer from upper extremity impairment. It has been proposed to assess the utilization of modular orthoses, as shown in Figs. 8.13, 8.14, and 8.15 to ascertain the benefits of modularity in contrast to conventional models (Poier et al. 2021). The wrist and forearm orthoses are also fabricated in the same way, as depicted in Figs. 8.16 and 8.17.

8.4.2 3D-Printed Prostheses

8.4.2.1 Prostheses for Lower Extremities

This includes the prostheses from and below hip joints such as trans-tibial (*also known as below knee*), as depicted in Figs. 8.18 and 8.19, trans-femoral (*also known*

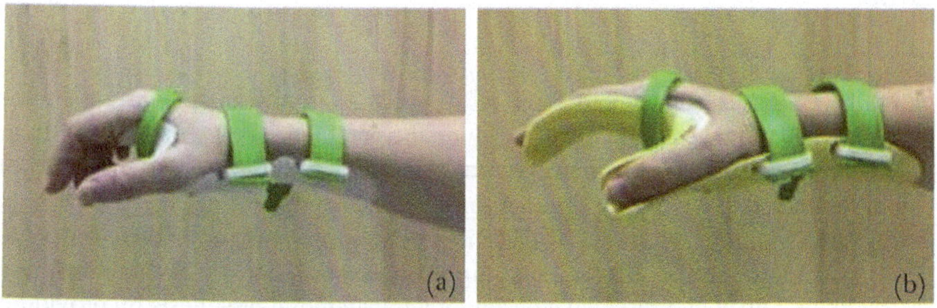

Fig. 8.12 Modular orthoses: (**a**) flexible and (**b**) rigid covered by flexible orthosis (Poier et al. 2021). (Re-use permission licensed under the CC-BY)

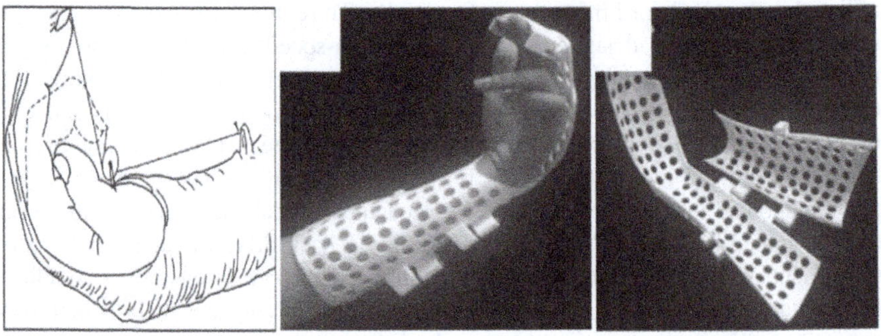

Fig. 8.13 3D printed modular architecture of flexor tendon injury (Li et al. 2022). (Re-use permission licensed under the CC-BY)

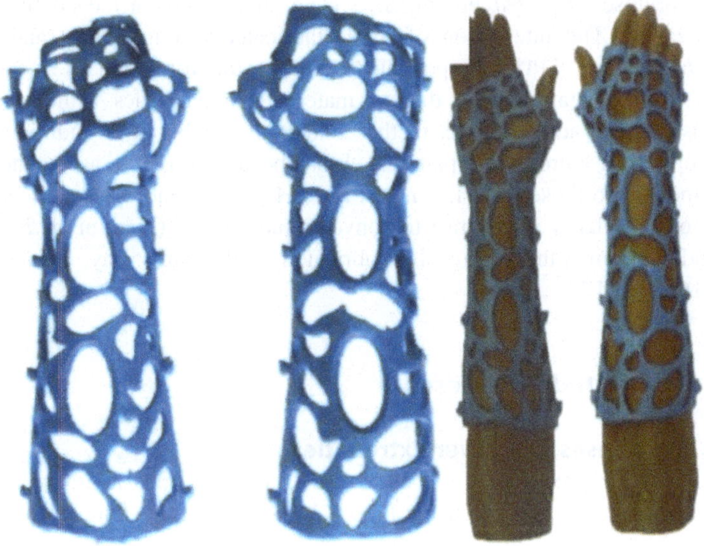

Fig. 8.14 Arm orthoses for fracture patients (Li et al. 2022). (Re-use permission licensed under the CC-BY)

as above knee), as depicted in Figs. 8.20 and 8.21, and trans-pelvic prostheses (hip-disarticulation). All individually include the prosthetic socket, pylon, and foot.

Studies have indicated that transfemoral amputees who utilize passive prostheses exhibit a metabolic energy expenditure of up to 60% greater than healthy persons during level walking. Additionally, these individuals may exert up to three times the power and torque at the affected-side hip (Waters et al. 1976). To address these issues, Frank Sup et al. presented a design of a transfemoral prosthesis by providing powered knee and ankle joints (Sup et al. 2008). (*The figure is not provided due to licencing constraints; however, the reference can be consulted for further*

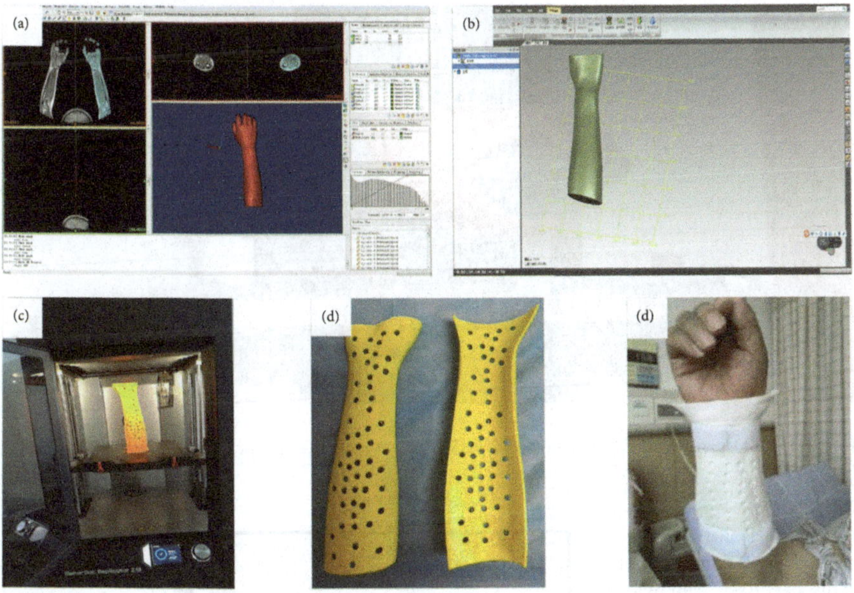

Fig. 8.15 3D-printed prostheses of the forearm and hand (**a**) 3D reconstruction of forearm and hand structure, (**b**) processing and entity modelling of 3D model of the orthosis, (**c**) 3D printing, (**d**) 3D printing physical model, and (**e**) 3D printed right orthosis (Li et al. 2022). (Re-use permission licensed under the CC-BY)

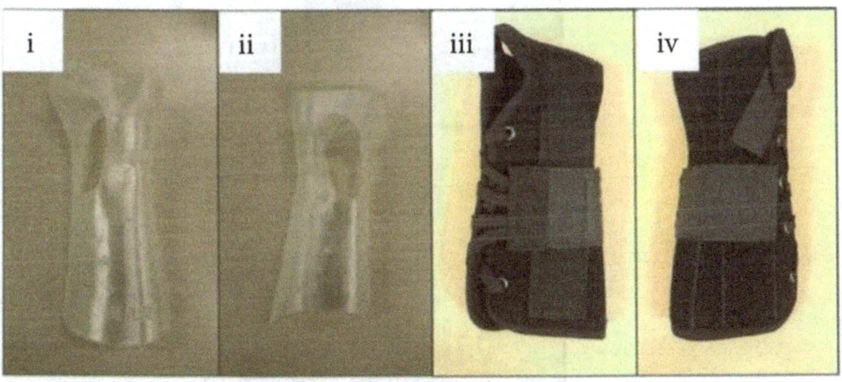

Fig. 8.16 Wrist orthoses (Li et al. 2022). (Re-use permission licensed under the CC-BY)

information.) The design is based on impedance control and implemented by Hogan Neville (Hogan 1985), also validated by David Winter, using regression analysis of gait data simple impedance model based on the joint toques, which is a function of joint angle and velocity (Winter 1987).

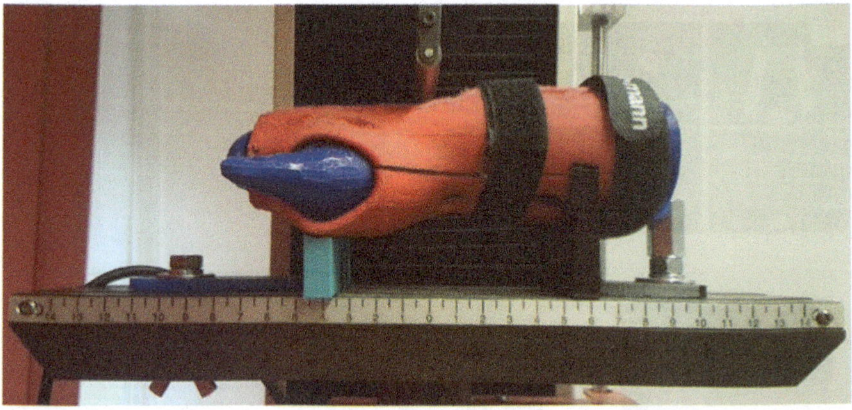

Fig. 8.17 3D-printed forearm orthoses (Górski et al. 2020). (Re-use permission licensed under the CC-BY)

Fig. 8.18 Transtibial prostheses (3D-printed foot and socket fixed with pylon) (van der Stelt et al. 2021). (Re-use permission licensed under the CC-BY)

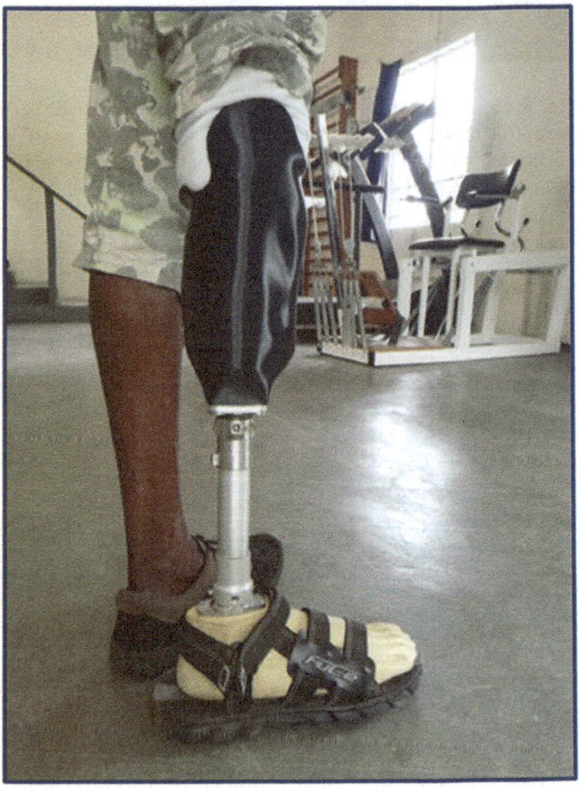

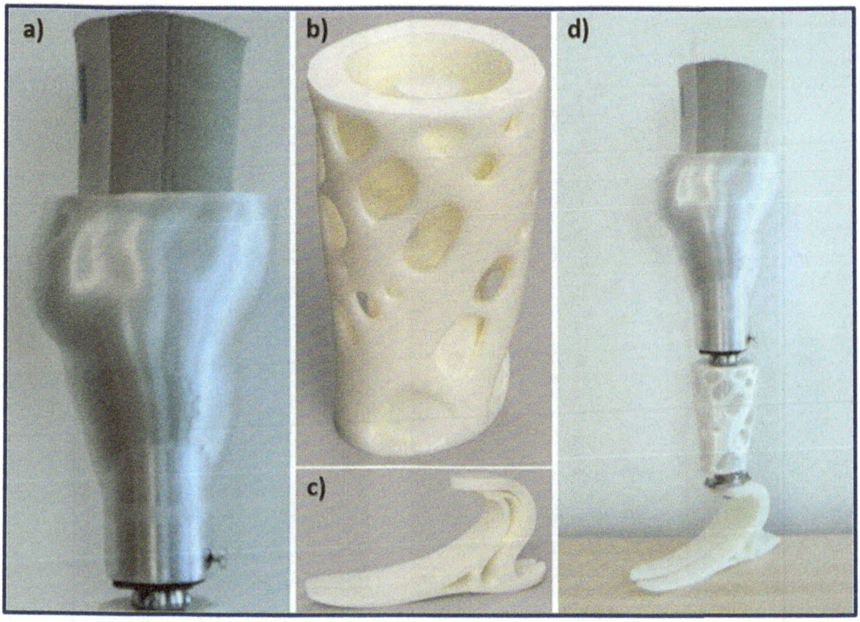

Fig. 8.19 Modular design of transtibial prostheses (**a**) socket with limb model, (**b**) tibial pylon section, (**c**) foot, and (**d**) a complete transtibial prostheses (Gabriele et al. 2021). (Re-use permission licensed under the CC-BY)

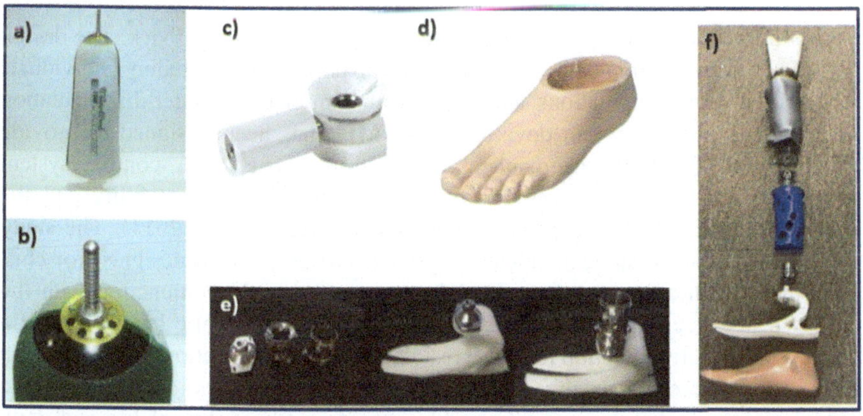

Fig. 8.20 Modular design of transfemoral prostheses (**a**) prosthetic socket, (**b**) socket-upper pylon connector, (**c**) knee-joint, (**d**) foot cover, (**e**) foot and ankle-joint, and (**f**) complete transfemoral prostheses (Gabriele et al. 2021). (Re-use permission licensed under the CC-BY)

8.4.2.2 Prostheses for Upper Extremities (Hand Prostheses)

M.M. Bridges et al. introduced the modular prosthetic limb (MPL), which is a limb with 17 degrees of freedom. The MPL's design specifications entail achieving performance metrics that closely approximate those of a natural limb, including

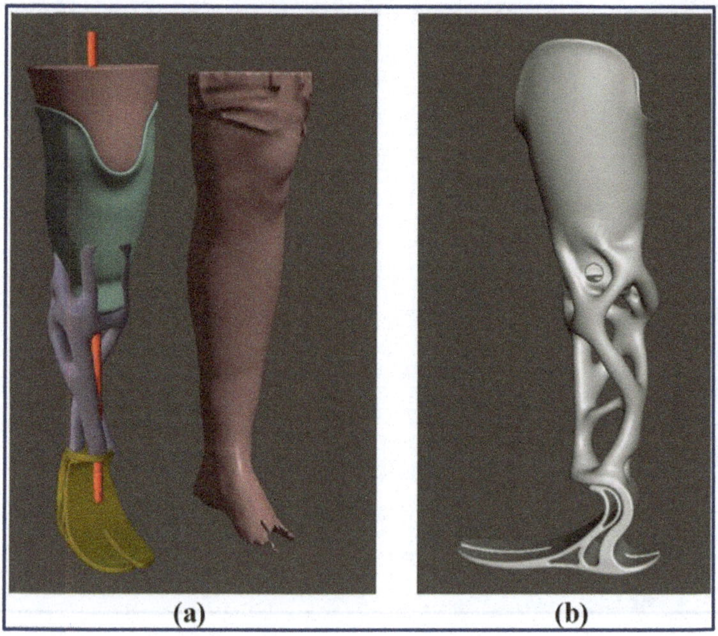

Fig. 8.21 Integral design of transtibial prostheses (**a**) Using the healthy leg scan and its mirrored model properly scale and align all components, and (**b**) Side view of final monocoque design (Gabriele et al. 2021). (Re-use permission licensed under the CC-BY)

but not limited to dexterity, strength, form factor, weight, and feedback. The design was required to accommodate a diverse patient population, including individuals with partial hand amputations and those with complete shoulder-disarticulation injuries. The control system devised for the MPL has been designed to provide patients with flexibility in managing their limbs. The MPL control system modularity has been developed to optimize the interface's adaptability and the control modularity at the disposal of the patient (Bridges et al. 2011). The study offers a depiction of an economical 3D-printed prosthetic hand designed for children, along with a suggested protocol for remote fitting. In conjunction with the proposed distance-fitting procedure, the Cyborg Beast prosthetic hand presents a viable, cost-effective solution for those residing in developing nations and those with limited or no access to healthcare professionals. The prosthetic device exhibits a considerable potential to have a favorable impact on the quality of life and daily functioning of the user. Subsequent investigations ought to scrutinize the operational efficacy, authenticity, and rate of non-acceptance of the economical 3D-printed hand design (Zuniga et al. 2015). The prosthetic hand must effectively embody the human hand's functional and visual attributes. A prosthetic hand's design necessitates considering the hand's dexterity, rotational motion, and manipulation, as depicted in Figs. 8.22 and 8.23. The hand's design must consider the joint mechanism of finger flexion and extension. The hand's design should consider the stresses caused by extension, hyperextension, and flexion. The utilization of anthropometric and

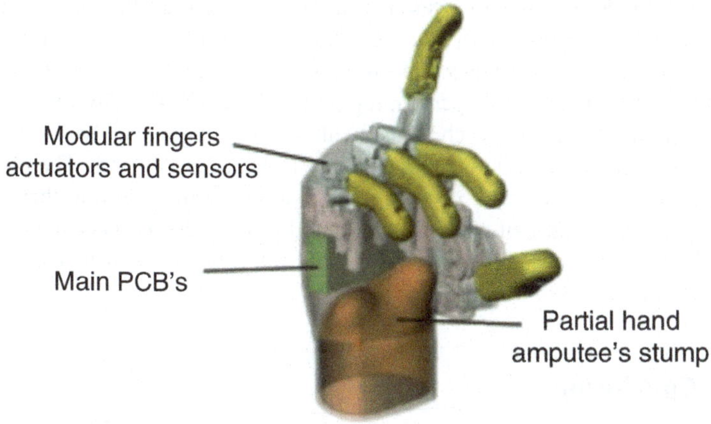

Fig. 8.22 A 3D-printed prosthetic hand (Mio et al. 2019). (Re-use permission licensed under the CC-BY)

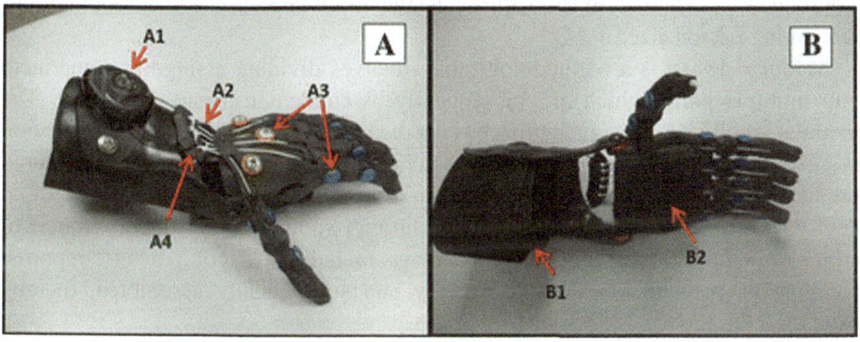

Fig. 8.23 Prosthetic hand: (**a**) top view and (**b**) bottom view (Zuniga et al. 2015). (Re-use permission licensed under the CC-BY)

operational analysis facilitates the determination of the mechanical parameters necessary for modeling a given system. The design variables are defined while designing the actuating forces, torque, and stress (Aryal and Pun 2022).

The Galileo Bionic Hand is a myoelectric upper-limb prosthesis designed for those who have undergone amputation below the elbow. It has an anthropomorphic design and is inexpensive and open-source. In addition, the prosthesis is under-actuated, which means it can perform various movements and functions with a limited number of actuators. The modular, parametric, and self-contained design of the device is intended to accommodate individuals with variable degrees of trans-radial amputation. The emergence of 3D printing technology has facilitated adhering to novel design principles. These principles prioritize simplicity while ensuring optimal performance in grasping capabilities, power consumption, and controllability. J. Fajardo et al. have proposed a functional design employing 3D printing technology to expedite manufacturing processes and reduce associated costs. The palm design encompasses gear motors that facilitate the movement of the thumb and fingers. Additionally, the PCB board controller comprises a microcontroller and three dual H-bridges. The fingers were designed to endure the strain induced by the actuators while performing routine tasks of everyday life. Nevertheless, it is noteworthy that each constituent of the finger can be conveniently reproduced and reconstructed using prevalent 3D printing polymers. The phalanges (proximal, intermediate, and distal) possess a parametric design that enables alterations in the length of the fingers (Fajardo et al. 2017). (*The figure is not provided due to licencing constraints, however the reference can be consulted for further information.*)

8.5 Conclusion

The market share of P&O is expected to increase in the future due to a rise in the number of patients with diabetes and locomotive impairments. The P&O devices necessitate complete customization as each patient possesses a unique body shape. Consequently, additive manufacturing is the most appropriate methodology for fabricating personalized P&O.

Modular design is a methodology that involves dividing a singular component into multiple parts, which are subsequently assembled in a partial manner. The modular architecture design approach is deemed most appropriate for the fabrication of customized P&O, given the product architecture, resulting in decreased overall product costs. Topology optimization can be utilized to decrease the weight of devices while maintaining their strength through simulation and incorporation of lattice structures. In the instance of damage to individual components, reported components may be fabricated separately and subsequently assembled, thereby extending the product's lifespan.

The chapter presents modular designs of certain P&O models, which offer a fundamental understanding of incorporating modular designs and the production of this design through additive manufacturing.

8.6 Future Challenges and Opportunities

The utilization of 3D printing technology has become prevalent in producing intricate and complex shapes, thereby enabling the fabrication of customized products. The preliminary expenses of establishing an AM setup are substantial, encompassing acquiring 3D scanning equipment, computer systems, design and slicing software, and the corresponding work cell. To enhance the production capabilities of AM, it is imperative to reduce costs and improve the dependability of the resultant product. To achieve a reduction in cost, it is necessary to decrease the product's overall weight. This can be accomplished through the implementation of optimized structures or a decrease in infill density. Decreasing the density of infill results in a reduction of the strength of the product. Thus, simulation-based optimization is a preferred approach for obtaining optimized results of frame and lattice structures. The incorporation of simulation software results in an additional increase in the initial cost. The implementation of modular design has the potential to decrease the total cost and enhance the dependability of the product. The primary task entails identifying components that can be detached from the overall design such that they can be readily replaced in the event of a malfunction.

Incorporating various materials in the production of P&O and optimizing their structures through graded material deposition can enhance patient comfort. Conventional manufacturing processes typically have single-material products that exhibit a rigid structural composition. The utilization of AM allows for the incorporation of adaptable materials, resulting in a decrease in wounds and ulcers. Currently, the aforementioned capability is not accessible. However, by utilizing multi-material systems and implementing software modifications, it is possible to accommodate the necessary specifications.

Implementing electrically powered and actuator-based devices, particularly in prosthetics, has gained significant attention. Transfemoral and trans-pelvic amputees exhibit significantly higher energy expenditure than trans-tibial amputees, with the former requiring 10 and 100 times more energy, respectively. Consequently, it is imperative to engage with the mechanisms of the crank and follower, linkages, and pneumatic and hydraulic actuators to supply the necessary energy to amputees.

Acknowledgments This work was conducted under the grant number SRG/2021/002204, funded by the Science and Engineering Research Board (SERB) grant, Department of Science and Technology (DST), Government of India.

References

Ali A, Fontanari V, Fontana M, Schmölz W (2021) Spinal deformities and advancement in corrective orthoses. Bioengineering 8(1):1–14. https://doi.org/10.3390/bioengineering8010002

Aryal MR, Pun S (2022) Additive manufacturing of prosthetic hands: a brief overview. Int J Interact Des Manuf 16(3):1099–1112. https://doi.org/10.1007/s12008-022-00857-6

Barbosa WS, Gioia MM, Temporão GP, Meggiolaro MA, Gouvea FC (2023) Impact of multi-lattice inner structures on FDM PLA 3D printed orthosis using Industry 4.0 concepts. Int J Interact Des Manuf 17(1):371–383. https://doi.org/10.1007/s12008-022-00962-6

Bridges MM, Para MP, Mashner MJ (2011) Control system architecture for the modular prosthetic limb. Johns Hopkins APL Technical Dig 30(3):217–222

Cha YH et al (2017) Ankle-foot orthosis made by 3D printing technique and automated design software. Appl Bionics Biomech 2017:1. https://doi.org/10.1155/2017/9610468

Chen RK, Jin Y, Wensman J, Shih A (2016) Additive manufacturing of custom orthoses and prostheses—a review. Addit Manuf 12:77–89. https://doi.org/10.1016/j.addma.2016.04.002

Comotti C, Regazzoni D, Rizzi C, Vitali A (2017) Additive manufacturing to advance functional design: an application in the medical field. J Comput Inf Sci Eng 17(3):1–9. https://doi.org/10.1115/1.4033994

Cook D, Gervasi V, Rizza R, Kamara S, Liu X (2010) Additive fabrication of custom pedorthoses for clubfoot correction. Rapid Prototyp J 16(3):189–193. https://doi.org/10.1108/13552541011034852

Coombes AGA, Greenwood CD, Shorter JJ (1996) Plastic Materials for External Prostheses and Orthoses. In: Wise DL, Trantolo DJ, Altobelli DE, Yaszemski MJ, Gresser JD (eds) Human Biomaterials Applications. Humana Press, Totowa, NJ. https://doi.org/10.1007/978-1-4757-2487-5_11

Fajardo J, Ferman V, Lemus A, Rohmer E (2017) An affordable open-source multifunctional upper-limb prosthesis with intrinsic actuation. IEEE workshop on advanced robotics and its cocial impacts (ARSO), Austin, TX, USA, pp. 1–6. https://doi.org/10.1109/ARSO.2017.8025206

Gabriele L, Nicoloso DV, Pelz J (2021) Towards 3D printing of a monocoque transtibial prosthesis using a bio-inspired design work flow. Rapid Prototyp J 11:67–80. https://doi.org/10.1108/RPJ-06-2021-0136

Górski F, Wichniarek R, Kuczko W, Zukowska M, Lulkiewicz M, Zawadzki P (2020) Experimental studies on 3D printing of automatically designed customized wrist-hand orthoses. Materials (Basel). 13(18). https://doi.org/10.3390/ma13184091

Górski F, Wichniarek R, Kuczko W, Żukowska M (2021) Study on properties of automatically designed 3d-printed customized prosthetic sockets. Materials (Basel) 14(18). https://doi.org/10.3390/ma14185240

Herbert N, Simpson D, Spence WD, Ion W (2005) A preliminary investigation into the development of 3-D printing of prosthetic sockets. J Rehabil Res Dev 42(2):141–146. https://doi.org/10.1682/JRRD.2004.08.0134

Hip P et al (2022) Enhancing voluntary motion with modular, backdrivable, powered hip and knee orthoses. IEEE Robot Autom Lett 7(3):6155–6162

Hogan N (1985) Impedance control: an approach to manipulation: part II—implementation. J Dyn Syst Meas Control 107(1):8–16. https://doi.org/10.1115/1.3140713

Jin Y, He Y, Shih A (2016, ISEM XVIII) Process planning for the fuse deposition modeling of ankle-foot-othoses. Proc CIRP 42:760–765. https://doi.org/10.1016/j.procir.2016.02.315

Kate J, Smit G, Breedveld P, Kate J, Smit G (2017) 3D-printed upper limb prostheses: a review. Disabil Rehabil Assist Technol 12:300. https://doi.org/10.1080/17483107.2016.1253117

Li J, Chen S, Shang X, Li N, Aiyiti W, Gao F (2022) Research Progress of rehabilitation orthoses based on 3D printing technology. Adv Mater Sci Eng 2022:1. https://doi.org/10.1155/2022/5321570

Mio R, Bustamante M, Salazar G, Elias DA (2019) A 3D-printed prosthetic hand with modular reconfigurable fingers. In: Interdisciplinary applications of kinematics. Springer, pp 93–102

Mirzaali MJ, Moosabeiki V, Rajaai SM, Zhou J (2022) Additive manufacturing of biomaterials—design principles and their implementation. Materials (Basel) 15:5457

Owen MK, DesJardins JD (2020) Transtibial prosthetic socket strength: the use of ISO 10328 in the comparison of standard and 3D-printed sockets. J Prosthet Orthot 32(2):93–100. https://doi.org/10.1097/JPO.0000000000000306

Poier PH, Arce RP, Rosenmann GC, Carvalho MGR, Ulbricht L, Foggiatto JA (2021) Development of modular wrist, hand and finger orthesis by additive manufacturing. Res Soc Dev 10(15): e333101522707. https://doi.org/10.33448/rsd-v10i15.22707

Pourfarzaneh A, Taghavi M, Helps T, Rossiter J (2019) Towards adaptive prosthetic sockets using 3D-printed variable-stiffness shape-memory structures, pp 1–6

Rai P et al (2022) Design and optimization of a 3D printed prosthetic socket for transtibial amputees. Mater Today Proc 70:454–464. https://doi.org/10.1016/j.matpr.2022.09.365

Rogers B et al (2007) Advanced trans-tibial socket fabrication using selective laser sintering. Prosthetics Orthot Int 31(1):88–100. https://doi.org/10.1080/03093640600983923

Saleh JM, Dalgarno KW (2009) Cost and benefit analysis of fused deposition modelling (FDM) technique and selective laser sintering (SLS) for fabrication of customized foot orthoses. In: Innovative developments in desing and manufacturing, 1st edn. Taylor & Francis, p 6

Saleh B et al (2020) 30 years of functionally graded materials: an overview of manufacturing methods, applications and future challenges. Compos Part B Eng 201:108376. https://doi.org/10.1016/j.compositesb.2020.108376

Silva M, Pinho IS, Covas JA, Alves NM, Paiva MC (2021) 3D printing of graphene-based polymeric nanocomposites for biomedical applications. Funct Composite Mater 2:8

SLS (2008) FO.pdf. Faustini MC, Neptune RR, Crawford RH, Stanhope SJ. Manufacture of Passive Dynamic ankle-foot orthoses using selective laser sintering. IEEE Trans Biomed Eng (2 Pt 1):784–790. https://doi.org/10.1109/TBME.2007.912638

Sup F, Bohara A, Goldfarb M (2008) Design and control of a powered transfemoral prosthesis. Int J Robot Res 27(2):263–273. https://doi.org/10.1177/0278364907084588

Ulrich K (1995) The role of product architecture in the manufacturing firm. Res Policy 24(3): 419–440. https://doi.org/10.1016/0048-7333(94)00775-3

van der Stelt M et al (2021) Pioneering low-cost 3D-printed transtibial prosthetics to serve a rural population in Sierra Leone—an observational cohort study. EClinicalMedicine 35:100874. https://doi.org/10.1016/j.eclinm.2021.100874

Walbran M, Turner K, McDaid AJ (2016) Customized 3D printed ankle-foot orthosis with adaptable carbon fibre composite spring joint. Cogent Eng 3(1). https://doi.org/10.1080/23311916.2016.1227022

Waters RL, Perry J, Antonelli D, Hislop H (1976) Energy cost of walking of amputees: the influence of level of amputation. JBJS 58(1):42. Available: https://journals.lww.com/jbjsjournal/Fulltext/1976/58010/Energy_cost_of_walking_of_amputees__the_influence.7.aspx

Winter DA (1987) The biomechanics and motor control of human gait: Normal, Elderly and Pathological. University of Waterloo Press. ISBN: 9780888981059. 1991. https://books.google.co.in/books?id=q_EHAQAAMAAJ

Zuniga J, Katsavelis D, Peck J, Stollberg J, Petrykowski M, Carson A (2015) Cyborg beast: a low-cost 3d-printed prosthetic hand for children with upper-limb differences. BMC Res Notes 8: 10. https://doi.org/10.1186/s13104-015-0971-9

Design and Development of 3D Printing on Bioinks and Biomaterials for Implants and Tissue Engineering

9

Murali Krishnan Ramachandran, Manigandan Kannan, Rajkumar Velu, and Paramasamy Shanmugam

Contents

M. K. Ramachandran (✉) · M. Kannan
Department of Mechanical Engineering, The University of Akron, Akron, OH, USA
e-mail: mr319@uakron.edu

R. Velu
Additive Manufacturing Research Laboratory, Mechanical Engineering, Indian Institute of Technology Jammu, Jammu, Jammu and Kashmir, India

P. Shanmugam
Department of Mechanical Engineering, Sethu Institute of Technology, Pulloor, Kariapatti, Tamil Nadu, India

R. Velu et al. (eds.), *Digital Design and Manufacturing of Medical Devices and Systems*, https://doi.org/10.1007/978-981-99-7100-8_9

Abstract

The capacity to produce complicated structures with high precision has made it possible to make personalized implants that fit the individual anatomy of the patient, improving outcomes and lowering risks. For drug testing and screening, 3D-printed tissue models have been employed, and current research is looking into how to fabricate intricate microstructures and drug delivery systems. This chapter explores how 3D printing has the potential to transform healthcare by making it possible to create patient-specific implants as well as useful tissues and organs for transplantation. It is important to consider aspects like biocompatibility, printability, mechanical qualities, degradability, and cost when choosing bioinks and biomaterials. In vitro testing is crucial to determine these materials' effectiveness, and it is used in the morphological, rheological, chemical, biocompatibility, and mechanical characterization of these materials. Finally, recent studies on bioinks and biomaterials using various 3D printing techniques are reviewed, including their limitations and implications for future research.

Keywords

3D bioprinting · Tissue engineering · Biomedical implants · Biomaterials

9.1 Introduction

Healthcare is one of the many areas that 3D printing, otherwise termed additive manufacturing, has the potential to disrupt. The capability to build highly intricate structures with an extraordinary degree of preciseness is one of the key advantages of 3D printing (Velu et al. 2020a). This has led to the development of patient-specific implants, such as hip and knee replacements, which can be designed to fit a patient's unique anatomy, resulting in improved outcomes and reduced risks. Moreover, tissue engineering has made use of 3D printing to produce 3D tissue models for drug testing and screening. The development of functional tissues and organs that may one day be utilized for transplantation has also been made possible using biomaterials and bioinks in 3D printing. Table 9.1 summarizes the types of 3D printing techniques and the materials commonly used in each technique (Velu et al. 2016, 2023a; Park et al. 2016):

Each type of 3D printing technology and material has its unique strengths and weaknesses, making it important to choose the right technology and material for a specific application. As 3D printing technology continues to advance, it is expected that new materials and improved methods will be developed, offering even greater capabilities and potential for various industries (Whenish et al. 2021). Recent studies have focused on the development of new and improved materials for 3D printing, as well as the optimization of printing techniques to enhance the 3D-printed structures' mechanical strengths. There is also ongoing research into the fabrication of complex microstructures and the development of new drug delivery systems via 3D printing.

Table 9.1 Types of commonly used 3D printing material, techniques, and benefits (Velu et al. 2016, 2023a; Park et al. 2016)

3D printing technology	Description	Materials	Benefits
Fused deposition modeling (FDM)	To construct a 3D part, the printer extrudes the filament layer by layer	• Acrylonitrile butadiene styrene (ABS) • Polylactic acid (PLA) • Nylon • Thermoplastic polyurethane (TPU) • Polyethylene terephthalate glycol (PETG) • Polycarbonate (PC) • Polyetheretherketone (PEEK).	• Affordable • Easy-to-use
Stereolithography (SLA)	A liquid resin that is cured using UV light to create 3D objects	• Photopolymers, resins • Acrylates • Epoxies	• High accuracy and precision • Ideal for applications that require intricate details
Selective laser sintering (SLS)	A laser to sinter powdered material, such as plastic or metal, to create 3D objects	• Polyamide 12 • Polyethylene terephthalate glycol (PETG) • Polycarbonate (PC) • Polyetheretherketone (PEEK) • Polypropylene	• The ability to produce complex geometry and functional parts
Digital light processing (DLP)	SLA-like, but using a projector rather than a laser to cure the liquid resin	• Photopolymers, resins • Acrylates • Epoxies	• High-resolution 3D objects with a smooth surface finish
Binder jetting (BJ)	Jetting a liquid binder onto a powder bed to create 3D objects	• Plaster • Ceramics • Sand • Metal powders	• A range of materials can be used including metals, ceramics, and plastics
Material jetting (MJ)	Inkjet printheads to jet liquid photopolymer material onto a build platform to create 3D objects	• Photopolymers • Resins • Acrylates • Epoxies	• High accuracy and ability to produce multiple materials in a single print
Directed energy deposition (DED)	Depositing melted material onto a substrate to create 3D objects	• Metals • Alloys • Composites	• Commonly used for metal additive manufacturing also possible to produce large and complex geometries

(continued)

Table 9.1 (continued)

3D printing technology	Description	Materials	Benefits
Extrusion based printing	It is like FDM but uses pneumatic pressure to extrude the material through a syringe or nozzle	• Bioinks • Hydrogels • Polymers	• Ability to print high-viscosity materials

This chapter discusses the factors to consider when selecting bioinks and biomaterials, including biocompatibility, mechanical properties, printability, degradability, and cost. Characterization techniques used for bioinks and biomaterials include morphological, rheological, chemical, biocompatibility, and mechanical testing. In vitro testing and analysis involve assessing biocompatibility, mechanical properties, and efficacy of 3D-printed constructs using biological systems such as cell cultures and tissues. Finally, recent studies on bioinks and biomaterials using various 3D printing techniques, their limitations, and implications of future research are discussed.

9.2 Bioinks and Biomaterials

Bioinks and biomaterials are key components in the field of 3D bioprinting, which involves using 3D printing technology to create biological tissue and organ constructs. Bioinks are specially formulated materials that can be used to create 3D-printed tissue constructs, while biomaterials are materials that are used in the body to replace or support damaged tissue.

Bioinks are typically made up of cells and a supportive matrix, which may include materials such as alginate, gelatin, hyaluronic acid, or collagen. These materials provide a scaffold for the cells to grow on and can be customized to promote specific cellular behaviors, such as proliferation or differentiation. Bioinks can be utilized with 3D bioprinting to produce functional tissue structures, such as skin, bone, and even organs. Biomaterials, on the other hand, are materials that are used in the body to support, augment, or replace tissue that has been damaged or lost. It can be expanded in medical applications, such as implants, drug delivery systems, and tissue engineering (Lee et al. 2021; Li et al. 2020).

The advancement of bioinks and biomaterials is an active area of research, with a focus on improving the biocompatibility, mechanical properties, and cellular response of these materials. As 3D bioprinting technology continues to advance, it is expected that new and improved bioinks and biomaterials will be developed, offering an even greater perspective for tissue engineering and re-forming medicine (Barrs et al. 2020; Das and Jang 2019).

9.2.1 Selection of Bioinks and Biomaterials

The choice of bioinks and biomaterials for 3D printing depends on several factors, including the type of tissue or implant being created, the properties of the bioink or biomaterial, and the 3D printing method being used. Below are some factors to consider when selecting bioinks and biomaterials for 3D printing (Lee et al. 2021; Li et al. 2020; Barrs et al. 2020; Das and Jang 2019; Shahbazi and Jäger 2020):

- Biocompatibility: Bioinks and biomaterials must be biocompatible, meaning they are not toxic and will not cause an adverse reaction in the body. They should also be able to support the growth and function of cells.
- Mechanical properties: Bioinks and biomaterials must have the appropriate mechanical properties for the intended application. For example, bone tissue requires a biomaterial with high compressive strength, while cartilage tissue requires a biomaterial with high elasticity.
- Printability: The bioink must be printable using the 3D printing method being used and must have the appropriate viscosity, surface tension, and other properties to ensure accurate and consistent printing.
- Degradability: In some cases, the bioink or biomaterial should be biodegradable, meaning it can be broken down and absorbed by the body over time.
- Cost: The cost of the bioink or biomaterial should also be considered, as it can have a significant impact on the overall cost of 3D printing.

9.2.2 Characterization of Bioinks

Characterization of 3D printing on bioinks and biomaterials for implants and tissue engineering is an important step to evaluate the properties and quality of the printed constructs. Here are some common techniques used for characterization (Iervolino 2019; Kumar et al. 2021a; Hsu et al. 2023):

- Morphological analysis: To analyze the surface and internal features of the printed constructs. This can be done using different imaging techniques, like scanning electron microscopy (SEM), confocal microscopy, and micro-CT.
- Rheological analysis: To investigate the flow and mechanical strengths of the bioinks. This is important for optimizing the printing parameters and ensuring the reproducibility of the printed constructs.
- Chemical analysis: To determine the composition and purity of the bioinks and biomaterials. This can be done using several approaches, such as Fourier-transform infrared spectroscopy (FTIR), Raman spectroscopy, and mass spectrometry.
- Biocompatibility analysis: To evaluate the potential toxicity and immune response of the printed constructs. This can be done using various techniques, including cell viability assays, cytokine analysis, and histopathological evaluation.

- Mechanical testing: To assess the mechanical strengths of the printed constructs, including their stiffness, strength, and elasticity. This is important for determining the suitability of the constructs for their intended application.

The overview of the different types of bioinks and biomaterials that have been selected and characterized for use in 3D printing for implants and tissue engineering is structured in Table 9.2 (Iervolino 2019; Kumar et al. 2021a; Hsu et al. 2023). It also includes the key benefits, highlighting the advantages and limitations of each bioink or biomaterial.

The flowchart of the summarization of characterization techniques is shown in Fig. 9.1 and further research can evaluate the properties and quality of the printed constructs and optimize their formulations for improved outcomes in implant and tissue engineering applications.

9.2.3 In Vitro Testing and Analysis

In vitro testing and analysis of 3D printing on bioinks and biomaterials heavily rely on the development and optimization of 3D printing techniques for implants and tissue engineering. In vitro studies involve the use of biological systems such as cell cultures and tissues to assess the biocompatibility, mechanical properties, and efficacy of 3D-printed constructs. Various tests can be performed to assess cell viability, proliferation, and differentiation within the 3D-printed constructs. Physical and mechanical tests such as tensile and compressive strength, modulus of elasticity, and degradation kinetics can be carried out to assess the mechanical strengths of the 3D-printed fabricates. Furthermore, to identify any potential issues with the 3D-printed constructs before they are implanted in vivo, thereby reducing the risk of adverse outcomes and improving the overall success of the printed fabricates for implants and tissue engineering. The following are some common techniques used for in vitro testing and analysis (Iervolino 2019; Kumar et al. 2021a):

- Cell viability assays: To assess the ability of the printed fabricates to back cell growth and survival. This can be done using various techniques, including MTT assay, AlamarBlue assay, and Live/Dead staining.
- Immunohistochemistry: To analyze the expression of specific proteins within the printed constructs. This can provide valuable information on the differentiation and function of the cells within the constructs.
- Gene expression analysis: To evaluate the changes in gene expression within the printed constructs over time. This can provide insight into the cellular response to the printed constructs and their potential for tissue regeneration.
- Mechanical testing: To determine the mechanical strengths of the printed constructs, including their stiffness, strength, and elasticity. This is important for determining the suitability of the constructs for their intended application.

Table 9.2 Overview of the types of bioinks and biomaterial for implants and tissue engineering via 3D printing (Iervolino 2019; Kumar et al. 2021a; Hsu et al. 2023)

Bioink/biomaterial	Source	Type	Properties	Advantages	Disadvantages
Gelatin methacryloyl (GelMA)	Gelatin	Protein-based	• Biodegradable • Biocompatible • Photocrosslinkable	• Mimics the extracellular matrix • Supports cell growth and differentiation	• Weak mechanical strength • Limited reproducibility • Potential for immune response
Fibrin	Fibrinogen	Protein-based	• Biodegradable • Biocompatible • Allows for cell attachment	• Supports cell proliferation • Angiogenesis • Wound healing	• Poor mechanical properties • Requires activation • Induce an immune response
Alginate	Seaweed	Polysaccharide-based	• Biodegradable • Biocompatible • Easily crosslinked	• High cell viability • Supports cell proliferation and differentiation	• Limited mechanical strength • Low print resolution • Potential for cell detachment
Polyethylene glycol (PEG)c	Synthetic	Hydrogel-based	• Biocompatible • Tunable properties • Can be modified with cell-adhesive peptides	• High print resolution • Customizable mechanical properties • Supports cell proliferation and differentiation	• Non-biodegradable • Low cell infiltration • Induce inflammation
Poly(lactic-co-glycolic acid) (PLGA)	Synthetic	Polymer-based	• Biodegradable • Biocompatible • Can be modified with bioactive molecules	• High mechanical strength • Customizable degradation rate • Supports cell proliferation and differentiation	• Low print resolution • Requires organic solvents

(continued)

Table 9.2 (continued)

Bioink/biomaterial	Source	Type	Properties	Advantages	Disadvantages
					• Induce inflammation
Hydroxyapatite (HA)	Mineral	Ceramics-based	• Biocompatible • Osteoconductive	• Promotes bone growth and integration • Mimics natural bone mineral	• Limited mechanical strength • Low print resolution • High sintering temperature
Collagen	Collagen	Protein-based	• Biodegradable • Biocompatible • Supports cell attachment and proliferation	• Mimics natural extracellular matrix • Supports tissue regeneration	• Low mechanical strength • Limited reproducibility • Induce immune response

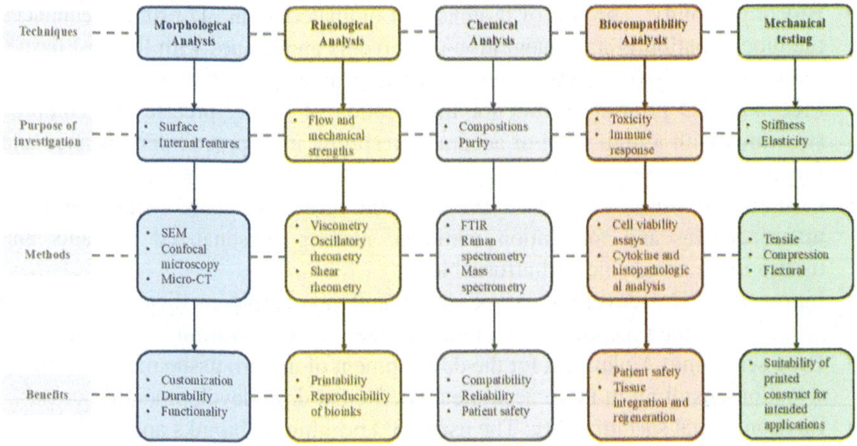

Fig. 9.1 The flowchart of various characterization techniques involved in 3D printing on bioinks/biomaterials

- Histomorphometry: To investigate the structure and composition of the printed constructs. This can provide insight into the organization of the cells and tissues within the constructs and their potential for functional tissue regeneration.

By performing these in vitro tests and analyses, researchers can evaluate the functionality and biocompatibility of the printed constructs and optimize their formulations for improved outcomes in implant and tissue engineering applications.

9.2.4 Significance of 3D Printing on Biomaterials

The purpose of 3D printing on bioinks and biomaterials for implants and tissue engineering is to develop novel and personalized medical devices and tissues that can imitate the arrangement and function of built-in tissues. The scope of the technology is broad, with applications ranging from the creation of patient-specific implants, such as bone, cartilage, and skin, to the fabrication of 3D tissue models for drug screening and testing. Technology also has the potential to revolutionize the field of regenerative medicine by providing new options for repairing and replacing damaged tissues and organs. Ongoing research in this area focuses on developing new and improved materials, optimizing printing techniques, and enhancing the performance and functionality of 3D-printed implants and tissues. 3D printing on bioinks and biomaterials for implants and tissue engineering is significant due to the following reasons (Kirillova et al. 2021; Moghaddam et al. 2021; Yin et al. 2022):

- Personalization: The creation of patient-specific implants and tissues that closely mimic the structure and function of native tissues, resulting in improved outcomes and reduced risks.

- Biocompatibility: The use of bioinks and biomaterials in 3D printing enhances the biocompatibility and integration of implants and tissues with the host tissue, reducing the risk of rejection and improving patient outcomes.
- Precision: 3D printing allows for the creation of highly precise and complex structures with a high level of accuracy, resulting in improved performance and functionality.
- Cost-effectiveness: To reduce the cost and time associated with traditional manufacturing and fabrication methods, making personalized implants and tissues more accessible and affordable.
- Innovation: The development of novel and innovative medical devices and tissues, with the potential to revolutionize the field of re-forming medicine.
- Drug screening: A platform for the development of in vitro tissue models for drug selection, resulting in more accurate and efficient drug development processes.
- Environmental sustainability: The use of 3D printing on bioinks and biomaterials can reduce waste and improve environmental sustainability by reducing the need for traditional manufacturing and fabrication processes.

9.3 3D Printing Techniques Using Bioinks and Biomaterials

Several 3D printing techniques can be used with bioinks and biomaterials. Here are some of the most common ones:

9.3.1 Extrusion-Based Printing

Extrusion-based 3D printing is one of the most used techniques in the field of tissue engineering and implant manufacturing using bioinks and biomaterials. It involves the extrusion of a viscous bioink or biomaterial through a nozzle, which is deposited layer by layer to create the final 3D construct (Velu et al. 2019a, 2020b). Figure 9.2 shows the schematics of extrusion-based 3D printing and its type on bioinks/biomaterial. There have been many research studies on extrusion-based printing with bioinks and biomaterials for these applications.

Jiannan Li et al. present that the addition of xanthan gum and polyethylene glycol dimethacrylate (PEGDMA) to the GelMA/alginate combination developed a room-temperature printable hydrogel bioink. The addition of PEGDMA makes it easier to tune the hydrogel's mechanical properties, whereas xanthan gum increases the hydrogel's viscosity which makes extrusion easier. The developed hydrogel exhibits good printability, broadly tunable mechanical, degradation, ionic solubility, and cytocompatibility properties and delivers excellent flexibility for bioprinting and tissue engineering (Li et al. 2023).

Hatai Jongprasitkul et al. developed an injectable hydrogel by two different crosslinking methods that used both ionic and photocrosslinkable bioinks. Methacrylate gellan gum (GGMA) was used as the biomaterial ink, which was altered to an extrudable hydrogel through the addition of an ionic crosslinker (Ca^{2+}), followed by

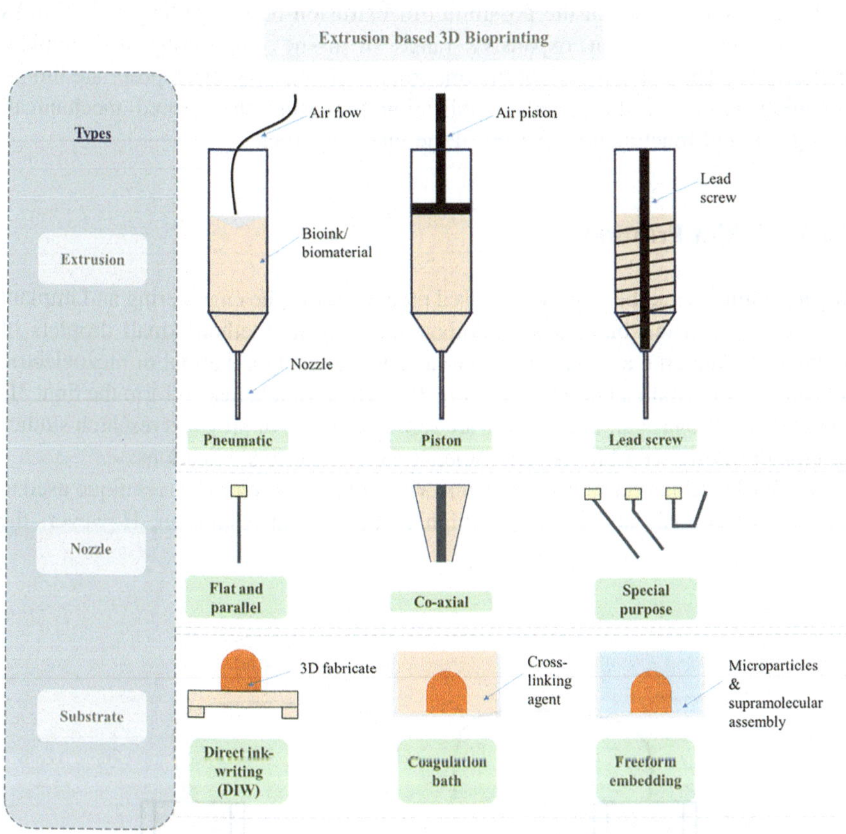

Fig. 9.2 The schematics of extrusion-based 3D printing and its type on bioinks/biomaterials

photocrosslinking. The optimized GGMA ink formulation demonstrated good printability during fabrication and was used to print 3D structures. Although the printed fabricates required greater resolution than control structures, the study shows that pre-crosslinked GGMA has the potential for an extensive range of bioprinting applications (Jongprasitkul et al. 2022).

Killian Flégeau et al. have developed granular hydrogel bioinks for 3D bioprinting cartilage tissue with improved porosity and modularity compared to traditional hydrogel-based bioinks. Enzymatically crosslinked hyaluronic acid (HA) microgels were used to form secondary crosslinked scaffolds with tunable porosity. Both in vitro and in vivo, the bioinks' exceptional rheological capabilities allowed for the creation of mature cartilage-like tissues, with thinner microgels creating stable structures with reduced immunogenicity and constant tissue development. The study provides a greater understanding of the foreign body response to the implantation of porous scaffolds (Flégeau et al. 2022).

These studies establish the possibility of extrusion-based printing with bioinks and biomaterials for an expansive range of tissue engineering and implant applications. They also highlight the importance of selecting the appropriate bioink and biomaterial for the specific application to ensure the desired mechanical, biological, and functional properties of the final construct.

9.3.2 Inkjet Printing

Inkjet printing is another commonly used practice for tissue engineering and implant manufacturing using bioinks and biomaterials. In this method, small droplets of bioink or biomaterial are deposited onto a substrate using a thermal or piezoelectric actuator inkjet printhead, as shown in Fig. 9.3. The droplets fuse to form the final 3D fabricate (Kirillova et al. 2021). Here are some examples of previous research studies on inkjet printing with bioinks and biomaterials for these applications:

Ratima Suntornnond et al. discuss material jetting bioprinting, a technique used to deposit biomaterials and cells with high precision and resolution. However, the

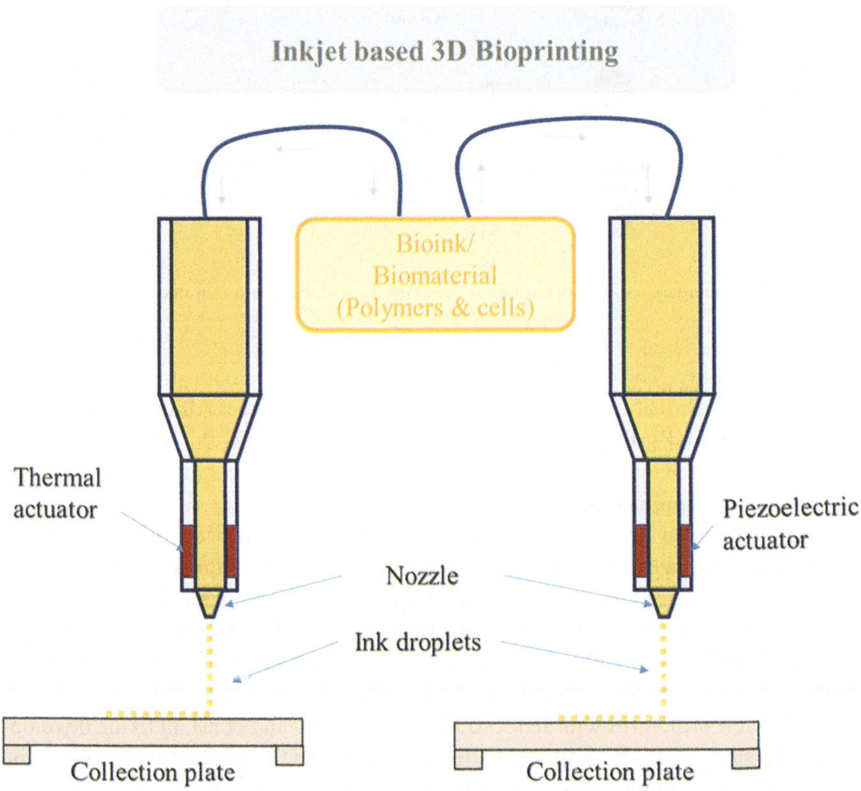

Fig. 9.3 Schematics of thermal and piezoelectric actuator printing setup

technique is limited by the series of the bio-printable hydrogel. To increase GelMA's printability, the article suggests adjustments that include saponification and heat treatment. The suggested method may be appropriate for basic cell and material interaction experiments (Suntornnond et al. 2022).

Elahe Masaeli et al. have developed a scaffold-free inkjet bioprinting system to create a layered retinal model for ocular tissue engineering that consists of bio-printed photoreceptor cells (PRs) over the bio-printed retinal pigment epithelium (RPE). Well-positioned structural layers and generated markers demonstrate a functional RPE monolayer and the potential to study sight-threatening diseases. The study highlights the benefits of carrier-free bioprinting for designing retinal therapies and maintaining layered complexity in ocular tissue engineering (Masaeli et al. 2020).

Hang Liu et al. developed ultrathin polycaprolactone scaffolds with an electrohydrodynamic jet (EHDJ) printing method for retinal pigment epithelial (RPE) cell culture, aiming to analyze retinal disorders including age-related macular degeneration (AMD). The scaffolds, resembling native human Bruch's membrane, showed high permeability and transepithelial potential difference and allowed RPE cells to form a polarized and functional monolayered epithelium. The findings suggest that the EHDJ-printed scaffolds can be a potential in vitro model for studying retinal diseases and treatment methods (Liu et al. 2022).

These studies prove the feasibility of inkjet printing with bioinks and biomaterials for an expansive range of tissue engineering and implant applications. They highlighted the modification to improve its printability for fundamental cells, to create a layered retinal model for ocular tissue engineering, demonstrating the potential to study sight-threatening diseases and finally suggesting a potential in vitro model for studying retinal diseases and treatment methods.

9.3.3 Laser-Assisted Printing

Laser-assisted printing is a relatively new technique for 3D printing with bioinks and biomaterials, but it has shown promise for tissue engineering and implant applications. This method uses a laser to solidify a liquid bioink or biomaterial layer by layer, creating the final 3D construct as shown in Fig. 9.4. Here are a few examples of previous research studies on laser-assisted printing with bioinks and biomaterials:

Olivia Kérourédan et al. utilized a pattern of tdTomato-labeled endothelial cells mixed with mesenchymal stem cells on a collagen hydrogel was created to form capillary-like structures using laser-assisted bioprinting. The formation and preservation of the capillary-like structures are the results of adding a collagen I hydrogel with vascular endothelial growth factor over the patterned cells. Tissue-engineered fabricates made of collagen hydrogel show that laser-assisted bioprinting may be used to create a vascular network with a specified design (Kérourédan et al. 2019).

Gerard Boix-Lemonche et al. reported a novel tissue-engineering technique for repairing corneal stroma utilizing 3D bio-printed hydrogel structures including

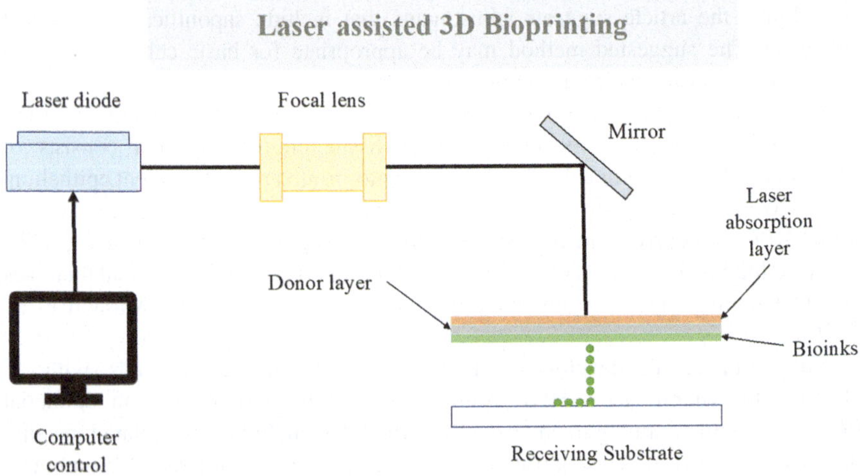

Fig. 9.4 The schematics of laser-assisted 3D printing using bioinks

mesenchymal stromal cells (MSCs). Using femtosecond laser-assisted intrastromal keratoplasty, these structures are transplanted into porcine corneas grown in organ culture. Throughout the observation time, the MSC-loaded bioprinted constructs remained intact, sustained cell survival, and contained extracellular matrix elements and moving cells. After day 14 post-implantation, optical coherence tomography imaging and immunofluorescent staining showed that the cellularized tissue equivalents had few or no cells (Boix-Lemonche et al. 2023).

Lothar Koch et al. produced tiny capillaries in predetermined patterns via Laser-based bioprinting. Since a functional vascular network is required for thicker tissues, they discovered that closed tubular structures with lumina could be printed, but the structures only lasted when other cell types were present to offer external stimulation (Koch et al. 2021).

Laser-assisted bioprinting using biomaterials is essential in tissue engineering as it enables the development of a vascular network with precise shapes and patterns in tissue-engineered fabricates. Additionally, it can be used to create small capillaries in predefined patterns, although determination of the printed tubular structures was attained only in tissue with external stimulation by other cell types.

9.3.4 Stereolithography

Stereolithography (SLA) is a 3D printing technique that utilizes photosensitive resin and a light source to create highly precise, detailed, and complex 3D structures. The technique uses a laser to polymerize a liquid photopolymer resin layer by layer to create the final 3D construct, as shown in Fig. 9.5. It is typically used for creating small, high-resolution structures. While it is a popular technique for rapid

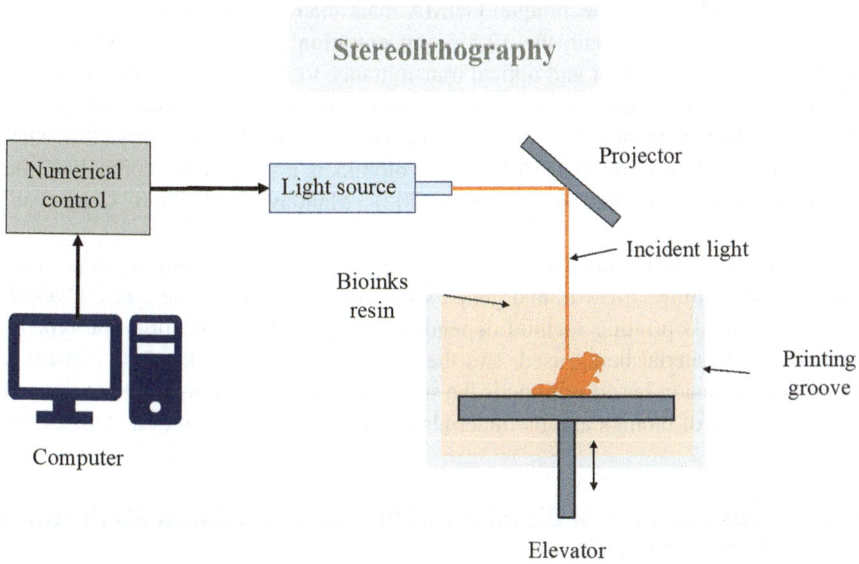

Fig. 9.5 The schematic of stereolithography using photocurable bioinks resin

prototyping and product development, it has also shown promise for tissue engineering and implant applications (Park et al. 2016). Here are a few examples of previous research studies on stereolithography with bioinks and biomaterials:

Lennard K. Shopperly et al. developed a biomimetic method to produce artificial cartilage-like tissue using stereolithographic bioprinting. Gelatin and methacrylate hyaluronic acid bioinks were mixed and layered to resemble the zonal structure of articular cartilage before being printed with porcine chondrocytes. The constructions were grown for 14 days before being examined for cellular viability, collagen and proteoglycan synthesis, and gene expression. The COL2A1 gene expression was significantly higher in the biomimetically stratified structures, which also maintained their gradient-like structure. With this method, cartilaginous tissue can potentially be more accurately modeled for use in in vitro or regenerative therapies (Boix-Lemonche et al. 2023; Shopperly et al. 2022).

To create slow sol-gel transition and visible light cross-linkable bioinks appropriate for digital light processing (DLP)-dependent stereolithography (SLA) bioprinting, Hitendra Kumar et al. improved the synthesis parameters of gelatin methacryloyl (GelMA). They identified eight GelMA arrangements that met for DLP-SLA bioprinting and discovered that the ones made with reverse osmosis purified water were best for high printing resolution. The bioinks showed excellent biocompatibility and allowed for the growth and integration of astrocytes and fibroblasts, highlighting their potential in tissue engineering and re-forming medicine applications (Moghaddam et al. 2021; Kumar et al. 2021b).

Sharareh Mahdavi et al. employed Gelatin methacrylate (GelMA) combined with corneal stromal cells as a bioink to 3D bioprint the human corneal stroma using the stereolithography (SLA) technique. GelMA macromer concentrations of 7.5% and 12.5% were evaluated, with the 12.5% concentration producing a stiffer scaffold with similar water content and optical transmittance to native corneal stroma tissue. Higher cytocompatibility, attachment, proliferation, and gene expression in the 12.5% GelMA scaffolds were seen in the encapsulated human corneal stromal cells, showing that using GelMA hydrogel bioinks is a strategy for corneal stroma tissue biofabrication (Moghaddam et al. 2021; Mahdavi et al. 2020; Ulag et al. 2021).

The use of various bioinks/biomaterials has shown promising results in promoting cellular viability, growth, and gene expression in various tissue types. Overall, the choice of 3D printing method depends on the specific application, the type of bioink or biomaterial being used, and the desired properties of the final construct. However, extrusion-based printing is the supreme technique due to its versatility and the wide range of bioinks and biomaterials that can be used with it (Yu et al. 2020).

9.4 Applications of Bioinks and Biomaterials Using 3D Printing Techniques

9.4.1 Overview of Implantable Medical Devices

3D printing is adapted in cochlear implants, as conventional cochlear implants use a standard electrode array that may not fit every patient's unique cochlear anatomy, reducing the implant's effectiveness. A personalized electrode array can be made for each patient via 3D printing, improving the chances of success. To increase biocompatibility and implant durability, scientists are looking into the use of biomaterials like poly(lactic-co-glycolic acid) (PLGA) and hydroxyapatite in the 3D printing process (Lehner et al. 2022).

Using 3D printing and biomaterials, neural/brain implants are also being created, such as brain–computer interfaces (BCIs). The printing of brain implants using biocompatible polymers like polycaprolactone (PCL) and polylactic acid (PLA) is one area of focus (Mao et al. 2023). These substances can be combined to produce a porous scaffold that aids in the regeneration of brain tissue and the integration of the implant. Furthermore, 3D printing enables the development of more intricate implant designs, such as electrodes with several contact points, which can increase the precision of neural signal stimulation and recording.

Another application for 3D printing and biomaterials is intraocular lens implants. There are few alternatives for vision correction with conventional lens implants, and there is a risk of problems like infection and inflammation. Nevertheless, 3D printing enables the production of personalized lens implants that can enhance biocompatibility and meet certain requirements for vision correction. The 3D printing method can also increase biocompatibility and encourage tissue integration with the implant by using bioinks like gelatin and collagen (Tan et al. 2022).

Bionic eye implants, which are designed to restore vision in individuals with retinal degenerative diseases, are also being developed using 3D printing and biomaterials. The use of biocompatible and electrically conductive materials, such as graphene and carbon nanotubes, in the implant's electrode array, is one area of focus (VijaiMeyyappan and Daniel 2022). These substances can lessen the possibility of negative responses while increasing the effectiveness of electrical signal transmission. Moreover, 3D printing enables the production of custom-fit implants that can increase stimulation precision and restore vision to a larger extent.

Spine implants, which are used to provide stability and support to the spine, are also being developed using 3D printing and biomaterials. The use of biodegradable materials, including magnesium alloys, in the 3D printing process, is one area of study (Shiri et al. 2022). These materials have the potential to deteriorate over time, decreasing the possibility of issues such as implant loosening and the requirement for revision surgeries. Furthermore, 3D printing makes it possible to build intricate implants that can increase implant stability and encourage bone formation surrounding the implant.

9.4.1.1 Organoids and Organ-on-Chip

Organoids are three-dimensional constructs that replicate the features of organs in a laboratory setting. They provide an excellent platform for research into the development of organs, the study of diseases, and the testing of pharmaceuticals. The size, complexity, and reproducibility of organoids are, however, constrained by current production techniques (Velasco et al. 2020). A potentially effective way to solve these problems is to use 3D printing technology. One of the key developments in 3D printing organoids is the creation of bioinks, substances used to create 3D structures that can support cell growth and differentiation. Hydrogels, extracellular matrix (ECM) components, and cell-rich materials are only a few examples of the materials that can be used to make bioinks. Because of their good biocompatibility, adaptable mechanical properties, and high-water content, hydrogels are frequently employed as bioinks for 3D printing (Da Silva et al. 2020). To improve cell adhesion and differentiation, bioinks have also been made with ECM components such as laminin and fibronectin. The creation of organ-on-a-chip models using microfluidic technology has also been investigated. These models have been created for several organs, including the liver, heart, and lung, and they have shown encouraging results in the testing of medications and the modeling of diseases. 3D printing organoids and organ-on-a-chip models utilizing bioinks can enhance our understanding of organ formation, disease mechanisms, and medication discovery with further improvements in this technology (Kogler et al. 2023).

9.4.1.2 Implants and Tissue Engineering

Bioinks and biomaterials are vital in 3D printing for implants and tissue engineering. The ability to create patient-specific implants and constructs with high accuracy has the potential to revolutionize healthcare. The selection of bioinks and biomaterials depends on various factors, such as biocompatibility, mechanical properties, printability, degradability, and cost (Velu et al. 2021). Research is ongoing to develop new and improved materials with better biocompatibility, mechanical properties, and cellular response. Extrusion-based printing is the supreme technique for tissue

Table 9.3 Bioinks and biomaterial using 3D printing techniques for implants and tissue engineering (Chun et al. 2018; Velu et al. 2019b; Velu and Singamneni 2014; Gopinathan and Noh 2018)

Bioinks/ biomaterial	Source	Type	Application	
			Implants	Tissue engineering
Hydroxyapatite	Synthetic	Biomaterial	• Dental • Cranial • Orthopedic	• Dental • Bone
Polycaprolactone	Synthetic	Biomaterial	• Cranial • Orthopedic • Facial	• Bone
PLA/PGA/ PLGA	Synthetic	Biomaterial	• Cranial • Orthopedic • Cardiovascular	• Cardiovascular
Collagen	Bovine, porcine, or human sources	Bioinks	• Dental • Facial • Prosthetic • Cardiovascular • Breast	• Bone • Cartilage • Skin
Gelatin	Bovine, porcine, or fish sources	Bioinks	• Prosthetic • Cardiovascular • Breast • Cranial • Orthopedic	• Cartilage
Alginate	Seaweed	Bioinks		• Cartilage • Skin
Fibrin	Fibrinogen	Bioinks		• Bone • Cartilage • Skin

engineering and implant applications, while inkjet printing is also showing great potential. The development of new and improved bioinks and biomaterials is expected to lead to even greater potential for tissue engineering, drug delivery systems, and other medical applications. Table 9.3 provides an overview of the applications of bioinks and biomaterials in 3D printing for implants and tissue engineering (Chun et al. 2018; Velu et al. 2019b; Velu and Singamneni 2014; Gopinathan and Noh 2018).

9.5 Conclusion

9.5.1 Summary

3D printing has the potential to revolutionize various industries, including healthcare, by creating highly complex structures with accuracy, making it ideal for creating patient-specific implants and tissue engineering. Bioinks and biomaterials are key components in 3D bioprinting, and their selection depends on various factors such as biocompatibility, mechanical properties, printability, degradability, and cost. Characterization of biomaterials is an important step to evaluate the properties and quality of printed constructs. Ongoing efforts aim to improve the biocompatibility, mechanical properties, and cellular response of these materials. Extrusion-based and inkjet printing methods are commonly used and have exhibited great prospects in tissue engineering and implant applications. The article presents research studies on the use of various bioinks and biomaterials with these techniques to create a range of tissue constructs. The article emphasizes the importance of selecting the appropriate bioinks and biomaterial for the specific application to ensure the desired mechanical, biological, and functional properties of the final construct.

9.5.2 Limitation

The design and development of 3D printing with bioinks and biomaterials for implants and tissue engineering face several limitations. One of the significant challenges is the lack of standardization in bioink and biomaterial characterization, which makes it difficult to compare different studies and materials. This is due to the diverse range of properties required for different tissues, including mechanical, biological, and functional properties, and the lack of consensus on how to evaluate these properties.

Another challenge is the limited availability of suitable biomaterials for 3D printing. While there has been substantial advancement in developing new biomaterials, few are suitable for use in 3D printing due to challenges such as printability, biocompatibility, and mechanical properties (Chun et al. 2018; Velu et al. 2023b). Moreover, the high cost of biomaterials also limits their availability and application. The resolution and accuracy of 3D printing also pose limitations, particularly for small features and structures. This can affect the functionality and viability of printed constructs, especially for tissues that require high precision and complexity, such as blood vessels and nerves.

Another limitation is the lack of knowledge of the long-term performance and safety of 3D-printed constructs in the body. The behavior of printed constructs in vivo is still not well understood, and the long-term biocompatibility and stability of these constructs remain a concern.

Overall, while 3D printing on bioinks and biomaterials has tremendous potential, there are still some challenges and limitations that need to be addressed to fully realize the potential of this technology in implants and tissue engineering.

9.5.3 Implications for Future Research

As 3D printing technology continues to advance, there are many future possibilities for the design and development of bioinks and biomaterials for implants and tissue engineering. The field of 3D bioprinting is anticipated to continue to grow, with more emphasis on the development of personalized treatments and complex structures (Fonseca et al. 2020).

One potential area for future research is the further exploration of stem cells in 3D bioprinting (Yun et al. 2019). Stem cells have the potential to differentiate into many different cell types, and they can be used to create complex tissues and organs. There is also potential for using 3D bioprinting to create organs for transplantation, which could help address the shortage of donor organs.

Another area for future research is the development of new bioinks and biomaterials with enhanced properties. For example, researchers are exploring the use of nanomaterials and smart materials in 3D bioprinting. These materials can respond to changes in their environment, such as temperature or pH, and could be used to create dynamic structures that can change over time.

There is also potential for combining 3D bioprinting with other technologies, such as microfluidics and robotics. This could enable the creation of more complex structures and could lead to new applications in areas including drug screening and tissue modeling.

In addition to technical advances, there is also a need for regulatory frameworks to govern the use of 3D bioprinting in healthcare. As personalized treatments become more common, there will be a need for standards and guidelines to ensure the safety and efficacy of these treatments.

Overall, future research on 3D printing on bioinks and biomaterials for implants and tissue engineering should focus on advancing the technology to advance the quality, functionality, and safety of printed fabricates, as well as addressing the regulatory and commercialization challenges.

References

Barrs RW, Jia J, Silver SE, Yost M, Mei Y (2020) Biomaterials for bioprinting microvasculature. Chem Rev 120(19):10887–10949

Boix-Lemonche G, Nagymihaly RM, Niemi EM, Josifovska N, Johansen S, Moe MC et al (2023) Intra-corneal implantation of 3D bioprinted scaffolds containing mesenchymal stromal cells using femtosecond-laser-assisted intrastromal keratoplasty. Macromol Biosci 23:2200422

Chun HJ, Park CH, Kwon IK, Khang G (eds) (2018) Cutting-edge enabling technologies for regenerative medicine. Springer, Singapore

Da Silva K, Kumar P, Choonara YE, du Toit LC, Pillay V (2020) Three-dimensional printing of extracellular matrix (ECM)-mimicking scaffolds: a critical review of the current ECM materials. J Biomed Mater Res A 108(12):2324–2350

Das S, Jang J (2019) Bioprinting vasculature. In: 3D bioprinting in medicine: technologies, bioinks, and applications. Springer, pp 127–148

Flégeau K, Puiggali-Jou A, Zenobi-Wong M (2022) Cartilage tissue engineering by extrusion bioprinting utilizing porous hyaluronic acid microgel bioinks. Biofabrication 14(3):034105

Fonseca AC, Melchels FP, Ferreira MJ, Moxon SR, Potjewyd G, Dargaville TR et al (2020) Emulating human tissues and organs: a bioprinting perspective toward personalized medicine. Chem Rev 120(19):11093–11139

Gopinathan J, Noh I (2018) Recent trends in bioinks for 3D printing. Biomater Res 22:1–15

Hsu CW, Williams T, Yu X (2023) Recent advancements and trends in 3D printing for biomedical applications. ChemRxiv. https://doi.org/10.26434/chemrxiv-2023-03c1m

Iervolino F (2019) Additive manufacturing of low and high temperature resistant thermoplastic composites and sandwich panels for sound absorption. Doctoral dissertation, Polytechnique Montréal

Jongprasitkul H, Turunen S, Parihar VS, Kellomäki M (2022) Two-step crosslinking to enhance the printability of methacrylated gellan gum biomaterial ink for extrusion-based 3D bioprinting. Bioprinting 25:e00185

Kérourédan O, Bourget JM, Rémy M, Crauste-Manciet S, Kalisky J, Catros S et al (2019) Micropatterning of endothelial cells to create a capillary-like network with defined architecture by laser-assisted bioprinting. J Mater Sci Mater Med 30:1–12

Kirillova A, Yeazel TR, Asheghali D, Petersen SR, Dort S, Gall K, Becker ML (2021) Fabrication of biomedical scaffolds using biodegradable polymers. Chem Rev 121(18):11238–11304

Koch L, Deiwick A, Chichkov B (2021) Capillary-like formations of endothelial cells in defined patterns generated by laser bioprinting. Micromachines 12(12):1538

Kogler S, Kømurcu KS, Olsen C, Shoji JY, Skottvoll FS, Krauss S et al (2023) Organoids, organ-on-a-chip, separation science and mass spectrometry: an update. TrAC Trends Anal Chem 161: 116996

Kumar A, Voicu SI, Thakur VK (2021a) 3D printable gel-inks for tissue engineering. Springer, Singapore

Kumar H, Sakthivel K, Mohamed MG, Boras E, Shin SR, Kim K (2021b) Designing gelatin methacryloyl (GelMA)-based bioinks for visible light stereolithographic 3D biofabrication. Macromol Biosci 21(1):2000317

Lee H, Jang TS, Han G, Kim HW, Jung HD (2021) Freeform 3D printing of vascularized tissues: challenges and strategies. J Tissue Eng 12:20417314211057236

Lehner E, Menzel M, Gündel D, Plontke SK, Mäder K, Klehm J et al (2022) Microimaging of a novel intracochlear drug delivery device in combination with cochlear implants in the human inner ear. Drug Deliv Transl Res 12:1–10

Li H, Fan W, Zhu X (2020) Three-dimensional printing: the potential technology widely used in medical fields. J Biomed Mater Res A 108(11):2217–2229

Li J, Moeinzadeh S, Kim C, Pan CC, Weale G, Kim S et al (2023) Development and systematic characterization of GelMA/alginate/PEGDMA/xanthan gum hydrogel bioink system for extrusion bioprinting. Biomaterials 293:121969

Liu H, Wu F, Chen R, Chen Y, Yao K, Liu Z et al (2022) Electrohydrodynamic jet-printed ultrathin polycaprolactone scaffolds mimicking Bruch's membrane for retinal pigment epithelial tissue engineering. Int J Bioprint 8(3):550

Mahdavi SS, Abdekhodaie MJ, Kumar H, Mashayekhan S, Baradaran-Rafii A, Kim K (2020) Stereolithography 3D bioprinting method for fabrication of human corneal stroma equivalent. Ann Biomed Eng 48:1955–1970

Mao X, Li T, Cheng J, Tao M, Li Z, Ma Y et al (2023) Nerve ECM and PLA-PCL based electrospun bilayer nerve conduit for nerve regeneration. Front Bioeng Biotechnol 11:1103435

Masaeli E, Forster V, Picaud S, Karamali F, Nasr-Esfahani MH, Marquette C (2020) Tissue engineering of retina through high resolution 3-dimensional inkjet bioprinting. Biofabrication 12(2):025006

Moghaddam AS, Khonakdar HA, Arjmand M, Jafari SH, Bagher Z, Moghaddam ZS et al (2021) Review of bioprinting in regenerative medicine: naturally derived bioinks and stem cells. ACS Appl Biomater 4(5):4049–4070

Park JY, Gao G, Jang J, Cho DW (2016) 3D printed structures for delivery of biomolecules and cells: tissue repair and regeneration. J Mater Chem B 4(47):7521–7539

Shahbazi M, Jäger H (2020) Current status in the utilization of biobased polymers for 3D printing process: a systematic review of the materials, processes, and challenges. ACS Appl Biomater 4(1):325–369

Shiri M, Jafari H, Singh R (2022) Effect of extrusion parameters on degradation of magnesium alloys for bioimplant applications: a review. Trans Nonferrous Metals Soc China 32(9): 2787–2813

Shopperly LK, Spinnen J, Krüger JP, Endres M, Sittinger M, Lam T et al (2022) Blends of gelatin and hyaluronic acid stratified by stereolithographic bioprinting approximate cartilaginous matrix gradients. J Biomed Mater Res B Appl Biomater 110(10):2310–2322

Suntornnond R, Ng WL, Huang X, Yeow CHE, Yeong WY (2022) Improving printability of hydrogel-based bio-inks for thermal inkjet bioprinting applications via saponification and heat treatment processes. J Mater Chem B 10(31):5989–6000

Tan G, Ioannou N, Mathew E, Tagalakis AD, Conceptualisation DAL, Conceptualisation CYWM (2022) 3D printing in ophthalmology: from medical implants to personalised medicine. Int J Pharm 625:122094

Ulag S, Uysal E, Bedir T, Sengor M, Ekren N, Ustundag CB et al (2021) Recent developments and characterization techniques in 3D printing of corneal stroma tissue. Polym Adv Technol 32(8): 3287–3296

Velasco V, Shariati SA, Esfandyarpour R (2020) Microtechnology-based methods for organoid models. Microsyst Nanoeng 6(1):76

Velu R, Singamneni S (2014) Selective laser sintering of polymer biocomposites based on polymethyl methacrylate. J Mater Res 29(17):1883–1892

Velu R, Fernyhough A, Smith DA, Guen M, Singamneni S (2016) Selective laser sintering of biocomposite materials. Lasers Eng Old City Publ 35:173

Velu R, Vaheed NM, Venkatesan C, Raspall F, Krishnan M (2019a) Experimental investigation on fabrication of thermoset prepreg composites using automated fibre placement process and 3D printed substrate. Proc CIRP 85:296–301

Velu R, Calais T, Jayakumar A, Raspall F (2019b) A comprehensive review on bio-nanomaterials for medical implants and feasibility studies on fabrication of such implants by additive manufacturing technique. Materials 13(1):92

Velu R, Vaheed NM, Venkatesan C, Raspall F, Krishnan M (2020a) Experimental investigation on fabrication of thermoset prepreg composites using automated fibre placement process and 3D printed substrate. Proc CIRP 85:293–298

Velu R, Vaheed N, Ramachandran MK, Raspall F (2020b) Experimental investigation of robotic 3D printing of high-performance thermoplastics (PEEK): a critical perspective to support automated fibre placement process. Int J Adv Manuf Technol 108:1007–1025

Velu R, Jayashankar DK, Subburaj K (2021) Additive processing of biopolymers for medical applications. In: Additive manufacturing. Elsevier, pp 635–659

Velu R, Ramachandran MK, Anand Kumar S (2023a) State-of-the-art overview and recent trends in additive manufacturing: opportunities, limitations, and current market. In: Nanotechnology-based additive manufacturing: product design, properties and applications, vol 1. Wiley, pp 1–25

Velu R, Tulasi R, Ramachandran MK (2023b) Environmental impact, challenges for industrial applications and future perspectives of additive manufacturing. In: Nanotechnology-based additive manufacturing: product design, properties and applications, vol 2. Wiley, pp 691–709

VijaiMeyyappan M, Daniel RJ (2022) Modelling, simulation and analysis of NPDA for sub-retinal implant using nano materials. In: IOP conference series: materials science and engineering, vol 1225(1). IOP Publishing, p 012010

Whenish R, Velu R, Anand Kumar S, Ramprasath LS (2021) Additive manufacturing technologies for biomedical implants using functional biocomposites. In: High-performance composite structures: additive manufacturing and processing. Springer, Singapore, pp 25–44

Yin Y, Xiao X, Peng L (2022) Prevention of venous thrombosis of lower limbs after cesarean section based on smart medical air pressure therapy instrument. BioMed Res Int 2022:1451881

Yu X, Zhang T, Li Y (2020) 3D printing and bioprinting nerve conduits for neural tissue engineering. Polymers 12(8):1637

Yun BG, Lee SH, Jeon JH, Kim SW, Jung CK, Park G et al (2019) Accelerated bone regeneration via three-dimensional cell-printed constructs containing human nasal turbinate-derived stem cells as a clinically applicable therapy. ACS Biomater Sci Eng 5(11):6171–6185

3D-Printed Smart Implants in Orthopedic Surgery

10

T. Pandelani, F. J. Nemavhola, and Anand Kumar Subramaniyan

Contents

T. Pandelani (✉)
Unisa Biomechanics Research Lab, Department of Mechanical Engineering, School of Engineering, College of Science Engineering and Technology, University of South Africa, Pretoria, South Africa

Department of Electrical and Electronic Engineering Science, University of Johannesburg, Johannesburg, South Africa

Faculty of Engineering and the Built Environment, Durban University of Technology, Durban, South Africa
e-mail: epandet@unisa.ac.za

F. J. Nemavhola
Faculty of Engineering and the Built Environment, Durban University of Technology, Durban, South Africa

A. K. Subramaniyan
Additive Manufacturing Research Laboratory, Mechanical Engineering, Indian Institute of Technology Jammu, Jammu, Jammu and Kashmir, India

R. Velu et al. (eds.), *Digital Design and Manufacturing of Medical Devices and Systems*, https://doi.org/10.1007/978-981-99-7100-8_10

Abstract

The field of orthopedic surgery has witnessed significant advancements in recent years, particularly with the emergence of 3D printing technology. 3D-printed smart implants have revolutionized the way orthopedic surgeries are approached, offering numerous benefits such as improved patient-specific customization, enhanced biocompatibility, and the integration of smart features. This chapter explores the current state of 3D-printed smart implants in orthopedic surgery, examining their applications, advantages, challenges, and future prospects. The development and implementation of 3D printing technology have revolutionized the field of biomedical engineering, particularly in the domain of smart implants. Smart implants, also known as intelligent implants or active implants, are advanced medical devices that integrate sensing, actuating, and feedback capabilities to enhance their functionality and improve patient outcomes. 3D printing enables the fabrication of complex implant geometries with high precision, personalized customization, and the incorporation of functional components, making it an ideal manufacturing technique for smart implants. This review aims to provide an overview of the current state of 3D-printed smart implants, their applications in various medical fields, and the challenges and future prospects in this rapidly evolving field.

Keywords

Smart implants · Orthopedic · 3D-printing · Biomaterials · Biocompatibility · Regulations

10.1 Introduction

Reconstructive surgery aims to restore tissue defects by replacing them with similar autologous tissue to achieve good clinical outcomes. 3D printing technology has several uses in different fields of application in biomedical engineering. In pre-operation planning for complex surgeries, the technology has enhanced success by enabling surgery visualization and understanding of complex patient-specific anatomy before the surgical operation. The technology has also helped educate trainee surgeons to understand the complex 3D anatomy of different organs. It also aids better communication across various hospital departments working on the same patient. Patients are also able to understand the risks involved in their surgical procedure.

In the development of medical devices, 3D printing technology has led to the fabrication of cost-effective patient-specific models and innovative dental implants. The process of creating 3D-printed custom implants begins with obtaining patient-specific imaging data, such as computed tomography (CT) scans or magnetic resonance imaging (MRI) images. Advanced imaging techniques allow for the accurate capture of the patient's bones, soft tissues, and blood vessels. These data are then converted into a detailed 3D model, which serves as the foundation for designing the custom implant (Wu et al. 2023).

The technology helps avoid material wastage and apparently manufacturing errors are less costly. Due to the low cost of consumables when anomalies arise. 3D printing technology has a huge impact in tissue engineering and organ bioprinting. The shortage of organ donors necessitates alternative ways of making organs available to patients. The evolution of 3D printing also shows that adding living cells and extracellular matrix to biomaterials aids tissue development and regeneration. This work has led to the development of organs as complex as the liver, which can further benefit drug discovery (Kizawa et al. 2017). Besides, innovative 3DP dressings have been developed to accelerate wound healing. The wound dressings automatically release healing biochemicals or cells into the broken skin area. Zhou and Vijayavenkataraman (2021) reviewed the potential of 3D printable conductive materials for tissue engineering and biomedical engineering applications, considering that they possess desirable properties such as conductivity, which can benefit the bioelectric potential of the engineering tissues. They found that ionic liquids have a huge potential for further research and development given their wide range of choices, excellent conductivity, and ability to tune their electrical and mechanical properties.

Drug delivery is another area of biomedical engineering that has benefitted from 3D printing technology. Some innovative drug delivery systems have been developed, such as wearable devices, capsules of different shapes, shape memory expandable delivery systems (Melocchi et al. 2019), and microneedles. Khatri et al. (2018) highlighted the various formulation strategies available for solid oral drug delivery, where they specifically concluded that these systems are beneficial only when customized for patients. Outwardly, using 3D printing allows for the manufacture of implants with complex geometries and internal architecture that more closely match the required clinical needs.

Polymers, ceramics, and metals have recently been as short- and long-term implantable medical devices due to their good mechanical properties, biocompatibility, and blood compatibility. They can be 3D printed to manufacture implants tailored to meet specific anatomical, mechanical, and biological requirements for biomedical applications, including catheters, cardiovascular devices, etc. Pore size, shape, and overall dimensions can be tailored to create the desired response in the host tissue. Such precise tailoring of the scaffold allows vascularization, oxygenation, and nutrient supply to be optimized to ensure a good outcome once implanted in the clinical setting. The ability to control the architecture is valuable for the biomedical field as it allows for manufacturing bespoke patient-specific implants or the repeatability and reproducibility of several implants.

However, the adoption of 3D-printed smart implants also presents challenges, such as ensuring long-term biocompatibility, reliability, and power supply for the embedded electronic components. As research and innovation progress, addressing these challenges will be crucial for the widespread adoption and successful implementation of this transformative technology.

3D-printed smart implants represent an exciting frontier in medical technology, merging the capabilities of 3D printing with advanced sensors and electronic components. By providing real-time data, responding dynamically to changes in the body, and promoting tissue regeneration, these implants have the potential to significantly improve patient care and outcomes across various medical specialties. As research and development in this area continue, the future of 3D-printed smart implants holds tremendous promise for the advancement of personalized medicine and transformative healthcare solutions.

Overall, this chapter addresses the current research on the current state of 3D printing techniques in orthopedic implant applications. The current challenges and future perspectives are also included. The role of sensors for bio-medical applications is a significant and emerging area in biomedical engineering, and sensors are also described. The application of sensors in biomedical diagnostics and bio instruments has brought a revolutionary change that may already have a positive impact on the quality of life and life-saving nature.

10.2 Introduction to 3D-Printing Process

10.2.1 Historical Background

The historical background of 3D printing traces the evolution and milestones in additive manufacturing, leading to its widespread adoption in various industries today. This review provides an overview of the key developments, technological advancements, and significant contributions that have shaped the field of 3D printing.

The origins of 3D printing can be traced back to the emergence of computer-aided design (CAD) in the 1960s and the pioneering work of Charles W. Hull, who introduced the concept of stereolithography in the 1980s (Hull 1986). Stereolithography served as the foundation for additive manufacturing techniques and marked the birth of 3D printing.

10.2.2 Rapid Prototyping and Industrial Adoption

The 1990s witnessed significant advancements in 3D printing technologies. The development of techniques like selective laser sintering (SLS) by Carl Deckard and fused deposition modeling (FDM) by Scott Crump opened new avenues for rapid prototyping and manufacturing (Deckard 1989; Crump 1989). These techniques allowed for the creation of complex and functional prototypes, revolutionizing the product development process (Hague et al. 2006).

Figure 10.1 shows the 3D printing technologies such as FDM and SLS. For the FDM (A): (a) coil reel; (b) plastic filament; (c) driving motor; (d) extruder; (e) molten paste chamber; (f) nozzle tip; (g) FDM printer bed and for SLS (B): (h) laser; (i) scanner system; (j) roller; (k) power bed.

The 2000s saw a shift toward open-source hardware and software in the 3D printing community. The RepRap project, initiated by Adrian Bowyer, introduced self-replicating 3D printers, enabling affordable and accessible desktop 3D printing (Bowyer 2004). This movement laid the foundation for the democratization of 3D printing technology and sparked a consumer-driven revolution. With the expansion of 3D printing applications, there have been significant advancements in printing materials and processes (Zhang et al. 2022). Innovations in high-resolution printing, multi-material printing, and the introduction of new materials such as metals, ceramics, and composites have broadened the possibilities for functional and end-use part production (Wohlers 2017).

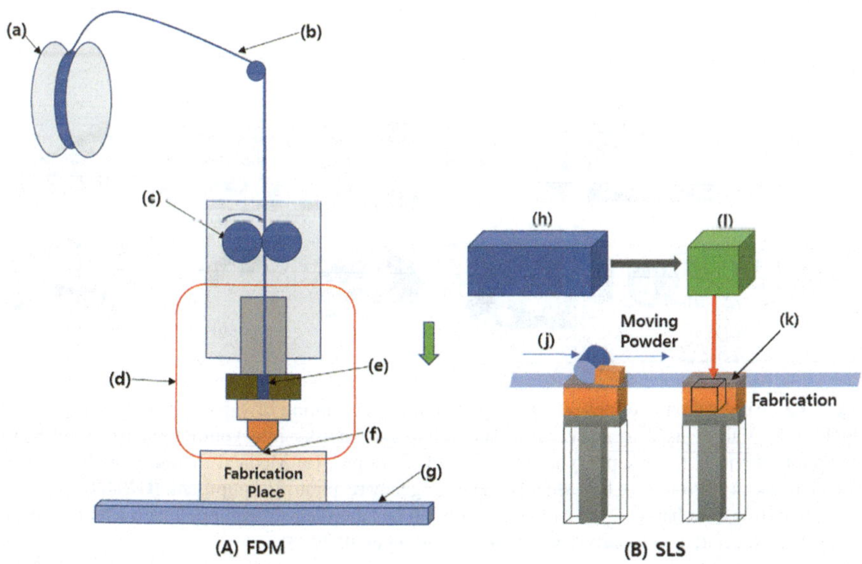

Fig. 10.1 3D printing technologies. (**A**) Fused deposition modeling and (**B**) selective laser sintering (SLS). (Reproduced with permission from Lee 2021)

In recent years, 3D printing has transitioned from a prototyping tool to an integral part of manufacturing processes. Increased precision, reliability, and scalability have led to its integration with traditional manufacturing techniques (Rahman et al. 2018). Industries such as aerospace, automotive, and healthcare have embraced 3D printing for its ability to create complex geometries, reduce costs, and enable customization.

10.2.3 3D Printing in the Medical Field

The medical field has witnessed remarkable advancements through 3D printing. From anatomical models and surgical guides to custom implants and prosthetics, 3D printing has transformed patient care and treatment (Ventola 2014). The process of creating 3D-printed custom implants begins with obtaining patient-specific imaging data, such as computed tomography (CT) scans or magnetic resonance imaging (MRI) images. Advanced imaging techniques allow for the accurate capture of the patient's bones, soft tissues, and blood vessels. These data are then converted into a detailed 3D model, which serves as the foundation for designing the custom implant.

Bioprinting and tissue engineering are emerging frontiers, with the potential to revolutionize regenerative medicine (Murphy and Atala 2014). Figure 10.2 shows the application overview. (a) Valves used to convert the snorkeling face masks into ventilators, (b) valves for respiratory devices, (c) nasopharyngeal swabs, (d) syringes, (e) medical manikins for swabs, (f) silicon masks, (g) protective face shields, (h) emergency respiratory equipment, (i) safety goggles, (j) contact-free door handles, (k) isolation wards, (l) isolation houses equipped with a bed, shower, and toilet.

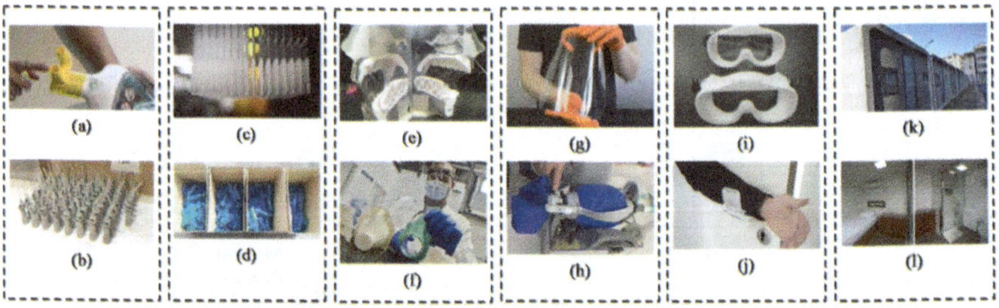

Fig. 10.2 Application overview shows application of 3D printing of valves, swabs, syringes, and shields, (**a**) Valves used to convert the snorkeling face masks into ventilators, (**b**) Valves for respiratory devices, (**c**) nasopharyngeal swabs, (**d**) Syringes, (**e**) Medical manikins for swabs, (**f**) Silicon masks, (**g**) Protective face shields, (**h**) Emergency respiratory equipment, (**i**) Safety goggles, (**j**) Contact-free door handles, (**k**) Isolation wards, (**l**) Isolation houses equipped with a bed, shower, and toilet. (Reprinted with permission from Rajendran et al. 2023)

10.2.4 Overview of the 3D Printing Workflow

The 3D printing workflow involves a series of steps that transform a digital design into a physical object. This overview provides a high-level understanding of the key stages in the 3D printing process. Figure 10.3 shows the 3D printing technology process.

The workflow begins with creating a three-dimensional digital model of the desired object using computer-aided design (CAD) software. The CAD software allows designers to design and manipulate the virtual model, incorporating precise dimensions, shapes, and features.

Once the digital design is finalized, it needs to be prepared for the 3D printing process. Specialized software is used to optimize the design file and slice it into thin cross-sectional layers. This slicing process divides the digital model into a series of 2D layers, which the 3D printer will later build upon (Campbell et al. 2011). Before printing can commence, the 3D printer must be properly set up and calibrated. This involves ensuring the printer is clean, the build platform is leveled, and the printing parameters, such as temperature and speed, are appropriately configured. Calibration ensures accurate and consistent printing results.

With the printer prepared, the 3D printing process begins. The printer follows the instructions generated during the slicing stage to sequentially deposit or solidify the material layer by layer based on the design specifications. As each layer is completed, the build platform is incrementally lowered to accommodate the next layer. Once the printing is finished, the physical object is typically subjected to post-processing steps. Post-processing can involve tasks such as removing support structures, sanding, polishing, or applying finishing touches to enhance the final appearance and functionality of the printed object.

After post-processing, the printed object undergoes a final inspection and evaluation to ensure it meets the desired quality standards. This may involve checking dimensions, surface finish, structural integrity, and other relevant criteria. Inspection and evaluation help identify any defects or issues that may require further adjustments or refinements.

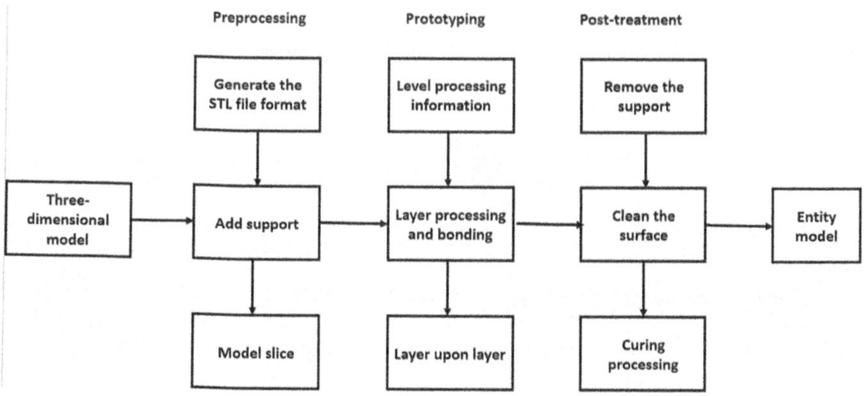

Fig. 10.3 The process flow of 3D printing technology. (Reprinted with permission from Hao and Lin 2020)

10.2.5 Comparison of 3D Printing with Traditional Manufacturing Methods

When 3D printing is compared with traditional manufacturing methods, including subtractive manufacturing and forming and casting processes, 3D printing is superior in design freedom due to the ability to fabricate complex geometries and intricate designs and reduced material waste since the parts are built layer by layer and only the required material is used, reducing waste significantly and lowering initial setup costs for small-batch production.

On the other hand, traditional manufacturing methods are faster and more cost-effective for mass production and offer a wider range of materials, including metals, plastics, composites, and ceramics, and proven mechanical properties. Figures 10.4 and 10.5 show the 3D printing and subtractive manufacturing process, respectively.

10.2.6 Types of 3D Printing Technologies

In the medical sector, different 3D printing techniques and materials are employed, depending on the specific applications. Figure 10.6 provides an illustration of the most frequently used 3D printing methods for medical device applications.

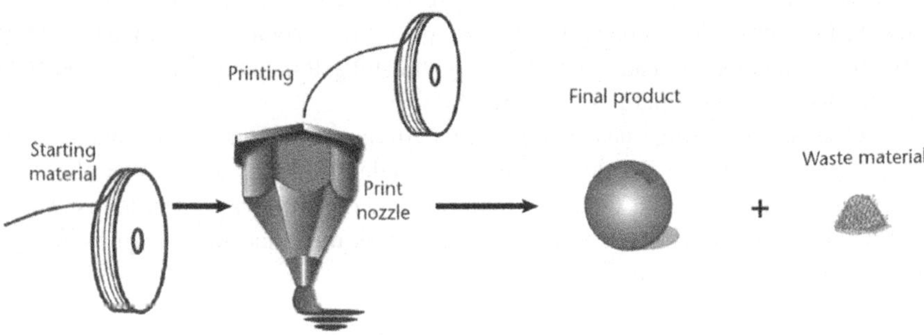

Fig. 10.4 3D printing manufacturing process (Levesque et al. 2020)

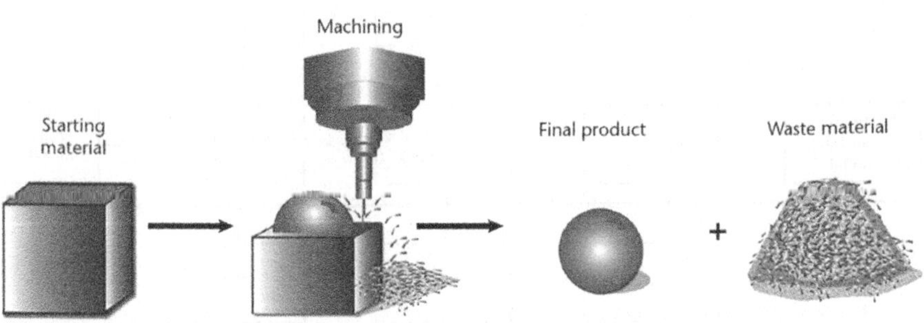

Fig. 10.5 Subtractive manufacturing process (Levesque et al. 2020)

Stereolithography (SLA) is an additive manufacturing process that uses a UV laser to selectively cure liquid photopolymer resin layer by layer. The UV laser solidifies the resin where it strikes, creating each layer of the object. SLA is known for its high-resolution prints and smooth surface finish, making it suitable for applications like dental models, jewelry, and highly detailed prototypes (Hull 1986).

Material extrusion, also known as fused deposition modeling (FDM) or fused filament fabrication (FFF), is one of the most popular 3D printing technologies. In this method, a thermoplastic filament is fed through a heated nozzle, which melts the material. The melted filament is then deposited layer by layer to build the object. FDM/FFF is widely used for rapid prototyping, functional parts, and hobbyist applications due to its affordability and accessibility.

Selective laser sintering (SLS) employs a high-power laser to selectively fuse powdered material, typically thermoplastics, metals, or ceramics, into a solid structure layer by layer. The un-sintered powder acts as support during the printing process. SLS technology is versatile, allowing for the production of complex geometries and functional end-use parts without the need for support structures (Deckard 1989).

Direct metal laser sintering (DMLS) is similar to SLS but uses metal powder as the material. A high-powered laser is employed to selectively fuse the metal particles to build the object layer by layer. DMLS is commonly used in aerospace, automotive, and medical industries for producing high-strength and complex metal components (Godbey 2007).

Electron beam melting (EBM) uses an electron beam to selectively melt metal powder in a high vacuum environment. EBM is particularly suitable for manufacturing high-strength, complex, and fully dense metal parts, and it is widely used in aerospace and medical applications (Cozzolino et al. 2023).

Digital light processing (DLP) is a 3D printing technology that uses a digital light projector to cure photopolymer resin layer by layer. DLP is similar to SLA but cures entire layers at once, resulting in faster print times. DLP is used for various applications, including dental models, jewelry, and customized prototypes (Hull 1986).

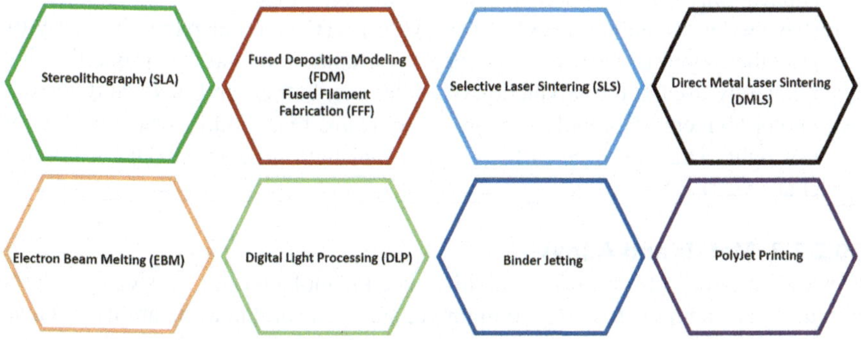

Fig. 10.6 3D printing methods for medical device applications

Binder jetting is an additive manufacturing process where a liquid binding agent is selectively jetted onto a powder bed, bonding the particles together to create the desired shape. The excess powder acts as support for the object. Binder jetting is used for metal, ceramic, and sand printing applications, such as creating metal parts, architectural models, and sand molds (Sachs et al. 1992).

PolyJet printing utilizes inkjet printing technology to deposit layers of photopolymer materials onto the build platform. Each layer is cured with UV light immediately after deposition. PolyJet technology can produce multi-material and multi-color parts with high accuracy and detailed surface finish, making it ideal for visual prototypes and realistic models (Huang et al. 2020).

10.2.7 Materials Used in 3D Printing

10.2.7.1 Polymers and Plastics

Polymers and plastics are widely utilized in 3D printing due to their versatility, affordability, and ease of processing. These materials are commonly employed in various 3D printing technologies, such as fused deposition modeling (FDM) and stereolithography (SLA). Some common polymers and plastics used in 3D printing include:

(a) Polylactic acid (PLA): PLA is a biodegradable and bio-based thermoplastic commonly derived from renewable resources like cornstarch or sugarcane. It is extensively used for 3D printing, educational purposes, and prototyping due to its ease of use and environmental friendliness (Tanrattanakul and Bunkaew 2014).

(b) Acrylonitrile butadiene styrene (ABS): ABS is a robust, impact-resistant thermoplastic known for its durability and ability to withstand higher temperatures. It finds applications in functional prototypes, automotive components, and consumer goods (Olivera et al. 2016).

(c) Polyamide (Nylon): Nylon is a tough and flexible thermoplastic with excellent mechanical properties. It is commonly used in 3D printing for engineering applications, such as functional parts, gears, and hinges.

(d) Polyethylene terephthalate glycol (PETG): PETG is a transparent and easy-to-print thermoplastic known for its impact resistance and food-safe properties. It is frequently used in the production of containers, bottles, and medical devices.

(e) Photopolymers: Photopolymers are liquid resins that solidify when exposed to UV light. They are used in SLA and digital light processing (DLP) (Fidanza et al. 2022).

10.2.7.2 Metals and Alloys

Metal 3D printing, also known as additive metal manufacturing, is extensively used in industries such as aerospace, automotive, and medical due to its ability to create complex and high-strength components (Horn and Harrysson 2012). Some common metals and alloys used in metal 3D printing include:

(a) Titanium: Titanium is a lightweight and biocompatible metal with excellent mechanical properties, making it ideal for medical implants, aerospace components, and high-performance applications.
(b) Stainless steel: Stainless steel is a versatile material with corrosion resistance and mechanical strength, used in a wide range of applications, including automotive, aerospace, and consumer goods.
(c) Aluminum: Aluminum is a lightweight metal with good thermal and electrical conductivity, making it suitable for industries such as aerospace and automotive.
(d) Cobalt-Chrome: Cobalt-chrome alloys are used in medical and dental applications, such as orthopedic implants and dental prosthetics, due to their biocompatibility and excellent wear resistance (Wong 2016).

10.2.7.3 Ceramics

Ceramic materials are valued for their high-temperature resistance, hardness, and biocompatibility. They are commonly used in dental and medical applications and as electrical insulators:

(a) Zirconia: Zirconia is a ceramic material known for its high strength and resistance to wear and chemical corrosion, making it suitable for dental crowns, bridges, and implants. Figure 10.7 shows the 3D-printed Zirconia crowns.
(b) Alumina: Alumina is a high-performance ceramic with excellent mechanical and thermal properties, used in applications such as cutting tools and medical implants.
(c) Multi-material 3D printing of ceramics: One of the most fascinating developments using ceramics is the emergence of multi-material 3D printing, where two innovative processes are combined: binder jetting (BJT) and material jetting (MJT) (ISO 2017).

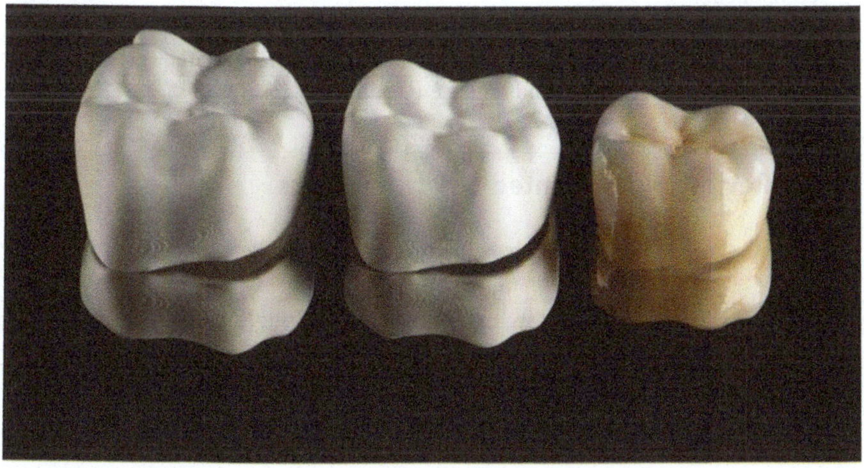

Fig. 10.7 3D printed zirconia crown (Schweiger et al. 2021)

In multi-material 3D printing, particle-filled inks are precisely applied directly to the powder bed via the print head. This technique allows for the integration of different materials within the same workpiece, providing unprecedented possibilities for altering the structural composition and functionality of the final product.

For instance, by selecting a different material for the ink, it becomes possible to create complex composite structures within the ceramic workpiece. Inks filled with metal particles can be injected into a ceramic powder bed, resulting in the creation of hybrid components. For example, an object made of silicate ceramics can now incorporate electrical conductor paths made of silver, allowing for the integration of electronic functionalities within ceramic parts.

This advancement has opened up a whole new realm of applications for ceramic 3D printing. The ability to combine multiple materials in a single printing process expands the design possibilities and functionality of ceramic components. Industries that heavily rely on ceramics, such as aerospace, electronics, and biomedical, can benefit significantly from multi-material 3D printing.

Orthopedic applications also stand to gain from multi-material ceramic 3D printing. By introducing biocompatible materials into ceramic structures, it becomes possible to fabricate complex medical implants that offer improved integration with the human body.

10.2.7.4 Composites

Composites are materials that combine two or more distinct components to achieve specific properties. In 3D printing, composites often involve mixing polymers or metals with reinforcing materials, such as carbon fiber, glass fiber, or metal particles. These composites offer improved strength, stiffness, and other desirable properties:

(a) Carbon fiber reinforced polymers (CFRP): CFRP composites are lightweight, strong, and widely used in aerospace and automotive industries for structural components.
(b) Metal matrix composites (MMCs): MMCs combine metals with ceramic or other materials, offering enhanced mechanical and thermal properties for applications in aerospace and defense (Godbey 2007).

10.3 Review of 3D-Printed Smart Implants

Orthopedic surgery has greatly benefited from the advancements in 3D printing technology, enabling the creation of patient-specific implants and surgical tools. The following sections provide insight into the use of 3D printing in orthopedic surgery.

10.3.1 Personalized Implants

3D printing allows for the fabrication of personalized implants tailored to individual patient anatomy. This customization improves the fit and function of implants, leading to better patient outcomes (Tack et al. 2016).

Moreover, 3D printing has revolutionized the production of prosthetics and orthotics. By utilizing patient-specific anatomical data, 3D-printed prosthetics and orthotics offer a precise fit, enhanced comfort, and improved functionality compared to traditional off-the-shelf solutions. This customization greatly benefits patients, providing them with better mobility and quality of life (Di Laura et al. 2023).

10.3.2 Complex Geometries

One of the significant advantages of 3D printing in orthopedic surgery is its capability to create complex implant geometries that were once challenging or even impossible to achieve using conventional techniques. Traditional methods, such as milling or casting, often struggle to produce implants with intricate designs due to the limitations of tooling and molding processes. 3D printing, however, utilizes a layer-by-layer additive approach, allowing for the precise fabrication of complex shapes and internal structures. As a result, orthopedic implants can be custom-designed to match the specific anatomy of each patient, promoting better fit, function, and long-term success (Bose et al. 2013).

The ability to achieve intricate designs through 3D printing translates into improved implant functionality and biomechanical properties. Research conducted by Bose et al. (2013) demonstrated that 3D printing enables the development of implants with optimized structural characteristics. By tailoring the internal architecture and porosity of the implant, engineers can enhance mechanical properties such as strength, flexibility, and load distribution. This level of customization ensures that the implant mimics the natural properties of the surrounding bone, reducing stress shielding and promoting better osseointegration, which is crucial for long-term implant success.

3D printing has transformed the field of orthopedic surgery by providing an unparalleled level of design flexibility, customization, and improved biomechanical properties for medical implants. The study conducted by Bose et al. (2013) highlights the potential of 3D printing to create implants with optimized structural characteristics, leading to better long-term outcomes for patients.

10.3.3 Surgical Guides

3D printing technology can be used to create surgical guides that assist surgeons in accurately placing implants during orthopedic procedures. These guides improve surgical precision, reduce operating time, and enhance overall surgical outcomes. Surgical guides, also known as patient-specific instrumentation (PSI) guides, are custom-designed tools created using 3D printing technology. These guides are tailored to match the unique anatomical features of each patient, providing a personalized and precise approach to surgery. The process starts with obtaining patient-specific imaging data, such as CT scans or MRI images. Advanced software then converts these data into a detailed 3D model of the patient's bone structure.

The 3D model serves as the foundation for designing the surgical guide, which is meticulously crafted to fit over the patient's bone during the surgical procedure. The guide includes specific pathways, holes, or slots that indicate the optimal locations for the surgeon to make incisions and place orthopedic implants. These guides act as a visual and tactile reference, allowing the surgeon to accurately navigate the surgical site and achieve precise alignment.

The use of surgical guides offers several key benefits for orthopedic procedures. First and foremost, they significantly improve surgical precision. By following the guide's pre-determined pathways, surgeons can ensure that the implant is placed at the correct angle and depth, reducing the likelihood of errors and complications. This level of accuracy is especially critical in joint replacements and spinal surgeries, where proper alignment directly impacts the patient's postoperative mobility and function.

Another advantage of surgical guides is their ability to streamline surgical workflows and reduce operating time. With a pre-designed guide, surgeons can avoid the need for time-consuming intraoperative measurements and adjustments. This not only saves valuable time during the procedure but also reduces the patient's exposure to anesthesia and the overall surgical risk.

Furthermore, the utilization of patient-specific surgical guides has been shown to improve overall surgical outcomes. Research conducted by Yuan et al. (2018) demonstrated that the use of 3D-printed surgical guides led to improved implant alignment and reduced malalignment rates in total knee arthroplasty. This study emphasizes the positive impact of 3D printing technology in orthopedic surgery, specifically in enhancing surgical precision and patient outcomes.

Figure 10.8 showcases an example of a customized neurosurgical guide created using selective laser sintering (SLS) with PA-12 powder. This figure illustrates the potential of 3D printing in producing patient-specific surgical guides for various orthopedic procedures, including neurosurgery.

10.3.4 Biomaterials and Implant Integration

The use of various biomaterials in 3D printing allows for the development of implants with improved biocompatibility and mechanical properties. Additionally, 3D-printed implants can be designed to incorporate drug delivery systems, sensors, and other advanced functionalities, further enhancing their therapeutic potential.

Another area where 3D printing technology has made a significant impact is in the field of tissue engineering and regenerative medicine. By utilizing 3D printing techniques, intricate scaffolds can be produced, providing a platform for cell growth and tissue regeneration. These scaffolds can be customized to match the specific

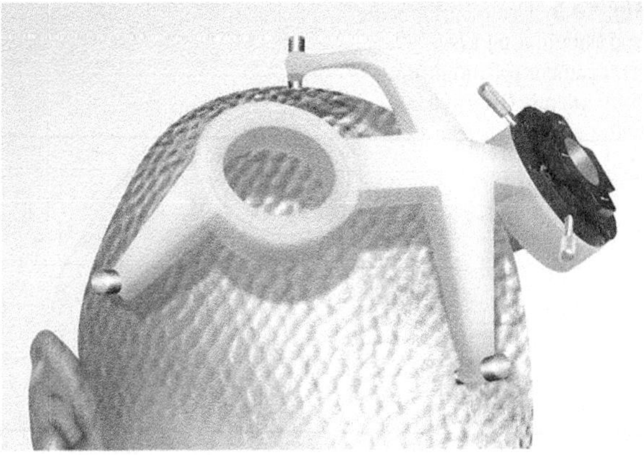

Fig. 10.8 Customized neurosurgical guide. (Reprinted with permission from Rajendran et al. 2023)

needs of patients, promoting bone healing and facilitating the integration of new tissue (Daly et al. 2018).

10.4 Smart Implants in Orthopedic Surgery

3D-printed smart implants have ushered in a new era of personalized and innovative medical solutions for knee, pelvic, and hip applications. By integrating intelligent technologies and capabilities, these implants offer real-time monitoring, remote tracking, adaptive functionalities, postoperative analysis, and improved implant longevity (Lal and Patralekh 2018).

10.4.1 Real-Time Monitoring

3D-printed smart implants equipped with sensors provide real-time monitoring of critical parameters such as implant stability, joint movement, and biomechanical forces. This dynamic feedback empowers healthcare providers with precise data on a patient's progress, enabling timely intervention and personalized treatment adjustments (Kelmers et al. 2022).

Figure 10.9 shows the components used to carry the diagnostic technology in orthopedic implants, showing the possible placement of sensors (S), electronics (E) and antenna (A) components within, and radiofrequency (RF) communications facilitate data collection from the implant.

10.4.2 Remote Monitoring

Wireless connectivity in 3D-printed smart implants enables remote monitoring of patients' conditions. Healthcare professionals can securely access patient data,

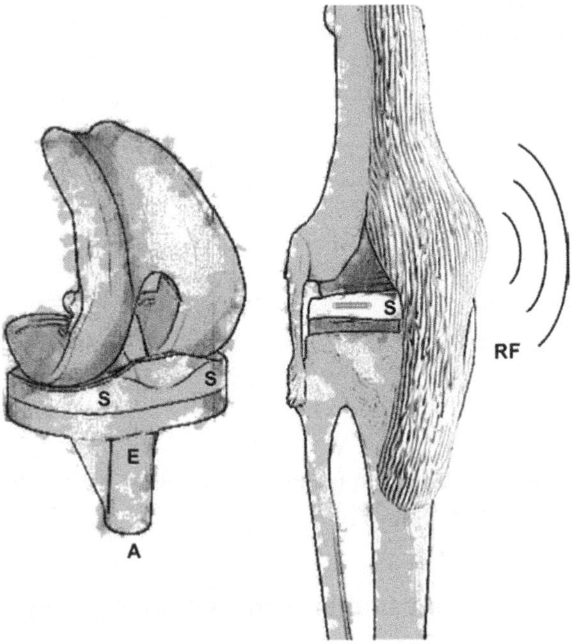

Fig. 10.9 Use of orthopedic implants in total knee replacement for monitoring components. (Reproduced with permission from Ledet et al. 2018)

ensuring that recovery progresses as intended, without the need for frequent in-person appointments. This streamlined approach enhances patient convenience and optimizes postoperative care (Young et al. 2021).

10.4.3 Adaptive Functionality

Smart implants leverage advanced algorithms and control mechanisms to offer adaptive functionality. Implants can respond to the patient's movements and needs, providing real-time support and adjustments. For instance, adaptive hip implants can adjust joint movement to facilitate varying activities, enhancing patient mobility and quality of life (Denecke and Baudoin 2022).

10.4.4 Postoperative Analysis

3D-printed smart implants enable postoperative analysis by collecting and analyzing data on joint movements, load distribution, and rehabilitation progress. This data-driven insight informs healthcare providers about the effectiveness of treatment plans, allowing for evidence-based decision-making and optimized patient outcomes (Żukowska et al. 2023).

10.4.5 Improved Implant Longevity

Through 3D printing technology, smart implants can be precisely customized to match individual anatomy. This accurate fit minimizes wear and stress on surrounding tissues, contributing to improved implant longevity. With better data-driven design and monitoring, smart knee implants can potentially extend the lifespan of the implant, reducing the need for revision surgeries and associated risks (Tan and van Arkel 2021).

10.4.6 Enhanced Stability and Load Distribution

Smart implants can provide real-time feedback on stability and load distribution within the implant and the surrounding tissue. This information can help surgeons ensure proper alignment and distribution of forces, reducing the risk of implant failure or complications.

10.4.7 Early Detection of Infection

Smart implants equipped with sensors can detect early signs of infection, such as changes in temperature or increased inflammation. Early detection allows for timely intervention, such as administering antibiotics or removing the infected implant, thereby reducing the risk of further complications.

10.4.8 Personalized Treatment

3D printing technology allows for patient-specific implants, tailored to an individual's unique anatomy. Smart implants can further enhance personalization by continuously monitoring the implant's performance and adapting treatment plans accordingly. This personalized approach can lead to improved patient outcomes and satisfaction. Figure 10.10 shows the pelvic and tibia customized implants.

10.4.9 Application of 3D-Printed Smart Implant Devices

The medical industry is facing a big challenge due to population growth and health problems. The supply is becoming low, and the demand for health products is high. The advancements in medical and dental applications have grown significantly over the recent years, intending to enhance clinical workflow via the use of state-of-the-art technology. The concept of additive manufacturing (3D printing) is indeed making a substantial contribution to the medical practices of developing countries. The production demands of medical implants perform right into 3D printing's functionalities, owing to the intrinsically complicated geometry of therapeutics,

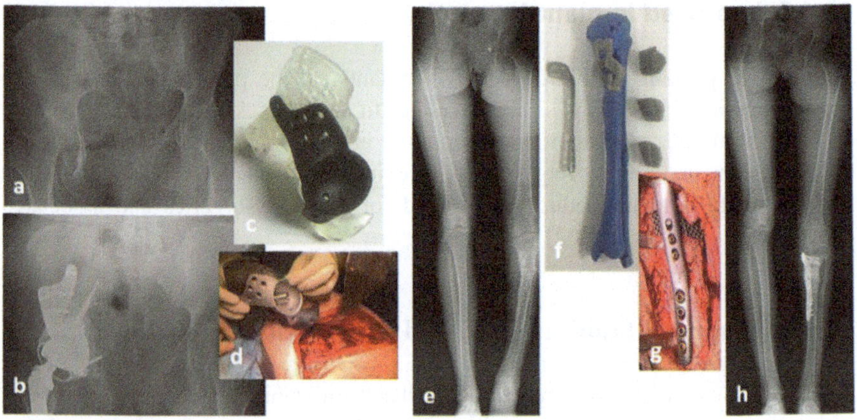

Fig. 10.10 Customized implants. Pelvic implant (**a–d**). Tibial implant (**e–h**) (Calvo-Haro et al. 2021, Copyright 2021. Reproduced with permission Springer Nature)

paired with the limited material compatibility. 3D printing is widely employed in the production of immensely customizable prosthetics and implants from a wide range of materials, including biomedical materials (including skin and bones). It is, paradoxically, enhancing orthopedic technology and treatment benefits utilizing polymers, ceramics, and metals. Both patients and manufacturers are beginning to experience significant enhancements in product quality and profitability. Undoubtedly, device designs that are more human-friendly—that are physically more similar to the natural bone—are a remarkable benefit. Furthermore, certain customized product designs are more cost-effective when produced by additive manufacturing.

It is also important to note that timescales for bespoke additive manufactured products are frequently lower than for conventional manufacturing, which benefits patients even more. A cost–benefit analysis of implementing 3D printing technology in medical facilities revealed that such advances improve complex procedures and would be a vital tool in alleviating time and budgetary strains for healthcare. In a nutshell, it is clear that the possibilities for 3D printing's application in the healthcare business are limitless, with the potential to improve society's quality of life, minimize healthcare expenditures, and also save lives.

Regarding the economy, 3D printing has the potential to increase output in the health industry over the next 10 years, with the overall commercial benefit of 3D printing-based on-shoring ranging from $60 to $90 billion. This indicates that the worldwide 3D Printed Medical Implants Industry is predicted to increase at a CAGR of 14.3% by 2027. Besides that, the opportunity for qualified job growth in developing countries is believed to be between 500,000 and 600,000. As an outcome, it is foreseen that the industry will continue to transform toward additive manufacturing as a significant component of any manufacturing process.

Biomaterials, in particular, play an important role in this frame of reference, as the worldwide biomaterials market is supposed to exceed $47.5 billion by 2025, up from

$35.5 billion in 2020, at a CAGR of 6.0% throughout the forecast timeframe, owing to skyrocketing demand for medical implants, and tissue repair implementations. The biomaterials market is categorized into four: metallic biomaterials, polymeric biomaterials, ceramic biomaterials, and natural biomaterials. In 2021, the metallic biomaterials category held the greatest proportion of the global market in the healthcare industry. Globally, the surging elderly population is likely to further boost growth in the forthcoming years.

10.4.10 Challenges of Smart Implants

10.4.10.1 Biocompatibility and Longevity

The materials used in 3D-printed smart implants must be biocompatible and safe for long-term implantation. Ensuring the longevity and stability of smart features, such as sensors or electronic components, can be challenging, as they need to withstand the harsh physiological environment and potential wear and tear (Calvo-Haro et al. 2021).

10.4.10.2 Reliability and Accuracy of Sensors

The reliability and accuracy of sensors integrated into smart implants are crucial for their effectiveness. These sensors must provide consistent and precise measurements, even in dynamic conditions, to ensure reliable monitoring and detection of abnormalities (Murr et al. 2012).

10.4.10.3 Power Supply and Energy Efficiency

Smart implants require a power source to operate their sensors or electronic components. Ensuring a stable power supply within the implant, without the need for frequent battery replacements, is a significant challenge. Developing energy-efficient systems or exploring alternative power sources, such as harvesting energy from body movements or utilizing wireless charging technologies, can help address this challenge.

10.4.10.4 Data Security and Privacy

Smart implants generate sensitive health data, and ensuring its security and privacy is of utmost importance. Protecting the transmission and storage of patient data from unauthorized access or cyber threats is a critical consideration in the development and implementation of smart implant systems.

10.4.10.5 Regulatory Approval and Standardization

The development and deployment of smart implants require regulatory approvals to ensure their safety, efficacy, and adherence to quality standards. Standardization of manufacturing processes, materials, and performance metrics is necessary to establish guidelines and benchmarks for smart implant technologies. Figure 10.11 illustrates the challenges of the 3D print implants for orthopedic applications (Wu et al. 2023).

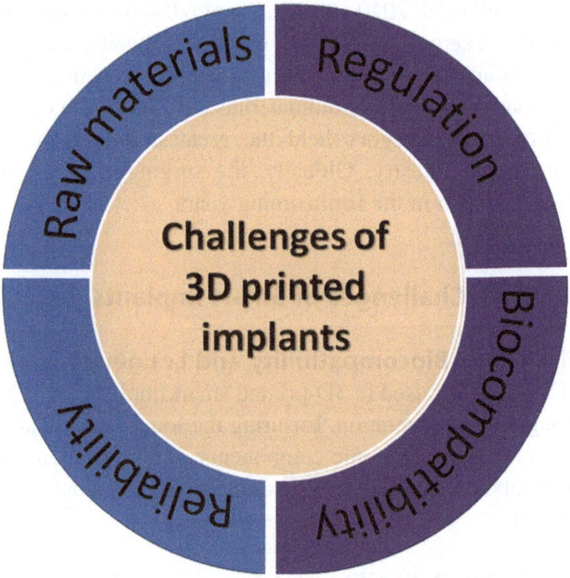

Fig. 10.11 Illustration of challenges of the 3D print implants for orthopedic applications

Despite these challenges, ongoing research and advancements in materials, sensors, power management, and data security are continuously addressing these issues. Smart implants have the potential to significantly improve patient care and outcomes in orthopedic surgery by providing real-time monitoring, personalized treatment, and early intervention.

10.5 Trends and Future Possibilities

The 3D printing technology has the ability to demonstrate functional, morphological, and mechanical qualities that are suitable for bone implant and biomedical applications. 3D printing has made it possible to create personalized prosthetic limbs, cranial implants, and orthopedic implants such as hips and knees. At the same time, its potential to modify the manufacture of medical products—particularly high-risk items like implants—could have an impact on patient safety, posing new hurdles for FDA regulation (Vasiliadis et al. 2022).

Custom implants may also be conceived and manufactured far more quickly. Patients will be able to obtain implants that are custom-made to match their bodies, leading to easier procedures and better health results (Fidanza et al. 2022). The capacity to design personalized implants for unique patients provides advantages throughout therapy. Many reconstructive treatments still need some handwork and creativity on the part of the physician. Procedures may be completed faster and less invasively, allowing patients to recover faster and have better health results. The use of a personalized, 3D-printed implant has the potential to save surgery time and

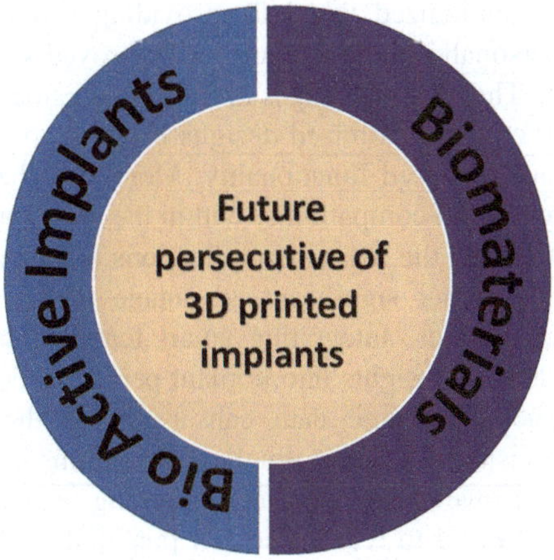

Fig. 10.12 Illustration of future perspectives of the 3D print implants for orthopedic applications

enhance implant fit. In addition to providing excellent stability and strength, 3D-printed implants have the potential to outlast traditional implants.

Bioactive implants' biological functions play a critical role in expediting the healing process and minimizing complications. Improving the biological functions of 3D printed implants through surface treatment and the incorporation of growth factors, functional molecules, peptides, or proteins in coatings offers a promising approach to shorten healing time and reduce complications. These advances hold significant potential to revolutionize medical implants, providing patients with more successful and safer solutions for various medical conditions.

Biomaterials also allow for radical design features and have shown a potential role in bone tissue regeneration and orthopedic implants, with exceptional rigid weight ratios, stimulated vascularization, tunable hydraulic penetration, and even increased surface volume ratios; the main benefit of this technology is its ability to produce a part with a curved layer of greater durability. Because human bones are really not flat and also have a curved surface, prosthetic bones must be manufactured using 5D printing to offer superior durability to bone implants. This technology has a significant deal of promise to meet this fundamental demand. As the healthcare industry's future, 3D printing will play an essential role in precision medicine and customized medicine. Multidimensional printing will become a bright point and vanity in the medical area in the future, promoting the worldwide growth of medical biology research. Figure 10.12 illustrates future perspectives of the 3D print implants for orthopedic applications such as bioactive implants and biomaterials.

10.6 Conclusion

In this chapter, we have explored the remarkable impact of 3D-printed smart implants on orthopedic surgery, showcasing their applications, benefits, and future prospects. The introduction of 3D printing technology has undoubtedly revolutionized the field, providing orthopedic surgeons with powerful tools for personalized patient care and improved surgical outcomes.

The key advantages of 3D-printed smart implants are evident through the ability to create customized designs based on patient-specific data, resulting in precise fit and enhanced functionality. Moreover, the use of biocompatible materials ensures long-term compatibility within the body, promoting successful osseointegration and reducing the risk of complications (Kadic et al. 2019).

Another significant advantage lies in the potential for real-time monitoring capabilities. Integrating smart features, such as embedded sensors, can provide valuable insights into implant performance, healing progress, and patient recovery. These real-time data can assist healthcare professionals in making informed decisions, ensuring timely interventions if necessary.

However, as with any emerging technology, there are challenges that must be addressed to realize the full potential of 3D-printed smart implants (Gibson et al. 2010, 2014). Regulatory considerations are crucial to ensure the safety and efficacy of these implants. Standardizing processes and materials is essential for reproducibility and widespread adoption in clinical practice. Additionally, cost-effectiveness remains a concern, as 3D printing technology and specialized materials can be expensive.

To overcome these challenges, continued collaboration between orthopedic surgeons, engineers, researchers, and regulatory bodies is imperative. Advancements in materials science, bioprinting techniques, and artificial intelligence integration hold tremendous promise for further improving 3D-printed smart implants' performance and capabilities.

In conclusion, 3D-printed smart implants have ushered in a new era in orthopedic surgery, providing personalized solutions and raising the bar for patient care. As research and technology advance, addressing the current challenges will open up new horizons for this transformative technology, benefiting patients and revolutionizing orthopedic surgical practice. With ongoing collaboration and dedication from the medical and engineering communities, 3D-printed smart implants are poised to play a pivotal role in the future of orthopedic surgery.

References

Bose S, Vahabzadeh S, Bandyopadhyay A (2013) Bone tissue engineering using 3D printing. Mater Today 16(12):496–504

Bowyer A (2004) The RepRap project. In: Gaskell G (ed) Rapid manufacturing: an industrial revolution for the digital age. Wiley, pp 143–162

Calvo-Haro JA, Pascau J, Mediavilla-Santos L, Sanz-Ruiz P, Sánchez-Pérez C, Vaquero-Martín J, Perez-Mananes R (2021) Conceptual evolution of 3D printing in orthopedic surgery and traumatology: from "do it yourself" to "point of care manufacturing". BMC Musculoskelet Disord 22:1–10

Campbell I, Bourell D, Gibson I (2011) Additive manufacturing: rapid prototyping comes of age. Rapid Prototyp J 17(2):148–149

Cozzolino E, Franchitti S, Borrelli R, Pirozzi C, Astarita A (2023) Energy consumption assessment in manufacturing Ti6Al4V electron beam melted parts post-processed by machining. Int J Adv Manuf Technol 125(3–4):1289–1303
Crump SS (1989) Apparatus and method for creating three-dimensional objects. U.S. Patent No. 5,121,329
Daly AC, Pitacco P, Nulty J, Cunniffe GM, Kelly DJ (2018) 3D printed microchannel networks to direct vascularisation during endochondral bone repair. Biomaterials 162:34–46
Deckard C (1989) Method and apparatus for producing parts by selective sintering. U.S. Patent No. 4,863,538
Denecke K, Baudoin CR (2022) A review of artificial intelligence and robotics in transformed health ecosystems. Front Med 9:795957
Di Laura A, Henckel J, Hart A (2023) Custom 3D-printed implants for acetabular reconstruction: intermediate-term functional and radiographic results. JB & JS Open Access 8(2):e22.00120. https://doi.org/10.2106/JBJS.OA.22.00120
Fidanza A, Perinetti T, Logroscino G, Saracco M (2022) 3D printing applications in orthopaedic surgery: clinical experience and opportunities. Appl Sci 12(7):3245
Gibson I, Rosen D, Stucker B (2010) Development of additive manufacturing technology. In: Additive manufacturing technologies. Springer, Boston, MA. https://doi.org/10.1007/978-1-4419-1120-9_2
Gibson I, Rosen DW, Stucker B (2014) Additive manufacturing technologies: 3D printing, rapid prototyping, and direct digital manufacturing. Springer
Godbey BB (2007) Surface finish control of three-dimensional printed metal tooling. Doctoral dissertation, Clemson University
Hague R, Dickens P, Hopkinson N (eds) (2006) Rapid manufacturing: an industrial revolution for the digital age. John Wiley & Sons
Hao B, Lin G (2020) 3D printing technology and its application in industrial manufacturing. In: IOP conference series: materials science and engineering, vol 782(2). IOP Publishing, p 022065
Horn TJ, Harrysson OL (2012) Overview of current additive manufacturing technologies and selected applications. Sci Prog 95(3):255–282
Huang J, Qin Q, Wang J (2020) A review of stereolithography: processes and systems. Processes 8(9):1138
Hull CW (1986) Apparatus for production of three-dimensional objects by stereolithography. U.-S. Patent No. 4,575,330
ISO/ASTM (2017) Additive manufacturing—general principles—terminology. Beuth, p 52900
Kadic M, Milton GW, van Hecke M, Wegener M (2019) 3D metamaterials. Nat Rev Phys 1(3): 198–210
Kelmers E, Szuba A, King SW, Palan J, Freear S, Pandit HG, van Duren BH (2022) Smart knee implants: an overview of current technologies and future possibilities. Indian J Orthop 57(5): 635–642. https://doi.org/10.1007/s43465-022-00810-5
Khatri P, Shah MK, Vora N (2018) Formulation strategies for solid oral dosage form using 3D printing technology: a mini-review. J Drug Deliv Sci Technol 46:148–155. https://doi.org/10.1016/j.jddst.2018.05.009
Kizawa H, Nagao E, Shimamura M, Zhang G, Torii H (2017) Scaffold-free 3D bioprinted human liver tissue stably maintains metabolic functions useful for drug discovery. Biochem Biophys Rep 10:186–191. https://doi.org/10.1016/j.bbrep.2017.04.004
Lal H, Patralekh MK (2018) 3D printing and its applications in orthopaedic trauma: a technological marvel. J Clin Orthop Trauma 9(3):260–268. https://doi.org/10.1016/j.jcot.2018.07.022

Ledet EH, Liddle B, Kradinova K, Harper S (2018) Smart implants in orthopedic surgery, improving patient outcomes: a review. Innov Entrepreneurship Health 5:41–51. https://doi.org/10.2147/IEH.S133518

Lee J (2021) A 3D food printing process for the new normal era: a review. Processes 9(9):1495

Levesque JN, Shah A, Ekhtiari S, Yan JR, Thornley P, Williams DS (2020) Three-dimensional printing in orthopaedic surgery: a scoping review. EFORT Open Rev 5(7):430–441

Melocchi A, Uboldi M, Inverardi N, Briatico-Vangosa F, Baldi F, Pandini S et al (2019) Expandable drug delivery system for gastric retention based on shape memory polymers: development via 4D printing and extrusion. Int J Pharm 571:118700

Murphy SV, Atala A (2014) 3D bioprinting of tissues and organs. Nat Biotechnol 32(8):773–785

Murr LE, Gaytan SM, Martinez E, Medina F, Wicker RB (2012) Next generation orthopaedic implants by additive manufacturing using electron beam melting. Int J Biomater 2012:1

Olivera S, Muralidhara HB, Venkatesh K, Gopalakrishna K, Vivek CS (2016) Plating on acrylonitrile–butadiene–styrene (ABS) plastic: a review. J Mater Sci 51:3657–3674

Rahman Z, Barakh Ali SF, Ozkan T, Charoo NA, Reddy IK, Khan MA (2018) Additive manufacturing with 3D printing: progress from bench to bedside. AAPS J 20(6):101. https://doi.org/10.1208/s12248-018-0225-6

Rajendran S, Palani G, Kanakaraj A, Shanmugam V, Veerasimman A, Gądek S, Korniejenko K, Marimuthu U (2023) Metal and polymer based composites manufactured using additive manufacturing—a brief review. Polymers 15(11):2564

Sachs E, Cima M, Williams P, Brancazio D, Cornie J (1992) Three-dimensional printing: rapid tooling and prototypes directly from a CAD model. J Manuf Sci Eng 114(4):481–488

Schweiger J, Edelhoff D, Güth JF (2021) 3D printing in digital prosthetic dentistry: an overview of recent developments in additive manufacturing. J Clin Med 10(9):2010

Tack P, Victor J, Gemmel P, Annemans L (2016) 3D-printing techniques in a medical setting: a systematic literature review. Biomed Eng Online 15:1–21

Tan N, van Arkel RJ (2021) Topology optimisation for compliant hip implant design and reduced strain shielding. Materials (Basel, Switzerland) 14(23):7184. https://doi.org/10.3390/ma14237184

Tanrattanakul V, Bunkaew P (2014) Effect of different plasticizers on the properties of bio-based thermoplastic elastomer containing poly (lactic acid) and natural rubber. Express Polym Lett 8(6):387

Vasiliadis AV, Koukoulias N, Katakalos K (2022) From three-dimensional (3D)-to 6D-printing technology in orthopedics: science fiction or scientific reality? J Funct Biomater 13(3):101

Ventola CL (2014) Medical applications for 3D printing: current and projected uses. Pharm Therap 39(10):704–711

Wohlers T (2017) Wohlers report 2017: 3D printing and additive manufacturing state of the industry. Wohlers Associates

Wong KC (2016) 3D-printed patient-specific applications in orthopedics. Orthop Res Rev 8:57–66

Wu Y, Liu J, Kang L, Tian J, Zhang X, Hu J, Wu Z (2023) An overview of 3D printed metal implants in orthopedic applications: present and future perspectives. Heliyon 9:e17718

Young C, Oliver ML, Gordon KD (2021) Design and validation of a novel 3D-printed wearable device for monitoring knee joint kinematics. Med Eng Phys 94:1–7. https://doi.org/10.1016/j.medengphy.2021.05.013

Yuan Z, Peng Z, Niu C, Yang Y (2018) Application of 3D printing technology in orthopedics: status quo and opportunities in China. Orthop Surg 10(3):185–194

Zhang LG, Leong K, Fisher JP (eds) (2022) 3D bioprinting and nanotechnology in tissue engineering and regenerative medicine. Academic Press

Zhou J, Vijayavenkataraman S (2021) 3D-printable conductive materials for tissue engineering and biomedical applications. Bioprinting 24:e00166

Żukowska M, Rad MA, Górski F (2023) Additive manufacturing of 3D anatomical models-review of processes, materials and applications. Materials (Basel, Switzerland) 16(2):880. https://doi.org/10.3390/ma16020880

Flexible and Embedded 3D-Printed Electronic Subsystems in Healthcare Products

11

G. Sahaya Dennish Babu, Saraswathi Nagaraj, Koyeli Girigoswami, C. Dhavamani, and Ahmed O. Mosleh

Contents

Abstract

3D-printed electronic subsystems can help healthcare product manufacturers create better more customized products at a lower cost and faster speed. This

G. S. D. Babu (✉)
Department of Physics, Chettinad College of Engineering and Technology, Karur, Tamil Nadu, India

S. Nagaraj · K. Girigoswami
Faculty of Allied Health Sciences, Chettinad Academy of Research and Education, Chettinad Hospital and Research Institute, Kelambakkam, Chennai, Tamil Nadu, India

C. Dhavamani
Department of Aeronautical Engineering, Mahendra Engineering College (Autonomous), Namakkal, Tamil Nadu, India

A. O. Mosleh
Faculty of Engineering, Benha University, Cairo, Egypt

R. Velu et al. (eds.), *Digital Design and Manufacturing of Medical Devices and Systems*, https://doi.org/10.1007/978-981-99-7100-8_11

can ultimately lead to improved patient outcomes and better healthcare overall. This is due to the features such as customization, faster prototyping, and improved functionality. Electronics and 3D printing work together to create new possibilities for creating specialized and individual medical equipment. An introduction to the fundamental concepts of electronics and 3D printing, including the many varieties of substances and printing techniques, follows at the beginning of the chapter. The necessity for specific tools and knowledge is then discussed, along with the potential and problems of incorporating semiconductors into 3D-printed structures. The uses of flexible and embedded 3D-printed electronic subsystems in healthcare items, such as medical implants, wearable technology, and sensors, are discussed in this chapter. A review of the prospects for flexible and incorporated 3D-printed electronics subsystems in healthcare items rounds off the chapter. This covers the potential for novel and cutting-edge products as well as the difficulties in expanding manufacturing and incorporating these items into current healthcare systems. This chapter gives a thorough review of the rapidly developing field of flexible and integrated 3D printing technology electronic subsystems in medical items and how it can change the healthcare sector.

Keywords

3D-printed electronics · Wearable healthcare devices · Flexible electronics · Embedded systems · Smart textiles · Biomedical sensors · Personalized healthcare

11.1 Introduction

One of the rapidly expanding technical disciplines with a better level of adaptability and dependability is printable electronics. Unfortunately, the little environmental impact of sustainable printing technology makes it necessary (Wong and Salleo 2009). Unlike conventional electronic devices made of rigid integrated circuit boards, hard silicon-based chips, resistors, and capacitors, flexible electronic devices made of organic polymers can retain electrical continuity both in their original condition and while being deformed. Due to their enhanced capacity to interact with human skin, these flexible electronic gadgets are not only portable for use in our daily lives but can also be utilized to monitor the body's health data (Corzo et al. 2020). This not only gives the devices a greater sensitivity to health indicators, but it also makes it possible for them to deliver health information at any time or place, which might improve people's quality of life and give rise to early warning systems in the field of digital health. Most flexible electrical gadgets, including frame relay, actuators, and transistors, only have simple planar topologies due to the limits of the technique used to fabricate electronic devices, such as coating, depositing, or inject printing. Flexible electronic devices that can meet individual demands and requirements have emerged as the next generation's development trend for applications including health monitoring, implantable, and biomimetic devices, thanks to the quick development of wearable technology (Gao et al. 2019; Chen et al. 2019).

While attaching antennas and basic conductive connections toward the exterior of 3D syringe plastic products has long been done using partly additive 3D electronics, new methods are now being utilized to add more complicated circuits to surfaces made of a range of materials. Whole circuits may also be embedded into an item thanks to in-mold electronics and 3D-printed electronics, which also have the advantages of streamlined production and innovative form factors (Wang et al. 2020). Using 3D electronics, it is no longer necessary to wire up the necessary switches, sensors, power sources, and other external components after embedding a rigid, flat Board into an item to provide electrical functionality. Fully 3D-printed electronics, which successively layer conducting materials and dielectric materials (often thermoplastics), are the least advanced technology (Liu et al. 2015; Caironi and Noh 2015). The main selling point is that each product and embedded circuit may be produced to a unique design without having to repeatedly produce masks and molds (Persad and Rocke 2022). As a result, fully 3D-printed electronics are ideally suited to applications where a variety of components need to be made quickly.

In fact, the US Army is testing a toughened 3D printer now to produce replacement parts during forward operating bases. The technique is particularly promising for medical equipment like hearing aids and prostheses, where a personalized form and even functionality are crucial. On-demand manufacturing may also be made possible by 3D-printed electronics' capacity to produce many components on the same machinery and the resulting separation of unit cost and volume (Espera et al. 2019; Tan et al. 2022; Rao et al. 2022). While the printing process may be sped up by employing several nozzles, it is best suited for uses where the flexibility to customize provides a noticeable benefit. Since post-hoc repairs are not possible with embedded circuits, ensuring dependability is another difficulty. One approach is to use image analysis to inspect each layer and make any necessary adjustments prior to the next one being deposited (Espalin et al. 2014). Compared to conventional, rigid alternatives, flexible electronics provide advantages in terms of size, weight, portability, and energy efficiency. Most importantly, they enable previously unimaginable designs and technology (such as wearable gadgets).

This book chapter discusses a new printing technique that enables the creation of complex 3D-printed electronic subsystems, improving the performance and safety of these devices or evaluating their efficacy in clinical settings. Such research would add to the existing body of knowledge in this field and contribute to developing innovative healthcare products that could improve patient outcomes.

11.2 Flexible Electronics

In general, a wide range of devices in the consumer, medical, and industrial sectors are increasingly created with printed flexible electronics. From Fig. 11.1, it is understood that the evolution and development of various functional materials for flexible electronics applications hold a valuable role in it. These goods include,

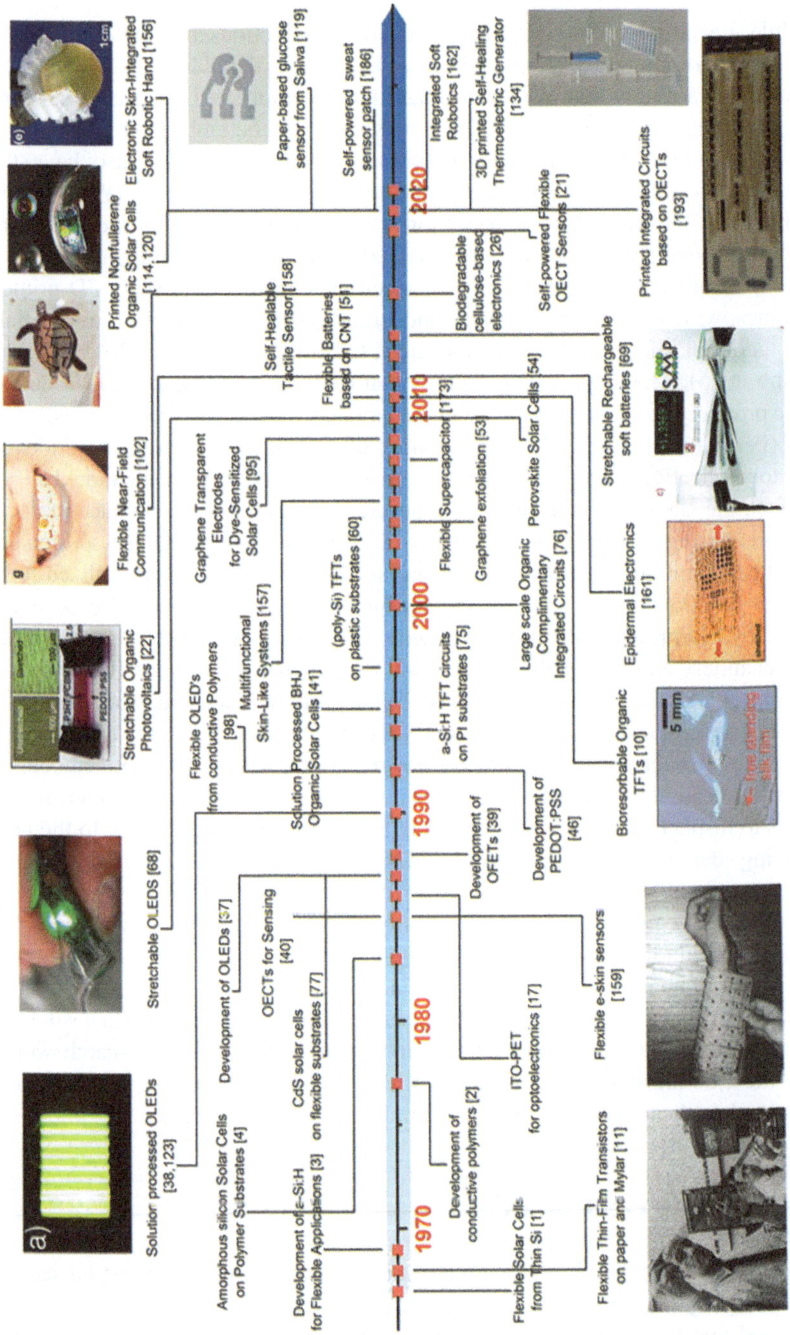

Fig. 11.1 Timeline of developments in materials, processing, and applications for flexible electronics. (Reproduced with permission from Corzo et al. 2020)

among others, soft robotics, array antennas, wearable electronics for human health and performance monitoring systems, structural health monitoring (roads, bridges, buildings, etc.), and soft robotics (Espalin et al. 2014; Espera et al. 2022; Park et al. 2022). Here, we have given some important types and their specifications of emerging flexible electronics-based technologies.

- Flexible electronics: Electronics made from stretchy or conformable materials, primarily plastic but also paper, metal foil, and flexible glass. Flexible electronics offer form factor and ease and may be utilized for a variety of purposes (Espalin et al. 2014).
- Flexible hybrid electronics: Devices that establish a new class of electronics by fusing the functionality of semiconductor devices with the adaptability and affordability of printed transparent plastic substrates. Stretchable, conformable, and flexible materials are substrates (Espera et al. 2022).
- Organic electronics: A branch of material science that deals with the conception, production, evaluation, and use of organic small molecules or polymers that exhibit desired electrical characteristics like conductivity. Generally, the increase of using different materials for organic electrical devices by discovering and producing novel high-conductivity materials (Park et al. 2022).
- Printed electronics: Functional electronics are created via additive manufacturing, which involves printing conductive lines using a variety of techniques, including screen, inkjet, gravure, flexography, and more. Printed circuit boards, which likewise employ printing techniques to link discrete active and passive components, are occasionally mistaken for printed electronics (Karahoca et al. 2018).

11.2.1 Flexible Electronics Based on 3D Printing Technologies

A type of electrical device known as flexible electronics frequently has substrates constructed of long or thin elastic materials. It may be folded, stretched, extended, rolled, or twisted to some extent to either adapt to certain harsh applications or to cause changes in electrical signals as a result of changes in stimuli, such as how a sensor operates. From the invention of the first electronic devices, the idea of a class of conformable electronics has been around. Its flexibility (more mechanical) when the application demands for it sets it different from any other electronics class. During the late 1970s, once flexible solar cells and thin-film transistors began to gain popularity, until their important contributions to biosensors in the last decade, the way they are made required a revolution in conventional production techniques (Espalin et al. 2014; Pravin and Sudhir 2018; Palo et al. 2017). Although the actual electrical component may still follow traditional methods for fabricating electronic devices, integrating it into its flexible substrate has always been difficult. As flexible electronics achieve popularity in the electronics sector, they also require "flexible" manufacturing methods that take an integrated approach to customization and application-specific requirements. The use of cutting-edge manufacturing techniques like 3D printing has been one creative way to push the boundaries of the production of flexible electronics. It opens a whole new manufacturing process and breed of products, such as wearables, biosensors, conformal antennas, and flexible energy harvesters and storage, that somehow respond to the demand for specialized, purpose-built devices from the fields of engineering, renewable energy, and medicine. New applications for these next-generation flexible electronics include flexible lighting and display technologies for consumer electronics, architecture, and textiles, wearables with sensors that track our habits and health, implantable electronics for better medical imaging and diagnostics, and enhancing the functionality of robots and unmanned aircraft with lightweight and conformable energy harvesting devices and sensor technology (Wiegard and Breitner 2019; Winters et al. 2003; Liu et al. 2019). Although conventional electronics are very capable of performing these tasks, flexible electronics are designed to increase the mechanical features to adhere to novel form factors through hybrid strategies, or as standalone solutions where the application does not call for high computation power. They are also meant to be extremely robust to deformation, low cost, thin, or disposable. Depending on the context, flexibility might mean several things.

Stretchable, wearable electrical devices may now be designed and printed digitally using a new technique called hybrid 3D printing, which combines soft, conductive inks with a material substrate. Beginning from scratch, the printer creates a complete stretchable circuit that combines the strong performance of off-the-shelf electronics with the mechanical durability of printed components (Persad and Rocke 2022; Tan et al. 2022; Consoli and Mina 2009). A digital file is used to produce a three-dimensional solid item in 3D printing, sometimes referred to as additive manufacturing. The "3D printer" sequentially deposits layers of material during the 3D printing process until the thing is fully constructed. In an additive process, the printer builds up layers of material until the desired item is "printed," producing 3D-printed things. Every layer of the printed object may be viewed as a thinly sliced cross-section. Using 3D printing, users can create intricate forms without using as much material as they would with conventional manufacturing techniques. The 3D printing process is the reverse of "subtractive manufacturing," in which the material is hollowed out or cut out using machinery like a milling machine. On the other hand, with additive manufacturing, physical items may be produced without the need of a mold or material block. Instead, it builds up and fuses together layers of material (Seider et al. 2009). Traditional manufacturing methods could not be as effective at creating complex geometries utilizing a variety of material types as 3D printing, which also provides quick product production, minimal initial fixed infrastructure costs, and these advantages. The concept of "rapid prototyping" gave rise to 3D printing. The phrase was used to describe the underlying technology when it was initially developed in the 1980s since, at the time, 3D printing could only be used to create prototypes rather than finished products. In actuality, the purpose of its invention was simply to speed up the production of new items through quick prototyping. Even though 3D printing has been around for a while, it has recently become extremely popular across sectors because of its improved simplicity, efficacy, and affordability. Prototypes are made using 3D printing in the healthcare

Table 11.1 Top industry problems for 3D printing

Consumer electronics	Healthcare	Heavy equipment
• Cost of pre- and post-processing • Cost of materials • Limited material selection	• Limited material selection • Cost of pre- and post-processing • Cost of system equipment	• Cost of pre- and post-processing • Cost of materials • Limited material selection
Automotive	**Industrial machines**	**Plastics and packaging**
• Limited material selection • Cost of pre- and post-processing • Technology limitations	• Cost of pre- and post-processing • No in-house expertise • Cost of system equipment	• Limited material selection • Cost of pre- and post-processing • Technology limitations

industry for the development of new medical and dental products (Murphy et al. 2020; Buga and Viana 2022). In dentistry, 3D printing is also useful for producing tools for making dental aligners and patterns for casting metal dental crowns. The answer is also useful for producing knee and hip implants directly, as well as other stock goods and patient-specific products like custom prostheses, hearing aids, and orthotic insoles. The potential for 3D-printed surgical guidance for specific surgeries, as well as drugs, bone, skin, tissue, and organs, is being investigated.

In general, 3D printing technology problems that bioprinting in general must overcome through these centers on developing new bioinks that are better suited for moving, shielding, and growing cells, as well as better bioprinting procedures, efficient crosslinking, and integration with microfluidic devices to offer a long-term and simulated physiological environment for cultivating bio-printed models (Liu et al. 2019; Consoli and Mina 2009; Seider et al. 2009; Murphy et al. 2020; Buga and Viana 2022; Luo et al. 2020). To best mimic the creation and infiltration of native tissues, the materials utilized to create tissue engineering scaffolds should be biocompatible, degradable, and absorbable. The direct synthesis of in vitro biological products utilized in medicines and regenerative medicine is made possible by 3D bioprinting. The 3D printing technology has recently been reached in biomedical applications, where designed organoids or micro-organs are built to create sophisticated in vitro living systems or micro-physiological systems. The flexibility of the substrate materials such as polyurethane (PU), silicone or polydimethylsiloxane (PDMS), natural rubber, and other thermoset and thermoplastic elastomer compositions that are used, should be emphasized as a vital component in flexible electronics (Buga and Viana 2022; Luo et al. 2020). The 3D printing sector also has difficulties with reproducibility, materials, post-processing, and equipment. Standards, design principles, and qualified people are also lacking. Prospective clients are also worried about environmental health and safety as well as sustainability. Table 11.1 summarizes the industrial-level problems faced by the industries for 3D printing of flexible electronics. Flexible electronics enable the development of these futuristic technologies. Each flexible electrical device is made up of the following four parts: substrate, backplane, front plane, and encapsulation. To accomplish this flexibility, each of these components must be equally adaptable and must not experience a loss or reduction in function.

It is suggested that the industries must shift the focus away from the technical advantages of additive manufacturing and toward its entire commercial value to overcome these obstacles. To evaluate how the technology may foster creativity and improve overall operations, businesses must examine their manufacturing strategy in addition to deciding which applications and parts to create using 3D printing (Chandrasekaran et al. 2022; Wang and Liu 2016; Zang et al. 2015). Make the technology suit the product and business model rather than looking for things that match the technology. It includes the following: economic low-volume production, cost-effective customization, improved environmental sustainability, optimized supply chains, manufacturing efficiency with more tools, jigs and fixtures, reduced inventory of spare parts, reduced lead times, and reduced raw material consumption.

11.3 Perspective of Structural Design of Healthcare Product

The process of creating the physical layout and medical equipment and gadgets used in the healthcare field is referred to as building system of healthcare products. This entails making a solution that is not just useful but also affordable, dependable, and safe. A sound structural plan may enhance treatment, decrease mistakes, and boost staff and patient satisfaction. Human factors engineering (HFE), which focuses on creating goods that are simple and intuitive to use, is one of the main viewpoints used in the structural design of healthcare devices (Wang et al. 2022; Khan et al. 2020). HFE guarantees that the product is intended to mitigate the chances of mistakes and accidents by considering the cognitive and physical capabilities of customers, including patients, physicians, and technicians. The application of cutting-edge materials and production methods is a crucial viewpoint. The strength, durability, and compatibility of the materials used in the product's construction must all be considered by structural designers (Righini et al. 2021). The creation of novel materials, such as shape-memory alloys and biocompatible polymers, has been facilitated by developments in materials science and has the potential to increase the safety and efficacy of healthcare products. In addition to functionality, cost is a crucial factor in the structural design of healthcare items. Designers must strike a balance between the demand for a high-quality product that satisfies the needs of patients and doctors and the expense of manufacturing and upkeep. A product will not be successful if it is cost-efficient but falls short of users' expectations (Ma et al. 2020; Liu et al. 2022; Sharma et al. 2021). Lastly, the architectural integrity of healthcare goods must take regulatory regulations into consideration. Strict regulatory criteria for safety, effectiveness, and quality, which might differ by nation and area, must be met by healthcare items. It is the responsibility of structural designers to guarantee that their work complies with all relevant rules. Regulatory standards, human aspects engineering, materials engineering, cost, and other considerations must all be considered while creating a healthcare product's structural framework. A sound structural plan may enhance treatment, decrease mistakes, and boost staff and patient satisfaction. The promise of structural design is broad and bright since it uses cutting-edge technology, materials, and methods.

Architectural integrity is more crucial than ever, given the rising need for dependable and environmentally friendly facilities in the context of global warming and rapid urbanization. To maximize designs and minimize environmental impact, the use of slashing technology and intelligent algorithms in building structure will be required in the future (Gu et al. 2020; Chiulan et al. 2017). The development of novel materials, such as self-healing pavement and three-dimensional steel, which will result in structures that are more efficient and durable, will alter the construction business. Generally, the discipline of structural design has a lot of possibilities for innovation and progress. Healthcare items' performance, safety, and usefulness all depend on their design. For many years, the design phase of healthcare items was a crucial factor, but with technological advancements, there is now and in the future room for fresh, creative ideas. The application of biomimicry is one growing field in the structural analysis of healthcare items. Designing goods that resemble the structure and operation of natural systems is known as biomimicry. A medical implant, for instance, may be made to resemble the structure of a bone to better blend in with the person's blood. This strategy may help healthcare goods operate better and last longer while also lowering the risk of problems (Ortiz-Acosta and Moore 2019). The use of innovative materials is another area with potential in the structural design of healthcare goods. Novel materials with special qualities, including graphene and nanocomposites, can be used to make goods that are more robust, lightweight, and long-lasting. As a result, there may be a less frequent need for replacements and improved performance over time. Also, the utilization of 3D printing for additive manufacturing is opening up new possibilities for design and construction in medical devices. Complex geometries and unique patterns may now be made with 3D printing that were previously impossible to make using conventional manufacturing techniques. Better performance, better patient outcomes, and lower costs can result from this.

11.4 Applications of Flexible Electronics in Healthcare Products

The market is generally moving toward greater digitalization in the healthcare industry. While remaining in constant contact with patients, digital health technologies like telehealth, telemedicine, and its subset, remote patient monitoring, deliver much-needed decentralization (keeping patients out of hospitals) (Ma et al. 2020; Gu et al. 2020; Ortiz-Acosta and Moore 2019). Continuous monitoring with linked medical devices, such as wearables, can offer better diagnostic capabilities and the chance to give preventative care, as opposed to discrete monitoring at each doctor visit. Overall, digital health offers traditional healthcare a cost-saving alternative while yet preserving a high standard of service. Patient compliance with medical procedures has historically been low, and this is also true of long-term usage of wearable technology. Options where the tests may run automatically as even the patient visits about their daily life are preferred since remote patient monitoring demands a high degree of compliance by the patient. In this situation, concepts like "fit and remember" or "every time monitoring" are advantageous. A person's everyday activities or devices that are implanted by a physician and remain in place might be choices to accomplish this. To optimize compliance, these devices must connect with the brain, be safe and pleasant to wear for an extended period, and not place an undue strain on the patient. The desire for flexible displays and smaller electronics is expanding the market for flexible electronics. Scientists are prepared to create new, flexible electrical gadgets for the future with this new approach to evaluating polymer conductivity.

11.4.1 Wearable Biosensors

Due to their advantages of having a large, exposed surface area and a greater affinity for water molecules than other active materials, functional inorganic nanomaterials including carbon, metal sulfides, and metal oxides stand out among other electrode materials for flexible humidity sensors (Xu et al. 2021; Gu et al. 2020). The flexible stability of a humidity sensor is another critical characteristic that is essential for practical applications. This characteristic calls for the use of sensing materials with the required mechanical compliance to guarantee consistent performance during measurements, particularly when the devices are attached to the skin or other curved surfaces. Metal oxide-based nanomaterials display hydrophilic properties for sensitive humidity sensors, much like metal sulfides do. Metal-oxide nanomaterials with outstanding electronic characteristics are mostly used for resistive or resistive stretchable humidity sensors due to their exceedingly small bandgap nature. The creation of wearable biosensors that can constantly monitor a patient's vital signs is another viable technique of wearable electronics in healthcare (Chiulan et al. 2017; Ortiz-Acosta and Moore 2019; Mpofu et al. 2014).

These biosensors can detect vital indications like pulse rate, breathing rate, and skin temperature and may be integrated into clothes or accessories like smartwatches or wristbands. Figure 11.2 gives the overview applications of sensors in multipurpose areas, including piezoelectric sensors used in (a) and (b) as haptic feedback actuators, (c) demonstrates the use and potential of piezoelectric sensors in detecting human motion detection, and (d) demonstrates the use of flexible wearable individualized health monitoring with piezoelectric sensors (Wu et al. 2021; Azahar et al. 2022). Healthcare professionals can utilize the information gathered by these sensors to monitor a patient's health and identify possible health issues before they become critical. The creation of implanted medical devices, including pacemakers, neurostimulators, and drug delivery systems, can also make use of flexible electronics. These devices can be made more comfortable for patients and less prone to difficulties by being made thinner, lighter, and more flexible. These devices can also include flexible electronic sensors that provide real-time monitoring and information collection that can be utilized to modify treatment programs. The creation of smart pills is another possible usage of wearable electronics in healthcare. These tablets have sensors that can detect a pill's position and movement throughout the digestive tract, providing important information about the medication's absorption and

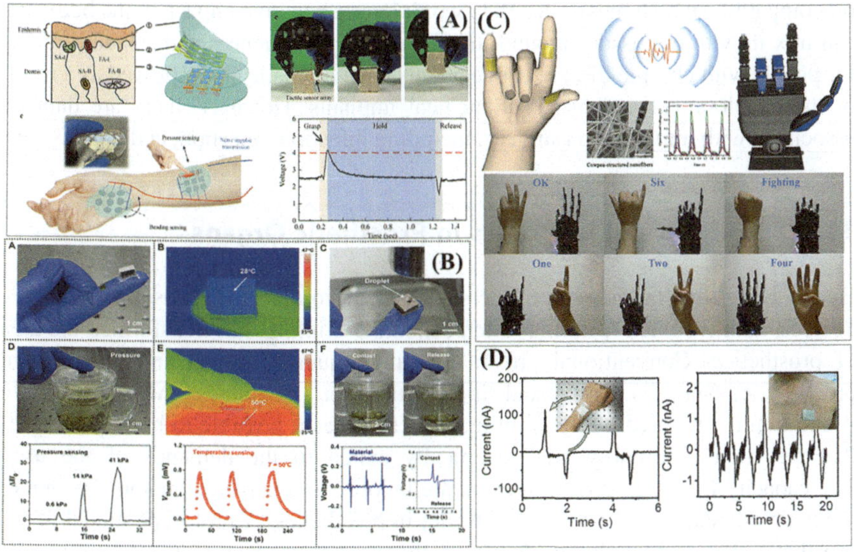

Fig. 11.2 Application of piezoelectric biosensors for detecting human motion detection. (Reproduced with permission from Wu et al. 2021)

effectiveness. This technology may enhance patient outcomes, lessen adverse effects, and enhance drug adherence.

11.4.2 Medical Implants

Transform medical implants and eliminate restrictions on customization. It requires a method to get there more quickly for the ready to boost productivity, encourage customization, and enhance patient safety. The forerunners of full metal additive manufacture are prepared to assist you when you're ready to supply orthopedic implants that are affordable and customized for each patient utilizing additive manufacturing technologies. Medical implants are items or tissues that are surgically inserted into the body to maintain biological structures, replace missing or damaged body parts, or offer therapeutic advantages. Typical medical implant kinds include: Orthopedic implants: These include bone plates and screws used to stabilize fractures, spinal implants, and joint replacement implants. Dental implants: These support dental prostheses like bridges and dentures and are used to replace lost teeth. Implants for the cardiovascular system include pacemakers, stents, and synthetic heart valves. Ophthalmic implants, such as the intraocular lenses used during cataract surgery, are used to treat visual issues. Neurological implants: These include spinal cord stimulators and deep brain stimulators for the treatment of Parkinson's disease and chronic pain, respectively. Metals, polymers, and ceramics are just a few of the materials used to make medical implants. They are intended to be biocompatible, which means that they won't have a negative impact on the body and can mix in with the tissues around them. Patients' experiences and standard of life for people with chronic diseases or accidents have dramatically improved as a result of the development and usage of medical implants. However, there are dangers associated with implantation surgery, including infection, rejection, and other issues.

11.5 3D-Printed Electronics in Prosthetic Organs

By enabling the fabrication of personalized, affordable, and useful prosthetic devices, additive manufacturing, often called 3D printing, has transformed the area of prosthetics. Conventional prosthetics are frequently pricey and may not fit precisely, causing discomfort and limiting the user's usefulness (Ma et al. 2020). A solution is provided by 3D printing, which makes it possible to build prostheses that are more affordably and specifically suited to the demands of the user. The capacity to design prostheses that are tailored to a person's anatomy is one of the main advantages of 3D manufacturing in prosthetics. A prototype model of the prosthetic device may be made using the precise measurements taken by 3D scanners of the remaining limb. This makes it possible to design prostheses that exactly suit the wearer's body, minimizing pain and enhancing functioning (Gu et al. 2020). The capacity to produce prosthetic devices rapidly and affordably with 3D printing is another advantage for prostheses. Conventional prosthetic devices can cost tens of thousands of dollars and take weeks or even months to produce. Prosthetics may now be produced quickly and cheaply using 3D printing in a couple of hours or days. This is crucial for people who lack access to reasonably priced prosthetic equipment since 3D printing can offer an economical substitute (Ortiz-Acosta and Moore 2019). Moreover, 3D printing makes it possible to design prostheses that are lighter and more comfortable than conventional prosthetics.

3D bioprinting is an emerging technology that involves the creation of three-dimensional structures using living cells. The process begins with the selection of a bioink, which is a substance that can support cell growth and promote tissue formation. The bioink is loaded into a 3D printer, which then creates a scaffold or structure layer by layer using the bioink and living cells. From Fig. 11.3, X-ray, computed tomography (CT), magnetic resonance imaging (MRI), and other scanning and reconstruction methods, as well as direct use of computer-aided design (CAD) software, can all be used to create 3D models. Next, using specialized software, 3D models would be cut into 2D horizontally slices with adjustable size and orientation (Xu et al. 2021; Chiulan et al. 2017). The various bioprinting techniques would further transform these data into particles or filaments. Cells, growth factors, biocompatible, and other materials should be carefully selected in accordance with the needs of printed structures and methodologies. The mixture of these materials is technically referred to as bioinks; however, they are typically just thought of as cell-filled hydrogels. To ensure biocompatibility, printability, and mechanical property, the choice of bioinks is essential. The living cells are carefully arranged to mimic the natural structure of the tissue being printed. Once the printing

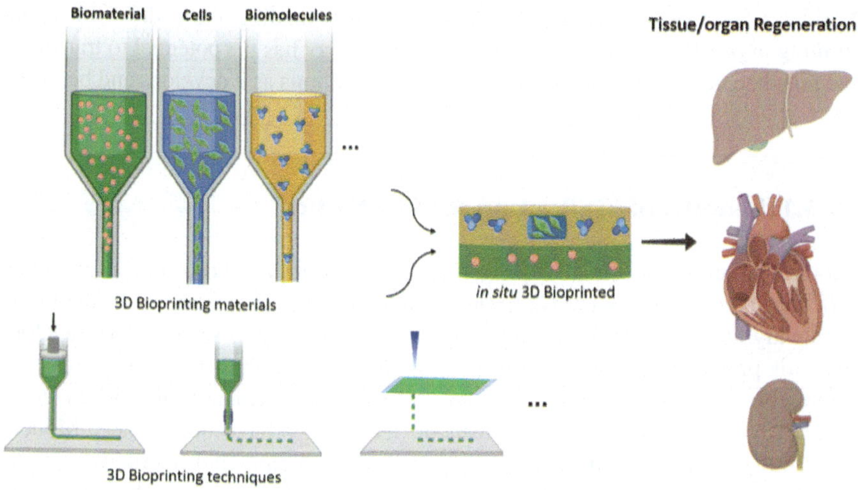

Fig. 11.3 3D bioprinting technology for tissue/organ regeneration

process is complete, the scaffold is placed in a bioreactor, where the cells can continue to grow and develop into functional tissue. This technology has the potential to revolutionize the field of regenerative medicine by enabling the creation of replacement tissues and organs (Seider et al. 2009; Liu et al. 2022; Ortiz-Acosta and Moore 2019). Conventional prostheses may be cumbersome and heavy, which may restrict movement and irritate the user. Prosthetics with distinctive characteristics and capabilities can also be made using 3D printing in addition to more conventional prosthetics. For instance, sensors and other electronics may be included into 3D-printed prostheses to offer input on pressure, temperature, and other variables. By doing this, the user may modify the prosthesis to make it more comfortable and useful. In order to build prosthetics that are both useful and visually beautiful, 3D printing may also be utilized to manufacture prostheses with intricate forms and patterns. The creation of children's prosthetic devices is a significant use of 3D printing in prosthetics. Children with deformities of the limbs frequently need prosthetics that can expand and change with them. As a person develops, prosthetic equipment may be quickly updated and altered thanks to 3D printing, which reduces the requirement for repeated replacements and lowers expenses.

Despite the numerous advantages of 3D printing for prostheses, certain issues still need to be resolved. Making sure 3D-printed prosthetic devices adhere to safety and quality requirements is one of the key issues. The user must feel comfortable and effective while using prosthetic equipment, which needs to be able to tolerate wear and tear. To maintain uniformity and dependability across many manufacturers, standardized standards for 3D-printed prosthetic devices are also required. Making sure that everyone who needs the technology can access it is a difficulty when it comes to employing 3D printing in prosthetics. Moreover, education and training on the use of 3D printing technology to produce prosthetic devices may be required for healthcare professionals and prosthetists. Notwithstanding these difficulties, 3D printing in prosthetics has a bright future. Technology has the potential to transform the prosthetics industry and enhance the lives of millions as it develops and becomes more widely available.

11.5.1 Benefits of 3D Printing for Prosthetics

People frequently envision 3D-printed jewelry, customized home décor, and even food when they think about 3D printing. However, many people are unaware of how frequently this technology is being employed in a variety of sectors. The development of prosthetic limbs for people who have lost a limb is one of the most impressive applications of this technology in the medical industry (Khan et al. 2020). Over time, advances in prosthetic technology have been made. Modern custom-fit prostheses with microprocessors and pneumatic and hydraulic controls to support natural movement have progressed from wooden toes in Ancient Egypt and hefty iron fingers in the sixteenth and seventeenth centuries. They demonstrate the continual advancement of the prosthetics sector, but it is crucial to emphasize that improvement is ongoing (Ortiz-Acosta and Moore 2019). The advent of 3D printing has completely changed the industry and transformed the life of ordinary folks, many of whom would never have been able to buy conventional, high-tech prostheses (Mpofu et al. 2014). In addition to this, benefits of 3D prosthetics must be led to focus on the following three aspects.

- Innovation: Be creative without being constrained by current production methods. Rapid prototyping has never been so simple thanks to 3D printers. Iterate your ideas and projects faster owing to this technology. Great future improvements will be made possible by going beyond conventional prosthesis manufacture.
- Personalization: Design modified prostheses. The most crucial argument in this case is the one about customization. The patients will benefit and have a better quality of life if a limb is lost if they receive adaptive equipment and prostheses. Thanks to 3D printers, it is now feasible to create customizable functioning prostheses.
- Cost: Once more, using conventional manufacturing methods is costly when creating a project as sophisticated as prostheses. Additive printing seems to be the most effective method for producing affordable prostheses, particularly if you want to customize it to the morphology of the patient. Making prosthetics in places where it is difficult or impossible to get such devices is turning into a life-changing answer. Custom-made prosthetics are superior and more effective. But, with traditional production, personalization is rather costly.

The most important thing is the 3D-printed prostheses' potential in the future Indeed, it is dazzling. The examples given in this article demonstrate how advantageous additive manufacturing is to the medical sector. Prosthetics are thousands of dollars less expensive thanks to 3D printing. They fit the limb perfectly, do not hurt the user, and are highly tailored, making them considerably more pleasant. Never has personalization been this high level.

11.6 Perspective on Human–Computer Interfaces

In the current modern age, physical education uses the Internet of Things (IoT) to instruct students and track their physical activity. Human–computer interface (HCI) is the multidisciplinary study of many aspects impacting this interaction (Wu et al. 2021). It is focused on the development, implementation, and assessment of interactive computer-based systems. The goal of HCI is to guarantee the security, usefulness, efficacy, and accessibility of such systems. The component of an interactive environment, program, or telematic service with which the user makes cognitive, perceptual, and physical contact is the user interface. The research and educational communities, as well as the information and technology and telecommunications (IT&T) business, have all given HCI a lot of attention recently. For IoT-based human–computer interaction in college physical education, the AI-based IoTS wearable technology is encouraged. The data needed by the pupils are recognized by the AI-IoTS. Use an IoT platform to collect cloud data, which AI will then process. The simulation approach of the proposed framework "AI-IoTS" demonstrated its independence in gathering and instructing pupils. Keyboards, speech recognition, motion sensors, and other devices that track certain sorts of information and extract data are examples of human–machine interface technology, which aids in integrating humans into sophisticated technological systems (Azahar et al. 2022; Singh et al. 2020; Kumar et al. 2021).

The user, task, tools or interface, and context are the four main components of HUI. The evaluation of observations made when the user is carrying out certain activities and the user's habits are both necessary for HCI research. The creation of interactive systems takes advantage of these data. The objective of HCI is to design a system that is user-friendly, useful, and secure. To do this, developers must have the following skills: the ability to empathize with consumers and foresee how they will use the technology provide instruments and methods that will enable best practices for creating an adequate system and create a productive, efficient, and secure exchange. In recent years, the area of human–computer interfaces (HCIs) with in medical industry has advanced quickly, and this trend is anticipated to continue in the years to come. Human–computer interaction, or HCI, is a term used to describe how humans communicate with computers as well as other electronic technologies. Use of the processing of natural language (NLP) technology is one of the most exciting developments in HCI. With the use of this technology, patients may communicate normally to a computer, which can then understand what they are saying and reply properly (Norcio and Stanley 1989; Heng et al. 2022; Patel and Kushniruk 1998). This may dramatically enhance the patient experience and assist medical personnel in diagnosing and treating patients more quickly and precisely, and it is clearly visible in Fig. 11.4.

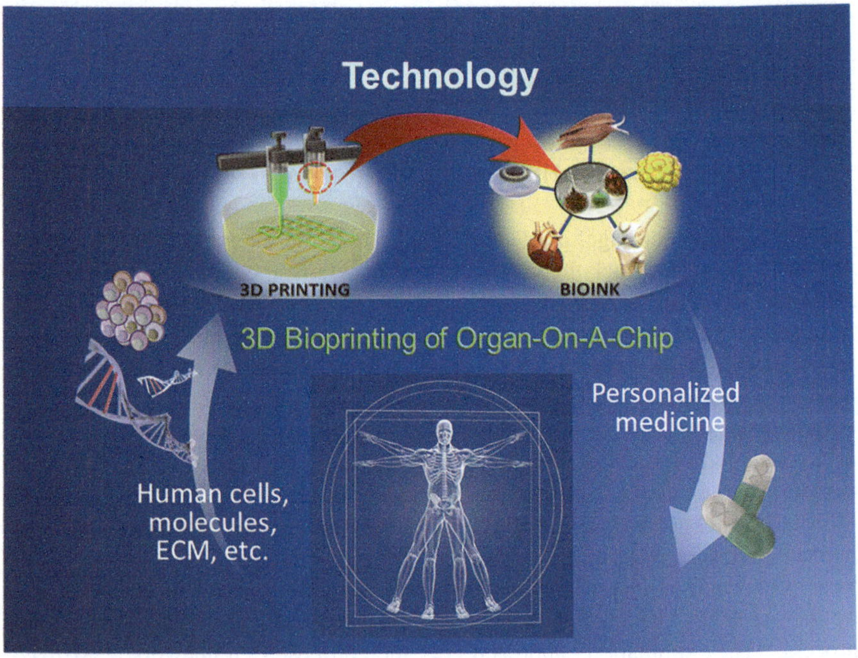

Fig. 11.4 Application of 3D bioprinting to organ-on-a-chip

The use of wearable technology to monitor patient health, including wearables and fitness trackers, is another area of emphasis in HCI. These gadgets may gather patient data on their heart rate, blood pressure, and other vital indicators, which can be sent to medical experts for study. As a result, more individualized treatment strategies and early detection of medical issues may be possible (Andreoni et al. 2007). It is also anticipated that augmented reality (AR) and virtual reality (VR) will play a bigger part in the medical industry. For medical students, virtual reality (VR) may be utilized to create immersive educational experiences that let them practice treatments in a genuine setting before applying them to actual patients (Wołczowski and Kurzyński 2010; Li et al. 2020; Zhang et al. 2022). Overall, the future of HCI in the medical field looks very promising, with many exciting developments on the horizon. As technology continues to advance, healthcare professionals will be able to provide more personalized, efficient, and effective care to their patients.

11.7 Conclusion and Future Outlook

By offering individualized and customized medical gadgets that are inexpensive and simple to produce, flexible and embedded 3D-printed electronic subsystems have the potential to transform the healthcare sector. The technique has a variety of benefits, including the capacity to design complicated forms, integrated functionality, and a decrease in the number of parts needed. The use of 3D printing technology in the medical sector is anticipated to increase over the next several years as demand for individualized treatment rises. Healthcare solutions that utilize flexible and integrated 3D-printed electronic subsystems may be able to diagnose and cure illnesses earlier, lower the risk of complications, and enhance patient outcomes. The creation of medical implants is one industry wherein 3D printer is already having an influence. The use of 3D printing enables the production of highly customized implants that precisely meet the anatomical requirements of a patient. This can lower the risk of problems and increase surgical success rates. Moreover, implants with distinctive forms and patterns that were previously impractical may now be made via additive manufacturing, improving patient outcomes. There are still obstacles to be addressed, though, including the demand for high-quality products and procedures, assuring legal compliance, and dealing with worries about data security and privacy. However, the price of 3D printing equipment and technology is still quite high, making it inaccessible to smaller healthcare institutions and providers. Notwithstanding these difficulties, there is hope for the future of flexible and integrated 3D-printed electrical subsystems in medical devices. It is anticipated that 3D printing will be utilized more often in the healthcare industry as technology develops and costs fall down, providing individualized, effective, and economical medical treatments.

Acknowledgments G.S.D.B. is grateful to the Management of Chettinad College of Engineering and Technology, Karur, for constant support and encouragement. S.N. and K.G. acknowledge the Management of Chettinad Academy of Research and Education (ChARE), Chennai, for their continuous support. C.D. acknowledges the Management of Mahendra Engineering College (Autonomous), Namakkal, for encouragement.

References

Andreoni G et al (2007) Human machine interface for healthcare and rehabilitation. In: Advanced computational intelligence paradigms in healthcare-2. Springer, pp 131–150

Azahar AM et al (2022) Recent advances in 3D printing of biomedical sensing devices. Adv Funct Mater 32(9):2107671

Buga CP, Viana JC (2022) The role of printed electronics and related technologies in the development of smart connected products. Flexible Print Electron 7:043001

Caironi M, Noh Y-Y (2015) Large area and flexible electronics. John Wiley & Sons

Chandrasekaran S et al (2022) A comprehensive review on printed electronics: a technology drift towards a sustainable future. Nanomaterials 12(23):4251

Chen X et al (2019) Materials chemistry in flexible electronics. Chem Soc Rev 48(6):1431–1433

Chiulan I et al (2017) Recent advances in 3D printing of aliphatic polyesters. Bioengineering 5(1):2

Consoli D, Mina A (2009) An evolutionary perspective on health innovation systems. J Evol Econ 19:297–319

Corzo D, Tostado-Blázquez G, Baran D (2020) Flexible electronics: status, challenges and opportunities. Front Electron 1:594003

Espalin D et al (2014) 3D printing multifunctionality: structures with electronics. Int J Adv Manuf Technol 72:963

Espera AH et al (2019) 3D-printing and advanced manufacturing for electronics. Progress Addit Manuf 4:245–267
Espera AH et al (2022) Advancing flexible electronics and additive manufacturing. Jpn J Appl Phys 61:SE0803
Gao W et al (2019) Flexible electronics toward wearable sensing. Acc Chem Res 52(3):523–533
Gu Z et al (2020) Development of 3D bioprinting: from printing methods to biomedical applications. Asian J Pharm Sci 15(5):529–557
Heng W, Solomon S, Gao W (2022) Flexible electronics and devices as human–machine interfaces for medical robotics. Adv Mater 34(16):2107902
Karahoca A, Karahoca D, Aksöz M (2018) Examining intention to adopt to internet of things in healthcare technology products. Kybernetes 47(4):742–770
Khan Y et al (2020) A new frontier of printed electronics: flexible hybrid electronics. Adv Mater 32(15):1905279
Kumar P et al (2021) 3D printing technology for biomedical practice: a review. J Mater Eng Perform 30(7):5342–5355
Li J et al (2020) 3D printing of hydrogels: rational design strategies and emerging biomedical applications. Mater Sci Eng R Rep 140:100543
Liu Z et al (2015) Flexible electronics based on inorganic nanowires. Chem Soc Rev 44(1):161–192
Liu J et al (2019) Current advances and future perspectives of 3D printing natural-derived biopolymers. Carbohydr Polym 207:297–316
Liu K et al (2022) Advances in flexible organic field-effect transistors and their applications for flexible electronics. npj Flexible Electron 6(1):1
Luo Y et al (2020) Devising materials manufacturing toward lab-to-fab translation of flexible electronics. Adv Mater 32(37):2001903
Ma Y et al (2020) Flexible hybrid electronics for digital healthcare. Adv Mater 32(15):1902062
Mpofu TP, Mawere C, Mukosera M (2014) The impact and application of 3D printing technology. Int J Sci Res 3:358
Murphy SV, De Coppi P, Atala A (2020) Opportunities and challenges of translational 3D bioprinting. Nat Biomed Eng 4(4):370–380
Norcio AF, Stanley J (1989) Adaptive human-computer interfaces: a literature survey and perspective. IEEE Trans Syst Man Cybern 19(2):399–408
Ortiz-Acosta D, Moore T (2019) Functional 3D printed polymeric materials. Funct Mater 9:1–5
Palo M et al (2017) 3D printed drug delivery devices: perspectives and technical challenges. Expert Rev Med Devices 14(9):685–696
Park Y-G et al (2022) High-resolution 3D printing for electronics. Adv Sci 9(8):2104623
Patel VL, Kushniruk AW (1998) Interface design for health care environments: the role of cognitive science. In: Proceedings of the AMIA symposium. American Medical Informatics Association
Persad J, Rocke S (2022) A survey of 3D printing technologies as applied to printed electronics. IEEE Access 10:27289–27319
Pravin S, Sudhir A (2018) Integration of 3D printing with dosage forms: a new perspective for modern healthcare. Biomed Pharmacother 107:146–154
Rao CH et al (2022) A review on printed electronics with digital 3D printing: fabrication techniques, materials, challenges and future opportunities. J Electron Mater 51(6):2747–2765
Righini GC et al (2021) From flexible electronics to flexible photonics: a brief overview. Opt Mater 115:111011
Seider WD et al (2009) Perspectives on chemical product and process design. Comput Chem Eng 33(5):930–935
Sharma A et al (2021) Wearable biosensors: an alternative and practical approach in healthcare and disease monitoring. Molecules 26(3):748
Singh T, Kumar S, Sehgal S (2020) 3D printing of engineering materials: a state of the art review. Mater Today Proc 28:1927–1931
Tan HW et al (2022) 3D printed electronics: processes, materials and future trends. Prog Mater Sci 127:100945

Wang X, Liu J (2016) Recent advancements in liquid metal flexible printed electronics: properties, technologies, and applications. Micromachines 7(12):206
Wang P et al (2020) The evolution of flexible electronics: from nature, beyond nature, and to nature. Adv Sci 7(20):2001116
Wang Z et al (2022) Advanced materials for flexible electronics. Mater Technol 37(12):1969–1970
Wiegard R-B, Breitner MH (2019) Smart services in healthcare: a risk-benefit-analysis of pay-as-you-live services from customer perspective in Germany. Electron Mark 29:107–123
Winters JM, Wang Y, Winters JM (2003) Wearable sensors and telerehabilitation. IEEE Eng Med Biol Mag 22(3):56–65
Wołczowski A, Kurzyński M (2010) Human–machine interface in bioprosthesis control using EMG signal classification. Expert Syst 27(1):53–70
Wong WS, Salleo A (eds) (2009) Flexible electronics: materials and applications, vol 11. Springer Science & Business Media
Wu Y et al (2021) Piezoelectric materials for flexible and wearable electronics: a review. Mater Des 211:110164
Xu J, Fang Y, Chen J (2021) Wearable biosensors for non-invasive sweat diagnostics. Biosensors 11(8):245
Zang Y et al (2015) Advances of flexible pressure sensors toward artificial intelligence and health care applications. Mater Horizons 2(2):140–156
Zhang L et al (2022) Nanomaterial integrated 3D printing for biomedical applications. J Mater Chem B 10(37):7473–7490

3D Printing of Pharmaceutical Products Using AI Technology

12

Brahmansh Kaushik, Anand Kumar Subramaniyan, Mitali Pareek, Sneha Sharma, and Rajkumar Velu

Contents

B. Kaushik
Department of Mechanical Engineering, Northwestern University, Evanston, IL, USA

A. K. Subramaniyan (✉) · R. Velu
Additive Manufacturing Research Laboratory, Mechanical Engineering, Indian Institute of Technology Jammu, Jammu, Jammu and Kashmir, India
e-mail: anand.subramaniyan@iitjammu.ac.in; rajkumar.v@iitjammu.ac.in

M. Pareek
Mahatma Gandhi Dental College and Hospital, Jaipur, Rajasthan, India

S. Sharma
The University of Texas at Dallas, Richardson, TX, USA

R. Velu et al. (eds.), *Digital Design and Manufacturing of Medical Devices and Systems*, https://doi.org/10.1007/978-981-99-7100-8_12

Abstract

The continuous development in the 3D printing (3DP) or additive manufacturing (AM) sector provides a faster and more customized product solution for every industry. The basic definition of 3D printing or additive manufacturing is a digital fabrication technology that can print an object by successive addition of material with the help of a computer-aided design (CAD) model. This CAD model allows the iteration of the product according to specific product needs. The other advantage of AM is to manufacture single or bulk products with the same ability to manipulate the outcome. Recent developments in AM technologies resulted in faster production and enabled multi-material manufacturing simultaneously. 3D printing is a potentially advancing technology in every sector, including the automotive, locomotive, agriculture, and healthcare industries. The pharmaceutical sector also takes advantage of this transforming technology of 3D printing. Due to its inherent versatility, unique ability to produce intricate designs, and relative cost-effectiveness compared to traditional mass manufacturing processes, this is often attributed to the success of the technology. Thus, it can enable the fabrication of personalized medicines, drug products, and appropriate drug dosing and delivery methods. 3D printing helps develop individualized drug products according to patient age, body weight, and lifestyle. These individualized drug products can prevent under and overdosing of the drug product due to unequal breaking in parts. Medical products like bio-composites, manufacturing tissues, and healthcare implants can also be well fabricated using digital fabrication technology. Despite all these advantages, 3D printing of drug products is a slow process and requires automation. Leveraging reforming digitalized technologies such as artificial intelligence (AI) into 3D printing can alleviate these gaps. Machine learning, a subset of AI, can accurately predict drug dosage and delivery processes and can help human expertise. Pharmaceutical management can be more streamlined with innovative drug design and precise quality control with the integration of the reforming technology of AI.

Moreover, due to the growth potential of AI in predicting and analyzing large datasets, it can reshape pharmaceutical management. In this work, an extensive review explores the potential of 3D printing pharmaceutical products using AI technology. Discussing the current limitations and their possible solutions with the possible future improvement is also incorporated. The potential conclusion that can be drawn from this work is that the integration of AI/ML proved to be an effective means of modeling the 3D printing workflow for the pharmaceutical industries.

Keywords

3D printing · Pharmaceutical products · Artificial intelligence · Personalized medicine

12.1 Introduction

In the early days of medication, plants and herbal remedies were used to treat various diseases and traumas. The origin of the pharmaceutical industry can be considered around the late nineteenth century. In the mid-twentieth century, the modern pharmaceutical industry originated, considered the Golden Age (Malerba and Orsenigo 2015). Today, there have been incredible advances in the pharmaceutical industry and a diverse range of drugs available to prevent, treat, and lessen the impact of ailments. The R&D in pharmaceutical products resulted in faster and safer drug development with the help of modern technologies, including advanced manufacturing and artificial intelligence. The advanced manufacturing included three-dimensional printing (3DP) of a product.

The market of pharmaceutical products is a multi-billion with several regulations at each step, from the manufacturing level to the patient level (Morton and Kyle 2011). These regulations must be followed by each product manufacturing firm. 3DP of pharmaceutical products has several challenges and opportunities to fit into this multi-billion market. In pharmaceutical markets, the cost of developing a drug is higher compared to replicating the same. This must be controlled by the proper claim of intellectual property rights about the formulation and technology designed (Grabowski 2002).

Pharmaceutical product manufacturing involves two major stages. The first stage is primary processing, which involves producing the active ingredient or drug. The second stage, known as secondary processing, entails converting the active drug into products suitable for human consumption (Reklaitis 2017). Initially, pharmaceutical products were made in batches without automation. Batch processing, as it is called, requires charging materials before processing and discharging the product after processing (Kleinebudde et al. 2017). However, this approach is resource-intensive and demands more human labor to operate and maintain the equipment regularly. Continuous automation transformed conventional production, resulting in a more efficient manufacturing process (Singh 2018). One of the limitations of batch manufacturing is the inability to customize pharmaceutical products, alter product specifications hourly or develop many products during constant production, and precisely control dose regimens based on patient characteristics. Moreover, there is a limit to the maximum dosage that conventional drug delivery devices can deliver, which affects their durability and ability to provide long-term delivery. Additive manufacturing (AM) has emerged as the most promising technology for personalized medicine and controlled drug delivery due to the limitations of the customization of products and current drug delivery systems (Wang et al. 2021).

Three-dimensional printing (3DP) is the process of manufacturing products by depositing successive layers. This method is also known as additive manufacturing (AM), rapid prototyping (RP), and solid free-form manufacturing. The layer-by-layer deposition allows for high dimensional accuracy and customization capabilities in product manufacturing. The extensive research and development in the field of 3DP made it be deployed in various industries, including automobile, aerospace, tool-making, cosmetics, and biomedical. The benefits of 3DP include

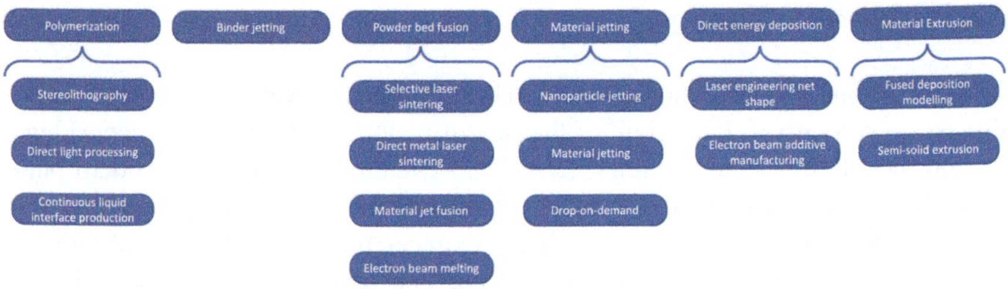

Fig. 12.1 Various 3D printing technologies

highly customized design, multi-material manufacturing, on-demand manufacturing, reduced ecological footprint, and cost-effective production. The biomedical industry has leveraged 3DP to manufacture pharmaceutical products, such as implants, drug development, and drug delivery systems (Rahman et al. 2018). The use of 3DP in pharmaceutical manufacturing allows for the development of personalized drugs, faster drug development, and on-demand manufacturing. The manufacturing technology used for pharmaceutical products includes selective laser sintering (SLS), sheet lamination, stereolithography (SLA), direct energy deposition (DED), and inkjet-based 3DP, as shown in Fig. 12.1 (Awad et al. 2018; Norman et al. 2017).

The use of 3DP in pharmaceutical industries is rapidly increasing, with research in the field growing exponentially. While 3DP has been utilized in pharmaceutical applications since the 1980s, recent advances have led to significant progress (Hurst 2016). Applications for 3DP in pharmaceuticals include tissue and organ fabrication, customized prosthetics, patient-oriented implants, bio-printing, patient-specific anatomical models, regenerative medicines, and more (Park et al. 2018; Liaw and Guvendiren 2017; Puls et al. 2021). One major advantage of 3DP in pharmaceuticals is the ability to produce customized formulations faster and more accurately, taking into account the patient's age, weight, and the severity of the disease. Other benefits of 3DP include flexible design, high precision and accuracy in fabricating complex dosage forms, on-demand manufacturing, increased productivity and cost-effectiveness, and less waste production (Eshkalak et al. 2020; Schubert et al. 2014). Additionally, artificial intelligence (AI) is helping to make more intelligent decisions about the product and manufacturing process, determining the appropriate parameters for 3D-printed products with optimal performance. 3D printing is a disruptive technology that can significantly impact the clinical field, improving medicine and healthcare and enabling affordable, accessible, and personalized medical care (Elbadawi et al. 2021). Furthermore, 3D printing is helping to deal with chronic diseases like osteoarthritis, cancer, and cardiovascular disease (CVD), as demonstrated in Fig. 12.2.

Despite its numerous potential benefits in medicine and economics, the implementation of 3DP technology is currently restricted by several technical challenges

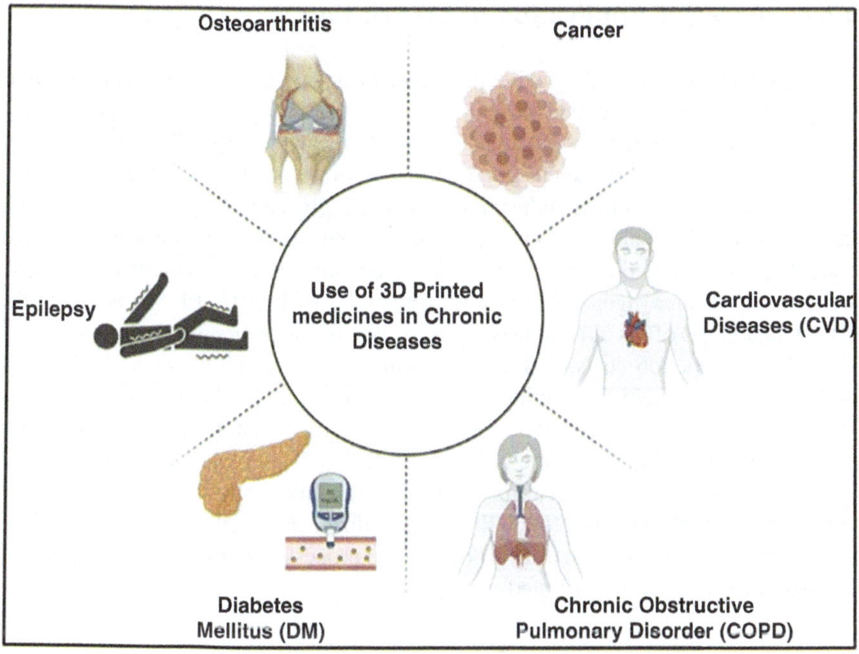

Fig. 12.2 Medicines from 3D printing used in the treatment of chronic disease (Varghese et al. 2022)

that impede its commercialization. These challenges include the limited availability of bio-compatible materials for 3DP printers, pharma-technical problems with current 3DP techniques, the capacity and reproducibility of processes, and the quality of final products. In addition, regulatory changes and considerations may be necessary to approve pharmaceutical products made by 3DP methods. Continual innovation and refinement of 3DP methods are necessary to overcome these regulatory and technical challenges, enabling the technology to be more widely used for various drug delivery systems in the future and facilitating the clinical use of more personalized dosage forms that are more patient-friendly (Roopavath and Kalaskar 2017).

This review work provides an overview of the present state and future potential of utilizing 3DP technology in the production of pharmaceutical products, with a detailed discussion of its various applications. Additionally, the paper highlights the growing role of artificial intelligence in improving the efficiency and intelligence of pharmaceutical production, including the development of new drug formulations and optimization of process parameters. Furthermore, the review suggests that the pharmaceutical industry can integrate AI with 3DP to facilitate decision-making related to dissolution behavior, printability, and formulation design.

12.2 Areas of Application of 3D Printing

Drug products, consisting of active pharmaceutical ingredients (APIs) and inactive excipients, can be formulated in various forms, such as pills, liquids, patches, or implants, with a need for sophisticated design to enable controlled drug release, long-term stability, and patient compliance (Bharate et al. 2010; Goyanes et al. 2015). The pharmaceutical industry has increasingly adopted 3D printing in the last decade due to its ability to fabricate complex objects and offer customization for patient-specific drug delivery devices based on physiological parameters such as weight, surface area, age, and gender (Prasad and Smyth 2016; El Aita et al. 2018). This technology offers advantages such as flexibility in geometrical shapes and sizes, low production costs, and minimal unit-to-unit variability. As a result, there is a growing interest in developing more robust and flexible 3D printing techniques (Jamróz et al. 2017). Common drugs like ibuprofen can be personalized with extrusion printing that shows the potential of 3DP to be deployed in the production of highly common drugs (Tabriz et al. 2022). This section discusses various applications of 3D printing, including personalized drug delivery, drug development, and data enrichment in drug products. The process flow for the development of a 3D-printed product is illustrated in Fig. 12.3.

12.2.1 Early Phase of Drug Development

In the initial stages of drug development, it is essential to create a suitable formulation of the active ingredient(s) for clinical trials. To achieve this, a thorough physiochemical analysis of the active ingredient(s) is necessary in order to develop a dosage form that can evaluate the drug's therapeutic efficacy. Using 3D printing technology during this phase can be advantageous as it allows for the creation of dosage forms quickly and with minimal investment of time, effort, and resources. This approach provides several benefits, such as the ability to produce dosage forms with high bioavailability and dose flexibility. In contrast, conventional manufacturing methods can be both labor-intensive and costly as they require larger batch sizes (Norman et al. 2017; Awad et al. 2018).

12.2.2 Data Enrichment Using 3D Printing

The 3DP printed pharmaceuticals are personalized as per the specific requirement. The production batch is also small, so the drug package labeling is inefficient. This problem can be solved by in-drug labeling proposed by Öblom et al. (2020). The proposal is to make data-enriched edible pharmaceuticals (DEEP) with a quick response (QR) encoded orodispersible film. The motivation for using the 3DP for the QR on the drug is to preserve the drug information and traceability, control abuse, maintain authenticity, and terminate the possibility of counterfeiting. This proposal shows the application of QR for medical cannabis drugs but can be

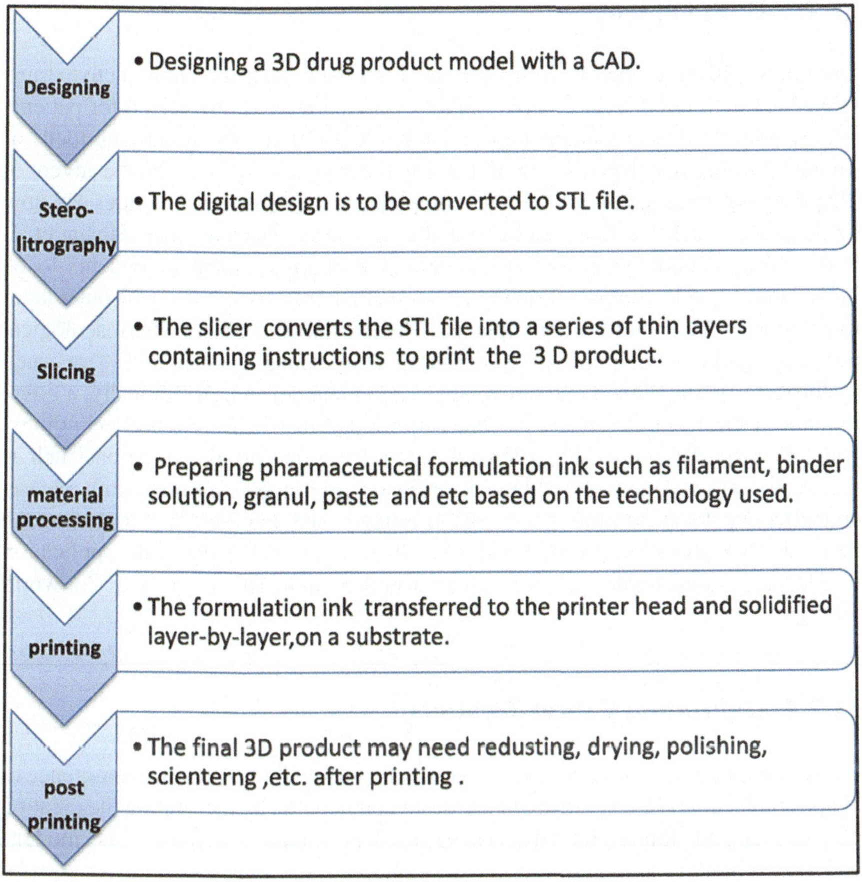

Fig. 12.3 A schematic of process flow involved in 3D printing (Samiei 2020)

Fig. 12.4 Schematic of data-enriched drug development

extended for other 3DP drugs. A similar approach is followed to keep track of and trace the medicine. Data enrichment also helps identify a counterfeit drug that helps identify a fake drug that helps ensure the uniqueness of the drug (Öblom et al. 2020). Figure 12.4 shows the proposed methodology of printing the QR code on the drug.

12.2.3 Drug Implant

Drug implants are a type of sustained-release dosage form that contains active drugs embedded within a delivery matrix, and they are particularly beneficial for patients who require long-term medication (Holländer et al. 2016). The traditional focus of implant development has been on prolonging the drug release, but with the advent of 3D printing technology, implants with complex micro and macro structures can now be designed to achieve more sophisticated drug release characteristics (Huang et al. 2007). This technology enables multiple active pharmaceutical ingredients to be loaded into a single implant, allowing for sequential drug release from the outer layer to the core. These multi-drug implants, which exhibit excellent pharmacological properties and cytocompatibility, show promise in managing chronic diseases such as chronic osteomyelitis, bone tuberculosis, and bone defects. Additionally, a novel implant in the form of a patch has been developed using 3D printing technology, which is designed to provide prolonged drug release for chronic conditions such as pancreatic cancer. Due to their high performance, prolonged controlled drug release, and effective local administration, 3D printing-based implants are becoming an increasingly viable dosage form for chronic disorders, which expands the application of 3D printing technology in the pharmaceutical industry (Dash and Cudworth 1998).

12.2.4 3D Printing Cancer Treatment

Cancer treatment is a highly complex issue in the medical field, but the emergence of 3D printing technology has brought about several benefits by facilitating the creation of personalized tumor models. These models include physical 3D models, bio-printed models, and tumor-on-chip models, which demonstrate superior correlation in vitro and in vivo, especially in areas such as drug screening, cancer metastasis, and prognosis studies. The use of 3D printing technology is significantly contributing to cancer modelling and research, providing valuable insights that can be applied to both treatment and diagnosis (Bhuskute et al. 2022).

12.2.5 3D Printed Tablets with Multiple Drugs

The development of a "polypill" through 3D extrusion-based printing allows for personalized medication based on patient profiles and comorbidities. A study focused on treating people with diabetes and hypertension combined the drugs captopril, nifedipine, and glipizide using an osmotic pump release method through a controlled porosity shell (captopril) and sustained release compartments/diffusion through gel layers (nifedipine and glipizide). The tablet was printed layer by layer, and various ratios of excipients were tested to ensure smooth printing and proper drug release. The HPMC barrier used a hydroalcoholic gel to avoid particle swelling and surface hydration. The tablet shell disintegrated within the first hour, splitting the pill into two parts with different release mechanisms. The study found no significant difference in drug release compared to individual drugs through X-ray powder diffraction data. The "polypill" has the potential to revolutionize the pharmaceutical industry by allowing for personalized treatment plans and modifications on the dose or method of delivery. Further optimization and calculations on the ratios of excipients and pastes used can create "polypills" that act identically to separate drugs (Khaled et al. 2015).

12.3 Applications and Advantages of Using AI

The AI program utilizes historical data for training, enabling it to be used for prediction and optimization once trained. Integrating AI into current manufacturing systems aims to automate and optimize the process. Machine learning (ML), a subset of AI, is widely used for prediction and classification, particularly in the pharmaceutical industry, where it can be used to predict optimized process parameters.

AI transforms 3D printing into a self-sufficient process by providing product prediction and analysis. In pharmaceutical product manufacturing, several AI algorithms, such as artificial neural networks (ANNs), principal component analysis (PCA), and linear regression, are frequently implemented to make the manufacturing process more efficient. In this section, various applications of AI are reviewed. They are categorized into three stages: the pre-manufacturing stage, the manufacturing stage, and the post-manufacturing stage. In each stage, AI can make the process autonomous and efficient. AI is also helping in the development of nanobots that are used in specific drug delivery and diagnosis. Figure 12.5 shows different types of nanobots (Jitendra et al. 2021)

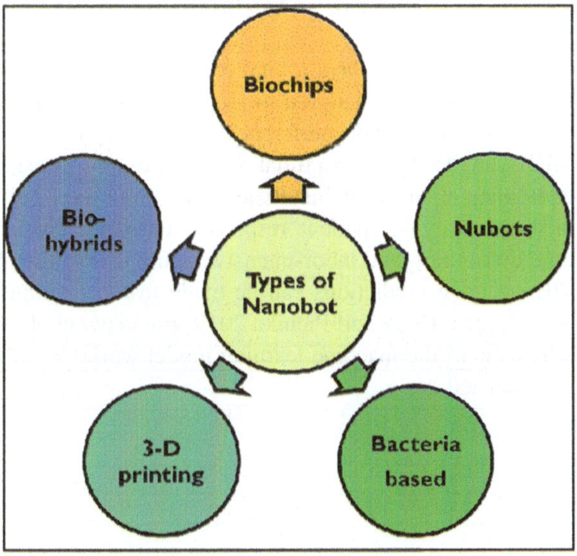

Fig. 12.5 Types of nanobots (Jitendra et al. 2021)

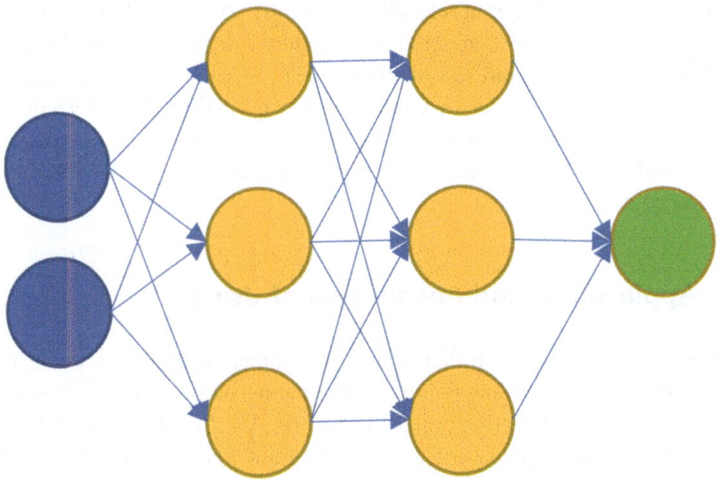

Fig. 12.6 A schematic of the neural network architecture model

A neural network is shown in Fig. 12.6. The blue color nodes are part of the input layer. The orange nodes are considered the hidden layer. The green is the output node. Each line in the neural network holds a mathematical weight determined by the backpropagation during the training of the network. These weights are optimized to reduce prediction's loss or mistakes. The model trained by historical data can be used in the prediction of desired attributes. AI is very helpful in the development of new drugs and testing the developed drugs.

12.3.1 AI in the Pre-manufacturing Stage

3D printing (3DP) plays a vital role in personalized drug development, where an ideal formulation is tailored to meet the patient's specific needs, including dosage size, age, sex, flavor preferences, and drug release kinetics. Machine learning (ML) can derive the optimal formulation by considering all these factors and correlating them with historical data. Moreover, ML is also applied to predict medicine stability, patient response, and drug kinetics, tasks that are otherwise time-consuming and labor-intensive using conventional methods. With the help of ML, accurate predictions can be made faster, making it an efficient tool for drug development (Mak and Pichika 2019; Elbadawi et al. 2020). Figure 12.7 shows the schematic of the machine learning model workflow of the parameter prediction for personalized drugs.

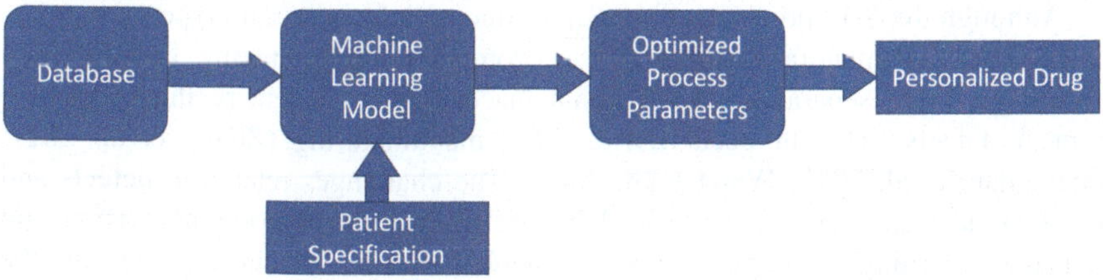

Fig. 12.7 A schematic of ML model workflow

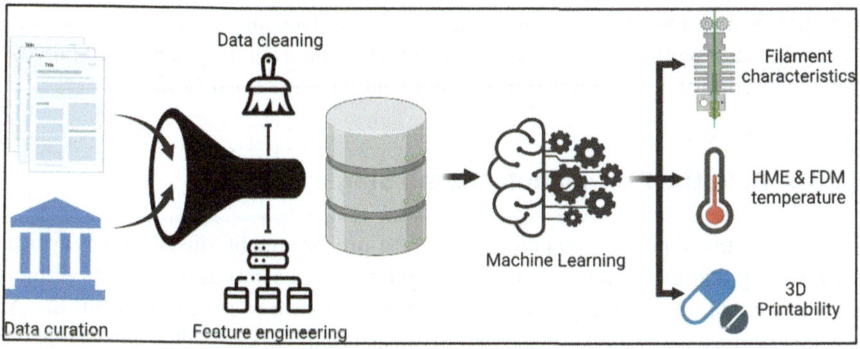

Fig. 12.8 A schematic of ML deployment in the 3D printing manufacturing process (Ong et al. 2022)

12.3.2 AI in the Manufacturing Stage

The inclination toward personalized drugs is increased, and in the manufacturing stage, it is difficult to change the process parameters after each product unit. Machine learning is helping automate the process by using algorithms like principal component analysis (PCA). These algorithms predict the process parameters depending on the product requirement and machine capabilities (Alhijjaj et al. 2019).

The use of machine learning is speeding up the 3D printing process by determining process parameters for hot melt extrusion (HME) and fused deposition modeling (FDM) based on available data. The application of ML algorithms occurs after data curation and filtration, which are important for predicting specific product needs. The data format must be easily interpretable and in accordance with process parameters. Once the data are curated, they undergo cleansing through various transformations, and uniform formatting is applied to all data points. Feature extraction is then performed on the cleaned data, which determines which data are most influential in the predictive model. The extracted features and corresponding data are used in conjunction with the ML algorithm, as illustrated in Fig. 12.8. The schematic shows that the trained model can predict filament characteristics, HME and FDM temperatures, and product printability (Ong et al. 2022).

Although the 3DP process is not entirely free of defects, certain types may occur in specific 3DP manufacturing processes. Porosities, under-melting, over-melting, shrinkage, layer separation, dimensional inaccuracy, and density fluctuation are typical defects that can occur during 3DP manufacturing (Zhang et al. 2017; Alafaghani et al. 2017; Wang et al. 2007). The challenges related to defects and dimensional accuracy can be solved by the integration of computer vision and machine learning. Computer vision enables in-situ monitoring during the manufacturing process. The in-situ monitoring gives insight into each deposited layer. The analysis contains dimensional accuracy, defect analysis, and process parameter optimization capabilities. AI helps in the decision of optimized process parameters and the classification of layers. To reduce the incidence of defects, researchers are working on incorporating in-situ monitoring and AI-enabled process parameter control, as mentioned in Kaushik and Anand Kumar (2023).

12.3.3 AI in the Post-manufacturing Stage

In pharmaceutical product manufacturing, post-process quality inspection is critical for ensuring that the final product meets regulatory and safety requirements. Principal component analysis (PCA) and regression are two powerful tools from the AI that can be used for non-destructive quality inspection purposes. This means that the inspection process does not damage or alter the product in any way, allowing for the examination and testing of multiple samples without compromising their integrity. PCA is often used as a non-destructive tool to visualize trends in the quality of the product. Specifically, it can be used to visualize the trend from the near-infrared (NIR) hyperspectral data obtained during the manufacturing process. Hyperspectral imaging is a powerful technique that can provide detailed information about the chemical composition of a product, and the NIR region of the electromagnetic spectrum is particularly useful for analyzing pharmaceutical products due to its ability to detect the presence of certain chemical functional groups. By applying PCA to the NIR hyperspectral data, manufacturers can identify patterns and trends in the predicted active pharmaceutical ingredient (API) and the real API to make informed decisions about the quality of the product. Regression analysis can then be used to model the relationship between these key features and the quality of the product. By analyzing these relationships, manufacturers can gain a better understanding of the factors that affect product quality and make adjustments to the manufacturing process as needed. This can help improve product consistency, reduce waste, and minimize the risk of quality issues. Overall, the combination of PCA and regression analysis provides a powerful toolset for post-process quality inspection in pharmaceutical product manufacturing (Trenfield et al. 2018, 2020; Vakili et al. 2015).

12.4 Conclusions

Technological advancements in the pharmaceutical field constantly improve, providing diverse methods to meet personalized drug therapy needs. Personalized medicine has gained significant attention, particularly about drug and dosage form personalization, which can benefit various patient groups, such as pediatrics and geriatrics. 3D printing or rapid prototyping can create patient-specific drug delivery devices (DDDs) and dosage forms. This technology has already been effective in producing small volumes of customized and complex designs that are difficult to fabricate through traditional means.

Despite the progress made in 3D printing technology, there is still a long way to go before it becomes standard practice in the pharmaceutical industry. General issues that can arise in most 3D printing methods include layer thickness variability, limited material choices, and unreacted raw materials. In addition to technical limitations, legal and regulatory challenges must also be addressed before these techniques can be applied in clinical settings. For 3D printing to become a mainstream clinical practice and improve patient care, it must use modern technologies.

Artificial intelligence can be combined with 3D printing, drug product development can be accelerated, quality control can be improved, and innovative dosage forms can be created. It can also aid the transition from "one size fits all" to personalized medicine through data-driven decisions. ML can potentially reduce costs, streamline and automate the 3D printing process, and enable more efficient drug delivery by generating accurate predictions for critical process and formulation parameters of drug-loaded products.

However, some challenges are associated with AI, including data availability, intellectual property rights, data protection, output interpretability, and professional liability. The ultimate goal is to digitally simulate the entire 3D printing workflow to move toward sustainable research, where operating costs and material waste are minimized. In conclusion, pharmaceutical industries are taking advantage of technological advancements and working toward more competent and more sustainable healthcare development.

12.5 Challenges and Future Prospects

The current 3DP methods require formal setup and CAD model-building training. The selection of a 3DP printer is also a complex task as the variety is increasing. The specificity of drugs is limited to a particular printing method, which hinders the scalability.

AI relies on large amounts of high-quality data to generate accurate predictions and insights. However, in the pharmaceutical industry, there may be limited availability of data or the data may be incomplete or inaccurate, making it difficult for AI systems to function effectively.

Contamination is a severe concern in edible product printing. The printer should be qualified sufficient to get cleaned easily to prevent contamination from the previous edible printing. The printer's parts need to get bacterial-resistant materials like stainless steel compared to the current material, which is brass for medical applications.

The quality of printed drugs depends on the dimensional accuracy. The generic 3DP tolerance is about ±1 mm. The tolerance decrement is related to the price of the printer; the lower the tolerance value, the higher the price.

Pharmaceutical manufacturing facilities often have a complex set of existing systems, equipment, and processes in place. Integrating AI systems into these existing systems can be challenging and require significant investment in both time and resources.

References

Alafaghani A, Qattawi A, Ablat MA (2017) Design consideration for additive manufacturing: fused deposition modelling. Open J Appl Sci 7(06):291–318. https://doi.org/10.4236/ojapps.2017.76024

Alhijjaj M, Nasereddin J, Belton P, Qi S (2019) Impact of processing parameters on the quality of pharmaceutical solid dosage forms produced by fused deposition modeling (fdm). Pharmaceutics 11(12). https://doi.org/10.3390/pharmaceutics11120633. ISSN: 1999-4923. https://www.mdpi.com/1999-4923/11/12/633

Awad A, Trenfield SJ, Goyanes A, Gaisford S, Basit AW (2018) Reshaping drug development using 3d printing. Drug Discov Today 23(8):1547–1555. https://doi.org/10.1016/j.drudis.2018.05.025. ISSN: 1359-6446. https://www.sciencedirect.com/science/article/pii/S1359644617305391

Bharate S, Bharate S, Bajaj A (2010) Incompatibilities of pharmaceutical excipients with active pharmaceutical ingredients: a comprehensive review. J Excipients Food Chem 1(3):3–26. ISSN: 21502668. https://ojs.abo.fi/ojs/index.php/jefc/article/view/26

Bhuskute H, Shende P, Prabhakar B (2022) 3D printed personalized medicine for cancer: applications for betterment of diagnosis, prognosis and treatment. AAPS PharmSciTech 23. https://doi.org/10.1208/s12249-021-02153-0

Dash AK, Cudworth GC (1998) Therapeutic applications of implantable drug delivery systems. J Pharmacol Toxicol Methods 40(1):1–12. https://doi.org/10.1016/S10568719(98)00027-6. ISSN: 1056-8719. https://www.sciencedirect.com/science/article/pii/S1056871998000276

El Aita I, Ponsar H, Quodbach J (2018) A critical review on 3d-printed dosage forms. Curr Pharm Des 25:12. https://doi.org/10.2174/1381612825666181206124206

Elbadawi M, Castro BM, Gavins FKH, Ong JJ, Gaisford S, Pérez G, Basit AW, Cabalar P, Goyanes A (2020) M3diseen: A novel machine learning approach for predicting the 3d printability of medicines. Int J Pharm 590:119837. https://doi.org/10.1016/j.ijpharm.2020.119837. ISSN: 0378-5173. https://www.sciencedirect.com/science/article/pii/S037851732030822X

Elbadawi M, McCoubrey LE, Gavins FKH, Ong JJ, Goyanes A, Gaisford S, Basit AW (2021) Disrupting 3d printing of medicines with machine learning. Trends Pharmacol Sci 42(9): 745–757. https://doi.org/10.1016/j.tips.2021.06.002. ISSN: 0165-6147. https://www.sciencedirect.com/science/article/pii/S016561472100119X

Eshkalak SK, Ghomi ER, Dai Y, Choudhury D, Ramakrishna S (2020) The role of three-dimensional printing in healthcare and medicine. Mater Des 194:108940. https://doi.org/10.1016/j.matdes.2020.108940. ISSN: 0264-1275. https://www.sciencedirect.com/science/article/pii/S0264127520304743

Goyanes A, Martinez PR, Buanz A, Basit AW, Gaisford S (2015) Effect of geometry on drug release from 3d printed tablets. Int J Pharm 494(2):657–663. https://doi.org/10.1016/j.ijpharm.

2015.04.069. ISSN: 03785173. https://www.sciencedirect.com/science/article/pii/S0378517315003890

Grabowski H (2002) Patents, innovation and access to new pharmaceuticals. J Int Econ Law 5(4): 849–860. https://doi.org/10.1093/jiel/5.4.849. ISSN: 1369-3034.

Holländer J, Genina N, Jukarainen H, Khajeheian M, Rosling A, Mäkilä E, Sandler N (2016) Three-dimensional printed PCL-based implantable prototypes of medical devices for controlled drug delivery. J Pharm Sci 105(9):2665–2676. https://doi.org/10.1016/j.xphs.2015.12.012. ISSN: 0022-3549. https://www.sciencedirect.com/science/article/pii/S0022354915002099

Huang W, Zheng Q, Sun W, Xu H, Yang X (2007) Levofloxacin implants with predefined microstructure fabricated by three-dimensional printing technique. Int J Pharm 339(1):33–38. https://doi.org/10.1016/j.ijpharm.2007.02.021. ISSN: 0378-5173. https://www.sciencedirect.com/science/article/pii/S037851730700169X

Hurst EJ (2016) 3d printing in healthcare: emerging applications. J Hosp Librariansh 16(3): 255–267. https://doi.org/10.1080/15323269.2016.1188042

Jamróz W, Kurek M, Łyszczarz E, Brniak W, Jachowicz R (2017) Printing techniques: recent developments in pharmaceutical technology. Acta Pol Pharm 74:753–763

Jitendra G, Reena G, Abhishek T (2021) Nanobot: artificial intelligence, drug delivery and diagnostic approach. J Pharm Res Int 33(59B):189–206. https://doi.org/10.9734/jpri/2021/v33i59B34369

Kaushik B, Anand Kumar S (2023) Chapter 10—Computer vision based online monitoring technique: part quality enhancement in the selective laser melting process. In: Kumar A, Mittal RK, Haleem A (eds) Advances in additive manufacturing, Additive manufacturing materials and technologies. Elsevier, pp 167–194. https://doi.org/10.1016/B978-0-323-91834-3.00007-7. ISBN: 978-0-323-91834-3. https://www.sciencedirect.com/science/article/pii/B9780323918343000077

Khaled SA, Burley JC, Alexander MR, Yang J, Roberts CJ (2015) 3D printing of tablets containing multiple drugs with defined release profiles. Int J Pharm 494(2):643–650. https://doi.org/10.1016/j.ijpharm.2015.07.067. ISSN: 0378-5173

Kleinebudde P, Khinast J, Rantanen J (2017) Continuous manufacturing of pharmaceuticals. John Wiley & Sons

Liaw C-Y, Guvendiren M (2017) Current and emerging applications of 3d printing in medicine. Biofabrication 9(2):024102. https://doi.org/10.1088/1758-5090/aa7279

Mak K-K, Pichika MR (2019) Artificial intelligence in drug development: present status and future prospects. Drug Discov Today 24(3):773–780. https://doi.org/10.1016/j.drudis.2018.11.014. ISSN: 1359-6446. https://www.sciencedirect.com/science/article/pii/S1359644618300916

Malerba F, Orsenigo L (2015) The evolution of the pharmaceutical industry. Bus Hist 57(5): 664–687. https://doi.org/10.1080/00076791.2014.975119

Morton FS, Kyle M (2011) Chapter 12 Markets for pharmaceutical products 11 the authors thank Tom McGuire for editorial advice and improvements and participants at the handbook conference for helpful suggestions. In: Pauly MV, Mcguire TG, Barros PP (eds) Handbook of health economics, vol 2. Elsevier, pp 763–823. https://doi.org/10.1016/B978-0-444-535924.00012-8. https://www.sciencedirect.com/science/article/pii/B9780444535924000128

Norman J, Madurawe RD, Moore CMV, Khan MA, Khairuzzaman A (2017) A new chapter in pharmaceutical manufacturing: 3d-printed drug products. Adv Drug Deliv Rev 108:39–50. https://doi.org/10.1016/j.addr.2016.03.001. https://www.sciencedirect.com/science/article/pii/S0169409X16300771. ISSN: 0169-409X. Editor's Collection 2016

Öblom H, Cornett C, Bøtker J, Frokjaer S, Hansen H, Rades T, Rantanen J, Genina N (2020) Data-enriched edible pharmaceuticals (deep) of medical cannabis by inkjet printing. Int J Pharm 589: 119866. https://doi.org/10.1016/j.ijpharm.2020.119866. ISSN: 0378-5173. https://www.sciencedirect.com/science/article/pii/S0378517320308516

Ong JJ, Castro BM, Gaisford S, Cabalar P, Basit AW, Pérez G, Goyanes A (2022) Accelerating 3D printing of pharmaceutical products using machine learning. Int J Pharm X 4:100120. https://doi.org/10.1016/j.ijpx.2022.100120. ISSN: 2590-1567

Park B, Choi H, Moon S, Kim S, Bajracharya R, Min J, Han H-K (2018) Pharmaceutical applications of 3d printing technology: current understanding and future perspectives. J Pharm Investig 49:10. https://doi.org/10.1007/s40005-018-00414-y

Prasad LK, Smyth H (2016) 3d printing technologies for drug delivery: a review. Drug Dev Ind Pharm 42(7):1019–1031. https://doi.org/10.3109/03639045.2015.1120743

Puls N, Carluccio D, Batstone MD, Novak JI (2021) The rise of additive manufacturing for ocular and orbital prostheses: a systematic literature review. Ann 3D Print Med 4:100036. https://doi.org/10.1016/j.stlm.2021.100036. ISSN: 2666-9641

Rahman Z, Barakh SF, Ali TO, Charoo NA, Reddy IK, Khan MA (2018) Additive manufacturing with 3d printing: progress from bench to bedside. AAPS J 20(6):101. https://doi.org/10.1208/s12248-018-0225-6. ISSN: 1550-7416.

Reklaitis G (2017) Prospects and challenges for process systems engineering in healthcare. Comput Aided Chem Eng 40:3–7

Roopavath UK, Kalaskar DM (2017) 1—Introduction to 3d printing in medicine. In: Kalaskar DM (ed) 3D printing in medicine. Woodhead Publishing, pp 1–20. https://doi.org/10.1016/B978-0-08-100717-4.00001-6. ISBN: 978-0-08-100717-4. https://www.sciencedirect.com/science/article/pii/B9780081007174000016

Samiei N (2020) Recent trends on applications of 3D printing technology on the design and manufacture of pharmaceutical oral formulation: a mini review. Beni-Suef Univ J Basic Appl Sci 9:12. https://doi.org/10.1186/s43088-020-00040-4

Schubert C, van Langeveld MC, Donoso LA (2014) Innovations in 3d printing: a 3d overview from optics to organs. Br J Ophthalmol 98(2):159–161. https://doi.org/10.1136/bjophthalmol-2013304446. ISSN: 0007-1161. https://bjo.bmj.com/content/98/2/159

Singh R (2018) Chapter 17—Automation of continuous pharmaceutical manufacturing process. In: Singh R, Yuan Z (eds) Process systems engineering for pharmaceutical manufacturing, Computer aided chemical engineering, vol 41. Elsevier, pp 431–446. https://doi.org/10.1016/B978-0-444-63963-9.00017-8. https://www.sciencedirect.com/science/article/pii/B9780444639639000178

Tabriz AG, Nandi U, Scoutaris N, Sanfo K, Alexander B, Gong Y, Hui H-W, Kumar S, Douroumis D (2022) Personalised paediatric chewable Ibuprofen tablets fabricated using 3D micro-extrusion printing technology. Int J Pharm 626:122135. https://doi.org/10.1016/j.ijpharm.2022.122135. ISSN: 0378-5173

Trenfield SJ, Goyanes A, Telford R, Wilsdon D, Rowland M, Gaisford S, Basit AW (2018) 3D printed drug products: non-destructive dose verification using a rapid point-and-shoot approach. Int J Pharm 549(1–2):283–292. https://doi.org/10.1016/j.ijpharm.2018.08.002. ISSN: 0378-5173.

Trenfield SJ, Tan HX, Goyanes A, Wilsdon D, Rowland M, Gaisford S, Basit AW (2020) Non-destructive dose verification of two drugs within 3D printed polyprintlets. Int J Pharm 577:119066. https://doi.org/10.1016/j.ijpharm.2020.119066. ISSN: 0378-5173

Vakili H, Kolakovic R, Genina N, Marmion M, Salo H, Ihalainen P, Peltonen J, Sandler N (2015) Hyperspectral imaging in quality control of inkjet printed personalised dosage forms. Int J Pharm 483(1–2):244–249. https://doi.org/10.1016/j.ijpharm.2014.12.034. ISSN: 0378-5173

Varghese R, Salvi S, Sood P, Karsiya J, Kumar D (2022) 3D printed medicine for the management of chronic diseases: the road less travelled. Ann 3D Print Med 5:100043. https://doi.org/10.1016/j.stlm.2021.100043. ISSN: 2666-9641

Wang R-J, Wang L, Zhao L, Liu Z (2007) Influence of process parameters on part shrinkage in SLS. Int J Adv Manuf Technol 33:498–504. https://doi.org/10.1007/s00170-006-0490x

Wang J, Yu Z, Aghda NH, Pillai AR, Thakkar R, Nokhodchi A, Maniruzzaman M (2021) Emerging 3d printing technologies for drug delivery devices: current status and future perspective. Adv Drug Deliv Rev 174:294–316. https://doi.org/10.1016/j.addr.2021.04.019. ISSN: 0169-409X. https://www.sciencedirect.com/science/article/pii/S0169409X21001472

Zhang B, Li Y, Bai Q (2017) Defect formation mechanisms in selective laser melting: a review. Chin J Mech Eng 30:515–527. https://doi.org/10.1007/s10033-017-0121-5

The manufacturer's authorised representative in the EU is Springer
Nature Customer Service Centre GmbH, Europaplatz 3, 69115 Heidelberg,
Germany. If you have any concerns regarding our products, please
contact ProductSafety@springernature.com

Printed and bound by CPI Group (UK) Ltd, Croydon, CR0 4YY
30/09/2026
02225319-0005